MINDFULNESS IN THE BIRTH SPHERE

Mindfulness in the Birth Sphere draws together and critically appraises a raft of emerging research around mindfulness in healthcare, looking especially at its relevance to pregnancy and childbirth.

Divided into three parts, this reflective book:

- Investigates the phenomena of mindfulness through discussions of neuroscience, an indigenous worldview and research methods.
- Develops the concept of mindfulness for use in practice with women/and babies across the continuum of childbirth. It includes chapters on birth environments, intrapartum care, mental health, fertility, breastfeeding and parenting among others.
- Explores mindfulness as a tool for birth practitioners and educators, promoting self-care, resilience and compassion.

Each chapter discusses specific research, evidence and experiences of mindfulness, including practical advice and an example of a mindfulness practice.

This is an essential read for all those interested in mindfulness in connection to pregnancy and childbirth, including midwives, doulas, doctors and birth activists, whether involved in practice, research or education.

Lorna Davies is a midwife, a mother and a grandmother, and is currently employed as an Associate Professor at Otago Polytechnic/Te Pukenga in Dunedin. Her PhD explored midwives' understanding of and attitudes towards the broad concept of sustainability within the context of midwifery practice. Her main research interest areas are sustainability in midwifery and healthcare, self-sustainability, inter-professional education and midwifery workforce issues.

Susan Crowther is currently a Professor of Midwifery at AUT University, Auckland, New Zealand. Her research interests are concerned with psycho-social, cultural and spiritual health around childbirth, rural maternity services and sustainable practice as well as a keen interest in meditative practices to enhance well-being and connection. Susan is on the review and editorial boards of a number of peer-reviewed journals and a member of the ICM research standing committee.

MINDFULNESS IN THE BIRTH SPHERE

Practice for Pre-conception to the Critical 1000 Days and Beyond

Edited by
Lorna Davies and Susan Crowther

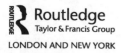
Routledge
Taylor & Francis Group

LONDON AND NEW YORK

Cover image credit: © Getty Images

First published 2023
by Routledge
4 Park Square, Milton Park, Abingdon, Oxon OX14 4RN

and by Routledge
605 Third Avenue, New York, NY 10158

Routledge is an imprint of the Taylor & Francis Group, an informa business

© 2023 selection and editorial matter, Lorna Davies and Susan Crowther; individual chapters, the contributors

British Library Cataloguing-in-Publication Data
A catalogue record for this book is available from the British Library

Library of Congress Cataloging-in-Publication Data
Names: Davies, Lorna, editor. | Crowther, Susan (Professor of midwifery) editor.
Title: Mindfulness in the birth sphere : practice for pre-conception to the critical 1000 days and beyond / edited by Lorna Davies and Susan Crowther.
Description: 1 Edition. | New York, NY : Routledge, 2023. | Includes bibliographical references and index. |
Identifiers: LCCN 2022028920 (print) | LCCN 2022028921 (ebook) | ISBN 9780367760366 (hardback) | ISBN 9780367760359 (paperback) | ISBN 9781003165200 (ebook)
Subjects: LCSH: Mind and body. | Conception. | Pregnancy.
Classification: LCC BF151 .M66 2023 (print) | LCC BF151 (ebook) | DDC 158.1—dc23/eng/20220921
LC record available at https://lccn.loc.gov/2022028920
LC ebook record available at https://lccn.loc.gov/2022028921

ISBN: 978-0-367-76036-6 (hbk)
ISBN: 978-0-367-76035-9 (pbk)
ISBN: 978-1-003-16520-0 (ebk)

DOI: 10.4324/9781003165200

Typeset in Bembo
by codeMantra

To the teachers and masters of old and recent who have shared their wisdom with grace and generosity so that humanity may benefit from their guidance.

To all women and their families, to all the midwives, doctors and allied health care providers practising in the maternity services globally – we dedicate this volume – may it gift solace and bring the light of compassion to self and others.

May all beings everywhere, whether near or far,
whether known to me or unknown, be happy.
May they be well.
May they be peaceful.
May they be free.

(Buddhist 'Metta' Lovingkindness prayer)

CONTENTS

FIGURES

TABLES

BOXES

CONTRIBUTORS

Doreen Balabanoff is an Artist/designer and a Professor Emerita (Design, OCAD University). Her research/practice focuses on the birth environment as an important global/local architectural project of our time. With international colleagues of the Birth Environment Design Network, she continues to work on transformational change for birth environment design. Two recently awarded SSHRC-funded grants are moving this project forward.

Anna Byrom has been a midwife for 20 years and worked across the UK as a case-load, team and birth centre midwife as well as a lecturer in midwifery education. Her PhD explored the influences of the Unicef UK Baby Friendly Initiative upon midwives and service-users. Anna is the publisher of *The Practising Midwife* and *The Student Midwife* journals and founding Director/CEO of the award winning All4Maternity.com supporting the learning, sharing and caring needs for all midwives and maternity workers.

Sheena Byrom is a midwife of 40 years standing, and was one of the UK's first consultant midwives Head of Midwifery in East Lancashire. Sheena is an international speaker and provides workshops and consultancy services on respectful maternity care. With her daughter Anna, she is joint owner of *The Practising Midwife* journal, and the online platform All4Maternity.com. Sheena was awarded an OBE in 2011 for services to midwifery and has received several honorary doctorates as well as being made an Honorary Fellow of the Royal College of Midwives in 2015.

Richard Chambers is a Clinical Psychologist, Mindfulness Consultant and an Adjunct Associate Professor at the Centre for Consciousness and Contemplative Studies, Monash University, Australia. Over the past ten years, he has led an initiative to embed mindfulness in the core curriculum for students.

Tracy Donegan is a Registered Midwife, author of *Mindful Pregnancy* and Founder of the GentleBirth Positive Birth App and FertileMind App. Tracy is a global advocate for humanized, positive birth experiences and has a special interest in mindfulness interventions for fertility, pregnancy and postpartum. Throughout her career, Tracy has led several maternity care improvement initiatives as a volunteer (Chair of Birth Matters Hospital Consumer group). Tracy is also a contributing writer for several European publications and is lead coordinator of the Irish Positive Birth conference held annually in Ireland.

Maralyn Foureur is the recently retired Professor of Nursing and Midwifery Research, and is now an Honorary Professor at University of Newcastle. She also holds Adjunct Professorial appointments at several Universities internationally. She is a leading Australian midwifery researcher with a national and international reputation established over a 40-year career in clinical practice and research. Her current research interests are in the areas of neuro-leadership, neurophysiology and genomics, and she is internationally regarded as an expert in the interdisciplinary field of Birth Unit Design.

Craig Hassed is a Professor at the Faculty of Medicine, Monash University. In 2021, he became the founding Director of Education at the Monash Centre for Consciousness and Contemplative Studies (M3CS). His teaching, research and clinical interests include mindfulness, mind–body medicine, lifestyle medicine, integrative medicine and medical ethics. In 2019, Craig was awarded the Medal of the Order of Australia (OAM) for services to Medicine.

Tracy Humphrey recently moved to take on the post of Head of School in the School of Nursing, Midwifery and Social Work, University of Queensland, Australia. As a Professor of Midwifery, she influenced and implemented national maternal and neonatal policies in Scotland through her research, practice and role as a government advisor. Her areas of research include reducing unnecessary interventions during childbirth and improving outcomes for women and families in remote and rural areas through educational and service improvement initiatives.

Lester Jones is a physiotherapist, educator and long-term advocate for better pain management. He has published on a wide range of topics including stress and pain, labour pain, pain associated with breastfeeding, pain in torture survivors, sports-related pain and clinical reasoning including the Pain and Movement Reasoning Model which he co-created. He has been active in pain-focused professional groups in UK, Australia and now Singapore, including as the inaugural chair of the National Pain Group (Australian Physiotherapy Association). He is currently based at the Singapore Institute of Technology.

Ira Kantrowitz-Gordon is an Associate Professor in the Department of Child, Family, and Population Health Nursing at the University of Washington School of Nursing, Seattle, Washington, USA, where he teaches nurse-midwifery. He has practiced nurse-midwifery for over 20 years, serving diverse populations. His research program focuses on (1) mindfulness interventions to help with perinatal stress and symptoms and (2) reducing the stigma of perinatal opioid use disorder.

Miriama Ketu-McKenzie is a Clinical Psychologist and mother of three, who specialises in working with Māori who have experienced trauma. Her clinical interests are in the areas of attachment, trauma and mind-body interventions, including mindfulness. She has research interests in the areas of attachment theory, epigenetics, intergenerational trauma transmission and psychoneuroendocrinology. She is a wāhine Māori of Ngāti Raukawa and Ngāti Tūwharetoa descent whose PhD research involved the successful adaptation of a mindfulness-based stress reduction programme for Māori women who had experienced stress in childhood.

Angus Macbeth is a Senior Lecturer in Clinical Psychology at the University of Edinburgh, Scotland. His research focuses on social determinants of mental health, specifically how mental health/psychological risk and resilience factors are transmitted intergenerationally, and how these can inform identification, treatment and recovery from mental health difficulties. He takes a lifespan approach to mental health, focused particularly on the perinatal period. This has the potential to lead to preventative or early intervention paradigms for mental health and well-being, alongside informing global health and societal priorities.

Kathleen Maki currently works as a Midwifery kaiako/Academic Lecturer at ARA Institute of Canterbury and is also the appointed Te Ara ō Hine – Tapu Ora Pacific Liaison for ARA School of Midwifery. Kathleen supported the development of the New Zealand Diploma in Pregnancy, Childbirth and Early Parenting Education while also teaching into the programme from its conception. As a Cook Island Māori/Tahitian midwife with almost 15 years of midwifery experience, Kathleen has worked across the Manawatu, Whanaganui-a-tara and Ōtautahi as a midwife within both hospital and community settings. Her research interests include Pacific Health and Leadership.

Valerie Malhotra Bentz works in the School of Leadership Studies at Fielding Graduate University, Santa Barbara, California. Her interests include phenomenology, somatics, social theory, consciousness development, contemplative research and Vedantic knowledge. She is engaged in collaborative research with alumni, students and colleagues leading to many publications including *Deathworlds into Lifeworlds: Collaboration with Strangers for Personal, Social and Ecological Transformation, Handbook of Transformative Phenomenology* and *Mindful Inquiry in Social Research*.

Janetti Marotta is a California-based private practice Clinical Psychologist who specializes in infertility and its treatment. Stemming from her own infertility experience, she became a long-time practitioner of meditation and mindfulness and is the author of *A Fertile Path: Guiding the Journey with Mindfulness and Compassion* and *50 Mindful Steps to Self-Esteem: Everyday Practices for Cultivating Self-Acceptance and Self-Compassion*.

Dan MacKay is a Neonatal Doctor near the end of my specialist training. Dan completed his Bachelor's degree in Psychology and Genetics (Canterbury), and an Honours degree in Molecular Genetics (ANU). After working for several years, Dan completed a medical degree (ANU) and basic training in Canberra before moving to Christchurch for Paediatric and Neonatal Intensive Care Training. His journey in mindfulness and compassion began as an elite ultra-endurance mountain biker and Cancer survivor. The time with his mentor Dr Maggie Meeks has brought increasing focus in it.

Maggie Meeks began her Paediatric career in the UK Royal Air Force (RAF) and believes that the RAF provided the foundation for her close relationship with human factors and simulation training. She emigrated to New Zealand in 2008 and continues to work clinically in neonatal paediatrics for Canterbury District Health Board (CDHB). She has more recently increasingly focused on her career in education with a specific focus on interprofessional education. Her interest in human psychology has led her recently to study in areas such as infant mental health and psychological counselling.

Christine Mellor has been a midwife since the early 1990s and is currently working as a Senior Midwifery Lecturer at AUT University. Her career so far has traversed various midwifery roles and settings, including practice and leadership roles, education and research. Her professional and research interests relate to maternal mental health and supporting physiological birth. Her growing interest in the significance of the mind-body dyad during pregnancy, labour and birth is born from a connection of these two areas of interest married with her experiences in practice.

Diane Menage is a Senior Lecturer of Midwifery at De Montfort University, Leicester, UK where she teaches research skills, evidence-based practice, and leadership. She is also a mother, grandmother, writer and feminist with a life-long interest in women's health and well-being. Her focus has always been on providing individualised evidence-based care through relationships. She has worked clinically in many settings including independent practice. Other research interests include a project to assess the impact of a mindfulness intervention on student midwives' stress levels and readiness to learn.

Liz Newnham is a Senior Lecturer and Director of Midwifery Programs at the University of Newcastle, Australia. Her research interests include cultural and political analysis of birthing practice, and the role of midwives in promoting physiological and humanised birth. Her key areas of study are birth culture and environment, midwifery practice to support birth physiology, birth technologies, pain in labour, maternity policy/politics and informed consent/bioethics.

Jenny Patterson is a UK Registered Midwife based in Edinburgh, Scotland. Jenny's work as a midwife since 2007, both independently and in the UK National Health Service, led to her particular interest in women's traumatic birth experiences and midwives work-related trauma. At present, Jenny is a Midwifery Lecturer at Edinburgh Napier University and her current research projects include exploring trauma management for student midwives, and processes of informed consent when language interpretation is required.

Aigli Raouna is a mixed-methods Clinical Psychology PhD candidate at the University of Edinburgh, Scotland. Her research focuses on the transition to parenthood and the identification of transactional risk and resilience pathways between parents and their babies. Alongside her research, she has been involved in several initiatives and research projects aimed at closing the gap between research and the public, advocating that research findings should be translatable and accessible to everyone and promoting the unique opportunity of prevention during the perinatal period.

Mo Tabib is a Midwifery Lecturer at Robert Gordon University and a student at the final stage of her PhD in Scotland. Over the last decade, her research interest and activities have been focused on implementing education on psychophysiological processes, and the relaxation practices that could influence these processes, in childbirth preparation programmes, as well as midwifery practice and education.

Melanie Welfare has a career in health that spans more than 40 years, both in the UK and Aotearoa/New Zealand. Her career began in the British Military as a nurse, and then a midwife, graduating from Bournemouth University. Her research interests include simulation for midwifery education, IPE, and professional sustainability. She is currently a PhD candidate at AUT researching virtual reality and midwifery education.

Laura Whitburn is a Senior Lecturer of Anatomy at La Trobe University, where she specialises in teaching neuroanatomy and pain science. Laura started her career as a physiotherapist before transitioning to tertiary education and research. Her early experiences of working with patients in pain led to a desire to better understand this human experience, in particular, the unique experience of pain associated with childbirth.

PREFACE

The subject of mindfulness has become increasingly visible and discussed within health services and education in recent years. Pre-conception through to the first 1,000 days of life is now acknowledged as pivotal to human growth and development. As midwives with more than half a century of midwifery practice between us, we appreciate the need and significance of women, families and communities reaching their full potential in order to flourish. As we move towards the ends of our own careers in midwifery, we are profoundly committed to ensuring a positive vision for childbirth for future generations. Furthermore, we both have mindfulness and medication practices that we use regularly. Our vision and mindfulness/meditation practices together have continually motivated us to seek out ways of caring and being with one another that promotes integrated human growth and personal development across the childbirth sphere in clinical, education, management and teaching. We have been concerned about the growing psychosocial impacts of practice arrangements and unsustainability of services. We were inspired to find ways to halt the escalating childbirth intervention rates and seek solutions that speak to the art of practice as well as the empirical supportive evidence. Moreover, we were eager to explore ways that safely and proactively address the worrying upward trend of perinatal mental health issues. As co-editors we contend that the current situation in the birth sphere is not sustainable for all involved and know that solutions to the current predicament exist and need to be put into practice. Unless the multidimensional qualities that constitute the birth sphere beyond purely measurable outcomes and biomedical model are honoured and addressed then we have sadly neglected something important. This 'something' dwells within the very core of our shared humanity, that is, the possibility to create anew and generate futures that are welcoming and just for all. We suggest that for any change to occur, all health care professionals involved in childbirth – women, families, midwives, medics and allied healthcare providers – need tools to enable them to attune in an appropriate and sustainable way.

This change beckons different styles and approaches to maternity care. This change is not just in the physical material structures and processes but also in the very way we comport ourselves to caring, how we interact, how we care for ourselves and how we attune to others in the inter-personal spaces of maternity organisations. We believe that mindfulness contributes and provides an opportunity to address this beckoning. Currently, there is a raft of research activity relating to mindfulness within healthcare, including areas related to psychosocial resilience; mental distress and health; compassionate and empathic care; self-care; sensitivity and tact in a technological age; psycho-neurobiology and emotional well-being. As we started to investigate this area, we realised that a resource that collated the empirical and experiential evidence in a usable and accessible format aimed at those experiencing childbirth and those working in maternity care was not available. Over the course of several months, we agreed that there needed to be some appraisal and critical discussion of the potential of mindfulness across the childbirth sphere from multiple perspectives. We agreed that any resource we created would have practical application and praxis weaved through the work. What you hold in your hands is the result.

As co-editors we interpret mindfulness as attunement to an intentional, attentive, reflective, deliberate, and conscious style of listening using all the senses. Through our own mindfulness and meditation practices, we saw how an attuned state provides an enhanced quality of perceived or lived-time experience for ourselves and others. We discovered, through practice and reading, that mindfulness is a state of being that evokes contemplation with purpose opening us to consideration of possibilities beyond our individual or/and siloed perspectives. We acknowledge that mindfulness is an ancient practice associated with Buddhism and other traditional cultures. We therefore stand in reverence to the teachers old and new who shared their wisdom. We also acknowledge that mindfulness holds spiritual and/or religious connections for some and is accepted by others as a purely secular practice. Either way, we as co-editors feel that mindfulness has the very real potential to improve our collective understanding of the birth sphere through the process of intentional inquiry into what matters most. In this book, you will discover how mindfulness facilitates the potential for all involved to act as change makers in the world of maternity care across the birth sphere. You will read how mindfulness encourages and reminds us to adopt an integral approach to childbirth that incorporates and invites creativity, wisdom and intuitional knowing. You will notice as you read through this book that these qualities invite connection with our inner guidance, a style of guidance that informs ways of communicating with care, love and compassion from a place of tenderness, non-judgement and acceptance. The content of this book asks different questions and invites different voices to the conversation and presents a series of sections and chapters that will take you on a journey of mindful inquiry that enlivens a fresh appreciation of what is possible in ways that disrupt the status quo and brings new energy and insight. As co-editors we carefully approached specific chapter authors to gift their time to proffer different horizons of understanding. Some chapters adopt an in-depth empirical scientific approach; others report their own research in the area of mindfulness. Others narrate their story in more auto-biographic and hermeneutic-styled accounts of mindfulness drawing us nearer into intimate spaces in which mindful inquiry surfaces the nuances of cultural interpretations. Others speak to the lived experience of practice, for example, the significance of mindfulness in breastfeeding, facilitating antenatal classes, the lived experiences of leading with compassionate mindfulness, and using mind-fulness as a tool to navigate crises and finding ways to cope in professional and personally challenging situations. All these new horizons together bring a new deeper understanding of the birth sphere through an extended epistemological appreciation that coalesces into an enlightened sustainable ecology of birth in the 21st century. Throughout the book, we encourage you to engage with each of the authors in a mindful dialogue as you read their words. Our wish is that the contents of this book more than merely pique your curiosity spur you to be proactive and apply the insights and recommendations proffered. We also hope that you will consider using the practical mindful practices suggested to support you on the journey of personal and organisational change so urgently called for across the birth sphere.

ACKNOWLEDGEMENTS

We acknowledge the chapter authors without whom this book would have never come to fruition. In a time of global pandemic and ongoing regional conflicts impacting on us all, we honour the time, efforts, and determination to get their chapters completed. As the rounds of drafted chapter iterations arrived, we heard stories of personal and professional challenges. The world has not been easy to navigate over the writing and editing of this book. We as co-editors are humbled by the fortitude of all the authors, who despite the external crises and personal difficulties confronting them produced works that are startling reflections of their idiosyncratic uniqueness and insightfulness. This book is a testament to the influences that mindfulness has had on all that contributed to these pages. Much gratitude to the chapter authors – your kindness, gifts of wisdom and insight will have untold impacts far and wide.

We also acknowledge the publishing team at Routledge. Deadlines needed to have a quality of plasticity due to the global unfolding situation. They were constantly accommodating and flexible; thank you for your patience – you had faith that we would get this done.

Acknowledgement must also go to our spouses, Tom (husband to Lorna) and Toby (husband to Susan), who waited for us to emerge from our offices late into evenings and across weekends as needed. Your ongoing supportive care and understanding is appreciated and very much noticed.

We also acknowledge each other as co-editors. Our lives too have been impacted by global and local crises. It has not always been an easy journey with many delays. With our own mindfulness practices, shared vision and passion, we were able to manifest this book. We honour the resonant connection we experienced in our co-editing; always done with loving kindness and compassion for each other it now gives us great pleasure to bring this book to you.

1

INTRODUCTION

Let judgements roll by, sit comfortably, and notice the breath

Lorna Davies and Susan Crowther

Pregnancy, childbirth, and transitioning to parenthood are significant life events and they should be times of joy, connection, personal growth, and discovery. Consequently, the care that pregnant, birthing, and postpartum women receive from health professionals during this time is meaningful and influential. Therefore, the carers who journey with the woman and her significant others during this period need to be empathic and compassionate and have enhanced levels of self-awareness. As US midwife and childbirth educator Nancy Bardacke, one of the earliest proponents of the use of mindfulness in preparation for childbirth courses, writes in her book on Mindful Birthing:

> They feel whatever we're feeling! If we're stressed out, they're stressed out! If we calm down, they calm down!
>
> *(Bardacke 2012)*

In many ways, this simple statement captures the essence and importance of mindfulness in the birth sphere. If those working within maternity services are able to provide care that leads to a calm and reflective state of being both for the providers and recipients of care, then all within and across the birth sphere are more likely to flourish. That is why this book is so important. Mindfulness has the potential to improve a collective 'orchestration' within the birth sphere by using a process of intentional inquiry into what matters most. A mindful approach facilitates the potential for all involved to act as change makers in the world of maternity care across the birth sphere.

DOI: 10.4324/9781003165200-1

Our stories

As co-editors of this textbook on mindfulness in the birth sphere, we have a fundamental belief that mindfulness offers the opportunity for the facilitation of such change. In our professional and personal lives, we both have a longstanding interest in mindfulness that has driven the desire to edit a book that explores the subject of mindfulness in maternity.

Lorna's story

I was introduced to yoga in my early twenties, and I dabbled with meditation for many years following. However, my real connection with mindfulness came after the series of significant earthquakes and aftershocks in Christchurch, New Zealand where I was living in 2010–2011. My stress response was extreme, and I went into the menopause overnight. I was shocked at this endocrine-based physical manifestation of my emotional and psychological state. I recognised that I needed some support, and I consulted a naturopath who suggested that I might be suffering from adrenal fatigue because of the stress relating to the many hundreds of aftershocks that followed the major quakes in the city. I followed her advice to commence a meditation practice and found solace almost immediately. Having experienced the benefits first hand, I became interested in the neurohormonal effects that led first to my crisis and then my recovery. It was not long before I was exploring the possibility of the benefits for women in the birth sphere. I enrolled for a mindfulness teaching qualification, and then with a colleague, designed and facilitated a preparation for childbirth and parenting course based around the principles of mindfulness. We were astounded at the difference that the approach appeared to make to the parents attending. I also supported the introduction of a mindfulness component into a Bachelor of Midwifery curriculum (see Chapter 13).

Susan's story

From age 11, I have had an interest in spiritual practices; an interest shaped by the cultural context of my youth. My childhood was mostly in England with sometime in Southeast Asia due to my father's Naval postings. As a child I became fascinated by the silence, calm, and prayer that I witnessed at the local Anglican church – these moments awakened something within me that has always remained. However, my time in Asia had ignited a desire to seek out the meaning of the Buddha statues and temples I visited. When I left home, I begun to explore this in earnest and returned to Asia where I immersed myself in both Buddhist and Yogic meditation practices. I attended retreats in both traditions from ten days of silence to many months and incorporated a blend of mindfulness and devotional practices. I remember at the time a meditation teacher saying to me – '*it is like having the top of your head removed and your mind freshened and re-organised.*' This proved so true, my early experiences of meditation were life altering. Since that time meditation practice continued to inform my midwifery practice and current academic role. For 36 years I have continued with a daily formal sit down meditation practice and seek out opportunities to sit with others when I can. Without doubt, meditation has helped me navigate some challenging personal and professional challenges over the years. For me, meditation and mindfulness draw forth a quality of awareness that is energizing, connecting and profoundly relational to self, others, and life.

The growth of the field of mindfulness

It sometimes feels as though the phenomenon of mindfulness is omnipresent in every facet of our lives. Every news outlet and popular media platform seems to be carrying an article or news story showcasing the practice and benefits of mindfulness. Businesses and educational establishments are increasingly incorporating mindfulness into their timetables and curricula (Pickert 2014). Mindfulness training and meditation classes are enjoying unprecedented popularity. A random search for 'mindfulness' on Google provided 228,000,000 links. The volume of research on mindfulness-related areas yields similar results on Google Scholar (786,000 research articles and papers) including a significant number of RCTs and systematic reviews evaluating the effects of mindfulness over the past few decades (Creswell 2017). Figure 1.1 illustrates the exponential nature of trends and developments in mindfulness research over 55 years.

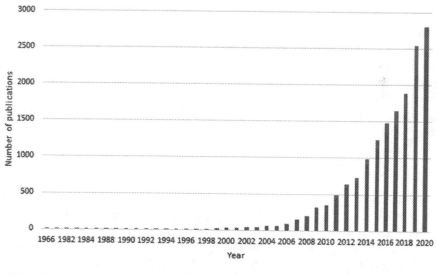

FIGURE 1.1 Trends and developments in mindfulness research over 55 years: a bibliometric analysis of publications indexed in Web of Science.

Source: Baminiwatta, A., and Solangaarachchi, I. (2021). Trends and Developments in Mindfulness Research over 55 Years: A Bibliometric Analysis of Publications Indexed in Web of Science. *Mindfulness* 12, 2099–2116. https://doi.org/10.1007/s12671-021-01681-x.

Perhaps as a result of this exponential growth, mindfulness has drawn criticism as a 'religion of the self' (Purser 2019). Purser and Loy coined the phrase 'McMindfulness' in a 2013 Huffington Post article which outlined how mindfulness has been fashioned by the ideology of neoliberalism. Žižek (2001) goes further by claiming that mindfulness offers itself as an ideological supplement to capitalism. Widdicombe (2015) argues that the commodification of mindfulness relegates it to an individualistic practice that is primarily for personal emotional regulation and self-improvement, which negates the value of mindfulness as a social activity. These critiques may not be unfounded, but they fail to acknowledge the many known benefits of the practice, which are grounded in health and well-being. As health professionals without commercial interest, we are in a strong position to support the more traditional values of mindfulness by encouraging more critically socially aware and engaged forms of mindfulness.

What is mindfulness?

The early origins of the practice of mindfulness are founded in meditation and are usually traced to Buddhist teachings dating back 2,600 years although documented images of meditation as early as 5,000 BC have been identified in Hinduism (Pickert 2014). Mindfulness can also be located in other Eastern ancient traditions such as Taoism and Jainism and even has roots in Judaism, Christianity, and Islam (Trousselard et al. 2014).

Although the earliest recorded Western scientific paper on the benefits of meditation was published in 1936, it was another three decades before it began to take on popular appeal within a Western context. Vietnamese Buddhist monk Thich Nhat Hahn [1926–2022] raised the profile of meditation in the United States during his publicised opposition to the Vietnamese war during the 1960s but it was Jon Kabut-Zinn, founder of the Center for Mindfulness at the Massachusetts Medical School, who primarily introduced the West to the concept of 'mindfulness' in the 1970s. Kabat Zinn developed a mindfulness program for use in clinical settings and named it mindfulness-based stress reduction (MBSR) and the scientific benefits of mindfulness became rooted in the field of psychology. MBSR used to treat conditions such as anxiety, stress and obsessive-compulsive disorder was followed by Mindfulness-based Cognitive Therapy (MBCT) which examines the role of mindfulness in treating depression and mood disorders. Mindfulness in a contemporary western setting is generally used to refer to "a set of techniques win which one gives deliberate sustained attention to presently occurring ambient, somatic or subjective phenomena" (Brazier 2013).

Mindfulness comes in many guises including yoga practice, formal meditation, or practising mindfulness in everyday activities such as mindful teeth brushing or dish washing. It can be practised individually or as part of a group practice. In terms of defining mindfulness, the most widely used definition can almost certainly be attributed to Jon Kabut-Zinn who describes mindfulness as "Paying attention in a particular way; on purpose, in the present moment, and non-judgmentally" (Kabat-Zinn 2005) This can be interpreted as attunement to an intentional, attentive, reflective, deliberate, and conscious style of listening using all the senses. This attuned state provides enhanced quality of perceived or lived-time experienced by self and others. Mindfulness is thus a state of being that evokes contemplation with a purpose that opens us to considering possibilities beyond individual or/and siloed perspectives.

There are many misconceptions and even mythical thinking around mindfulness (Iglesias 2019). Table 1.1 presents some of the prevailing assumptions alongside the authentic principles of mindfulness practice.

Meditation and mindfulness

Meditation and mindfulness often get conflated and become used interchangeably. However, although meditation and mindfulness weave within each other they can be explored and understood separately. Mindfulness is concerned with non-judgemental detached awareness and is a quality or aspect of meditation. Meditation has many forms and myriad of practices. Some would contend that mindfulness is a quality and meditation a practice – but that may be too simplistic

TABLE 1.1 What Mindfulness Is and What Mindfulness Is Not

What Mindfulness: Is Not	• *What Mindfulness Is*
A mystical or mysterious state of mind	Awareness; attention; choosing to focus on something without judgement
Pushing away or blocking a thought or feeling	Noticing a thought or feeling (then maybe choosing to focus on something else)
A quick fix or panacea for all ills	A part of living an effective life; often a first step in using other skills
A skill that is easily learned	A skill that requires much practice
Something that only spiritual people do	A capacity everyone has (whether you know it yet or not)
Having perfect focus; never getting distracted	Choosing to try to keep your focus even though distractions will probably arise again and again. Mindfulness involves noticing the wandering and gently guiding your attention back to your chosen focus
A relaxation exercise	An exercise that involves full participation and acceptance of "what is," which at any given time could be a state of tension
Something that will change who you are	A non-judgemental acceptance of reality (even though it may lead you to make changes)
Something that will Solve our problems	Enables us to relate in a new way to the things that trouble us, rather than trying to make them go away

Adapted from Lynch and Bronner (2006).

and abstract. Mindfulness is certainly an important part of meditation practice. According to Walsh and Shapiro (2006), meditation is,

> ...a practice where an individual uses a technique – such as mindfulness or focusing the mind on a particular object, thought, or activity – to train attention and awareness, and achieve a mentally clear and emotionally calm and stable state
>
> *(pp. 228–229)*

In some meditation practices visualisations are used, for example seeing deities with the mind through concentration, or mantras spoken internally in relation to the movement of the breath. Some may use prayer, comforting phrases, or a spiritual self-questioning, such as 'who am I?' in their meditation. Some meditations cultivate qualities like compassion, lovingkindness, or devotion to a form(s) of divinity involving concentration, rather than being mindful as things are. In Zen meditation practice, the goal is to eliminate the sense of self through strict discipline. Conversely, mindfulness is a practice that nurtures a mindful self in everyday life activities. What is evident is that meditation is a practice involving concentration and mindfulness which involves specific focus that considers and contemplates something thoughtfully. That focus may have a powerful religious and spiritual intent, such as devotional meditation or a non-religious psycho-spiritual purpose. What we speak about in this book is mindfulness, a practice of being present in the moment in a state of non-judgemental awareness of one's thoughts, feelings, body, self, others, and environment.

The value of mindfulness

As previously identified, there are literally thousands of studies that explore the use of mindfulness-based interventions and as a result the body of evidence to support the benefits of using mindfulness is extensive. Although much of the work is grounded in psychological studies, epidemiological research relationship exploring the association between mindfulness and health is also increasing. However, further evidence from large and more broadly representative population samples are required in order to establish the benefits of mindfulness at a population level (Bartlett et al. 2021).

Table 1.2 highlights a small selection of the many studies and reviews that have produced data relating to the beneficial effects of mindfulness-based interventions as a psychological therapy or as a self-help method for improved self-awareness and self-improvement. This list is far from definitive, but interventions have shown to be effective in promoting resilience and well-being, reducing stress, and treating mental and physical health issues like depression, anxiety, and chronic pain (Klingbeil et al. 2017; Zenner, Herrnleben-Kurz, and Walach 2014).

TABLE 1.2 Benefits of Mindfulness

Increases attention and consciousness of experience	Chambers, Gullone, and Allen (2009) Garland et al. (2017)
Reduces autonomic reactivity	Crane et al. (2017)
Stress relief	Goyal et al. (2014) Grossman et al. (2004) Khoury et al. (2015)
Treating anxiety and depression	Orme-Johnson and Barnes (2014) Hofmann and Gómez (2017) Creswell (2017)
Encourages creativity	CAPURSO, Fabbro, and Crescentini (2014)
Lengthens attention span	Norris et al. (2018) Tsai et al. (2018)
Treating addictive behaviour	Garland et al. (2017) Katterman et al. (2014)
Sleep improvement	Ong et al. (2014)
Reliving pain	Hilton et al. (2017) Davis et al. (2015)

An existential crisis

To fully appreciate the potential benefits of mindfulness within the birth sphere, we need to contextualise contemporary delivery of care and the current state of the workforce. As we previously alluded to, maternity care is in an intensifying state of crisis. The State of the Worlds Midwifery Report advises that the world needs 900,000 more midwives which represents a third of the global midwifery workforce (Nove et al. 2021) In many countries an exodus of experienced midwives coinciding with a drop in the recruitment of student midwives is creating staffing problems. Stress and burnout seem to feature evermore regularly in the professional literature. Likewise, there is a growing shortage of obstetricians internationally in both low- and medium-resource countries (Hoyler et al. 2014) and also, in high-income countries such as the United States (Stonehocker, Muruthi, and Rayburn 2017). A growing reliance on medicalisation and technology in a risk averse, over-litigious world challenges those working in the field and can lead to defensive practice that impacts those accessing care. As a result of these challenges, many of those within maternity systems, both caregivers and those accessing maternity services, report feeling distress rather than its antonym of eustress (McCarthy, Houghton, and Matvienko-Sikar 2021; Ockenden Review 2022). In the face of such apparent adversity, it might be easy to lose faith and simply feel a sense of despair. However, it is important to acknowledge that these problems are not unique to maternity care and need to be situated in a broader societal context.

Some theorists and philosophers advocate that we are living in an unprecedented state of existential crisis which leads us to question the intrinsic meaning of life. Parfit (2011) mooted that we are 'living at the "hinge" of history' (p.616) during possibly the most influential period in human terms, that could set the fate of our species. If we consider just some of the 'wicked' problems that humanity is currently grappling with, which might include a global pandemic; the increasingly urgent threat of climate change; technological insurgency; economic uncertainty; and the death and destruction of war, it is easy to understand how feelings of unease about meaning and purpose may arise. Additionally, existential crises occur on a more personal level following life events such as birth or changing life circumstances. At both a macro and a micro level, an existential crisis has the potential to uproot us from a place of safety and familiarity into a place of uncertainty and unpredictability.

However, in contrast to leaving us feeling adrift and afraid, an existential crisis can provide us with the opportunity grow and develop. It has the potential to move us closer to our authentic self, lead us to question our purpose in life and even provide direction. As Nietzsche philosophised "there has never been such a new dawn and clear horizon, and such an open sea" (Nietzsche et al. 2001)

Meaning and purpose have been found to have a positive association with mindfulness. Greater self-awareness and self-worth could give life greater meaning. Additionally, mindfulness can help to make sense when adverse events threaten to bring us down (Hanley et al. 2015). Having a strong sense of purpose in life has been identified as a significant factor in relation to well-being and health-related outcomes (McKnight and Kashdan 2009). So, in a world where it can sometimes feel as though we have no control or influence, mindfulness may be able to provide a bridge between existential crisis and personal growth and healing. Mindfulness is also said to enhance social connection by creating positive emotions that lead to decreased social isolation thus improving our mental health and well-being as well as our sense of agency (Adair et al. 2018; Crego et al. 2021). Moreover, Jon Kabat-Zinn claims that there is a fundamental social element to mindfulness (Kabat-Zinn 2003).

Mindfulness in the birth sphere

The benefits of mindfulness apply to those experiencing pregnancy, birth, and new parenting as much as they do to others within the general population. However, there are specific attributes that emerge from a mindful approach that have significance for this community. These include reducing the incidence of antenatal depression, ameliorating the fear of labour and birth, lowering the risk of postnatal depression, increasing attachment with the baby, and increasing the likelihood of effective lactation.

The pre-conceptual period through to the first 1,000 days of life is now acknowledged as pivotal to human growth and development. When a pregnant woman is supported to achieve their full potential during this period, they are able to flourish, and integrated human growth and development is facilitated. This also requires that the health care professionals involved are attuned in an appropriate and sustainable way. However, many would contend that the birth sphere in its current state is not sustainable unless the multidimensional qualities beyond purely measurable outcomes and biomedical model are honoured and addressed.

This recognition beckons different styles and broader approaches, and mindfulness contributes and provides opportunity to address this beckoning. As we have determined, there is a raft of research activity relating to mindfulness within healthcare generally (Table 1.2) There is a similar exponential growth in the number of research studies relating to the childbirth continuum. However, to date any evidence within the domain of maternity care has not been collated into an evidence-based usable and accessible format aimed at those experiencing childbirth and those working in the area. It is evident that there needs to be some appraisal and critical discussion as well as practical application and praxis.

Outlining the book

Mindfulness encourages and reminds us to adopt an integral approach to childbirth that incorporates and invites creativity, wisdom, intuitional knowing allowing us to connect with our inner guidance for everyone to communicate with care, love, and compassion. The content of this book asks different questions and invites different voices to the conversation and presents a series of sections and chapters that takes the reader on a journey of mindful inquiry that enlivens a fresh appreciation of what is possible in ways that disrupt the status quo and bring new energy and insight. Each of the chapter authors and co-editors proffers different horizons of understanding that coalesce and inform a new understanding of the birth sphere with suggestions for personal and organisational mindful practices.

The book draws upon an interdisciplinary body of knowledge, including physiology, midwifery, medicine, nursing, psychology, and sociology. The chapters are principally an assembly of compositions that represent a broad range of perspectives. The authors bring ontological and epistemological standpoints from their own areas of knowledge and weave the principles of mindfulness into their discipline areas. In so doing, they proffer different horizons of understanding that inform and contribute to new understandings of the birth sphere along with suggestions for personal and organisational mindful practices.

The chapters within the book are presented within three distinct sections. **Section 1** begins by introducing the reader to the conceptual underpinnings of mindfulness. Australian researchers Craig Hassed and Richard Chambers set the scene by introducing mindfulness as a type of meta-skill that underpins other essential self-care and clinical skills. They explore the why and how of mindfulness and its applications by the practitioner in the birth sphere. Diane Menage and Jenny Patterson two midwifery academics, then unpack the concepts of compassion, empathy, and resilience in relation to birth trauma to show how mindful and compassionate midwifery care can reduce fear and increase feelings of safety. Miriama Ketu-McKenzie is a clinical psychologist and academic who presents an indigenous perspective analysing how the concepts in mindfulness and the concepts in the Māori worldview (te ao Māori) converge. She also explores the relevance that mindfulness practice has for Māori women. Mindful Inquiry is introduced by Valerie Bentz in Chapter 5 as a deeply reflexive research methodology which offers a powerful way of understanding and making meaning from personal experience by using an autobiographical approach.

Section 2 draws our focus to the application of mindfulness within the many contexts of practice across the birth sphere. In Chapter 6, Janetti Marotta, a clinical psychologist who specialises in fertility, uses mindfulness in her practice to work with what she describes as the 'overwhelming challenges of infertility'. Susan Crowther and Christine Mellor present the findings from an antenatal educational programme that focuses on the interrelatedness of mind and body in childbirth in order to improve birthing outcomes for those attending. In Chapter 9, Doreen Balabanoff and Maralyn Foureur move us into the intrapartum space by considering how best to create mindful birthing environments and conclude that mindfulness in the design approach is essential in order to enable women to immerse themselves mindfully in the birthing process. Mo Tabib and Tracy Humphrey consider how meditation and relaxation can bring presence to labour and birth and mitigate the effects of fear and anxiety that are so common during pregnancy and childbirth. In Chapter 10, Laura Whitburn, Liz Newnham, and Lester Jones explore the association between the relevance of pain and the concept of a state of mindfulness with a specific focus on pain in labour. In the postnatal context, Maggie Meeks and Dan who are both neonatologists, deliberate on the value of mindfulness as a tool in the neonatal setting and how its use could provide a vehicle for change in the medicalised and highly technological world of neonatal intensive care. The chapter by Angus MacBeth and Aigli Raouna explores the relevance of, and evidence for mindfulness-based interventions as a psychological intervention option for perinatal mental health in both the ante- and postnatal periods. Tracy Donegan also spans the whole of the childbirth continuum in her chapter on mindfulness during situations of crisis. Finally, lactation is presented in Chapter 11 where Anna Byrom and Ira Kantrowitz-Gordon consider how mindfulness could be used to improve breast-feeding rates.

Section 3 accommodates the final chapters of the book, where governance, leadership, and education are reflected upon in relation to the value of mindfulness in the birth sphere. These chapters also outline strategies that may help to introduce mindfulness at a more strategic level. Lorna Davies, Melanie Welfare, and Kathleen Mahy present a case study on how mindfulness was incorporated into a Bachelor of Midwifery programme in Aotearoa/New Zealand and how the principles could be adopted for use in other settings. In Chapter 16, Sheena Byrom uses a reflexive approach to explore the importance of mindful leadership in maternity care and calls for action for leaders to nurture compassion within the organisations and departments where they are based. In the final concluding chapter, Susan Crowther and Lorna Davies revisit the key insights of the proceeding chapters through the lens of an ecology of birth. They highlight the need to open our gaze and notice the multifaceted qualities that inform and influence the childbirth sphere and present the reader with the attributes of a mindful practitioner.

In conclusion

The incorporation of a mindful approach has the potential to provide significant benefits during the important transitional period of maternity. However, becoming more mindful necessitates a shift in attitude and levels of self-awareness. If we are to support those we serve during pregnancy, birth and in early parenting to achieve a state of mindfulness during this time, we need to learn to embrace the values of mindfulness and to experience the benefits of mindfulness first hand. We hope that by taking the time to look at this book that you are exploring ways to consider how you can make your own clinical practice more mindful. A state of mindful self-awareness is a powerful one and has the potential to release us from existing assumptions and transform both our lives as practitioners and the lives of those that we serve within the birth sphere.

References

Adair, Kathryn C., Barbara L. Fredrickson, Laura Castro-Schilo, Sumi Kim, and Stephania Sidberry. 2018. "Present with You: Does Cultivated Mindfulness Predict Greater Social Connection through Gains in Decentering and Reductions in Negative Emotions?" *Mindfulness* 9 (3): 737–749. https://doi.org/10.1007/s12671-017-0811-1.

Bardacke, Nancy. 2012. *Mindful Birthing: Training the Mind, Body, and Heart for Childbirth and Beyond*. Harper Collins.

Bartlett, Larissa, Marie-Jeanne Buscot, Aidan Bindoff, Richard Chambers, and Craig Hassed. 2021. "Mindfulness Is Associated With Lower Stress and Higher Work Engagement in a Large Sample of MOOC Participants." *Frontiers in Psychology* 12. https://www.frontiersin.org/article/10.3389/fpsyg.2021.724126.

Brazier, David. 2013. "Mindfulness Reconsidered." *European Journal of Psychotherapy & Counselling* 15 (2): 116–126. https://doi.org/10.1080/13642537.2013.795335.

Capurso, Viviana, Franco Fabbro, and Cristiano Crescentini. 2014. "Mindful Creativity: The Influence of Mindfulness Meditation on Creative Thinking." *Frontiers in Psychology* 4. https://www.frontiersin.org/article/10.3389/fpsyg.2013.01020.

Chambers, Richard, Eleonora Gullone, and Nicholas B. Allen. 2009. "Mindful Emotion Regulation: An Integrative Review." *Clinical Psychology Review* 29 (6): 560–572. https://doi.org/10.1016/j.cpr.2009.06.005.

Crane, R. S., J. Brewer, C. Feldman, J. Kabat-Zinn, S. Santorelli, J. M. G. Williams, and W. Kuyken. 2017. "What Defines Mindfulness-Based Programs? The Warp and the Weft." *Psychological Medicine* 47 (6): 990–999. https://doi.org/10.1017/S0033291716003317.

Crego, Antonio, José Ramón Yela, María Ángeles Gómez-Martínez, Pablo Riesco-Matías, and Cristina Petisco-Rodríguez. 2021. "Relationships between Mindfulness,

Purpose in Life, Happiness, Anxiety, and Depression: Testing a Mediation Model in a Sample of Women." *International Journal of Environmental Research and Public Health* 18 (3): 925. https://doi.org/10.3390/ijerph18030925.

Creswell, J. David. 2017. "Mindfulness Interventions." *Annual Review of Psychology* 68 (January): 491–516. https://doi.org/10.1146/annurev-psych-042716-051139.

Davis, Mary C., Alex J. Zautra, Laurie D. Wolf, Howard Tennen, and Ellen W. Yeung. 2015. "Mindfulness and Cognitive-Behavioral Interventions for Chronic Pain: Differential Effects on Daily Pain Reactivity and Stress Reactivity." *Journal of Consulting and Clinical Psychology* 83 (1): 24–35. https://doi.org/10.1037/a0038200.

Garland, Eric L., Adam W. Hanley, Phillipe R. Goldin, and James J. Gross. 2017. "Testing the Mindfulness-to-Meaning Theory: Evidence for Mindful Positive Emotion Regulation from a Reanalysis of Longitudinal Data." *PLoS One* 12 (12): e0187727. https://doi.org/10.1371/journal.pone.0187727.

Goyal, Madhav, Sonal Singh, Erica M. S. Sibinga, Neda F. Gould, Anastasia Rowland-Seymour, Ritu Sharma, Zackary Berger, et al. 2014. "Meditation Programs for Psychological Stress and Well-Being: A Systematic Review and Meta-Analysis." *JAMA Internal Medicine* 174 (3): 357–368. https://doi.org/10.1001/jamainternmed.2013.13018.

Grossman, Paul, Ludger Niemann, Stefan Schmidt, and Harald Walach. 2004. "Mindfulness-Based Stress Reduction and Health Benefits: A Meta-Analysis." *Journal of Psychosomatic Research* 57 (1): 35–43. https://doi.org/10.1016/S0022-3999(03)00573-7.

Hanley, Adam W., Gary W. Peterson, Angela I. Canto, and Eric L. Garland. 2015. "The Relationship between Mindfulness and Posttraumatic Growth with Respect to Contemplative Practice Engagement." *Mindfulness* 6 (3): 654–662. https://doi.org/10.1007/s12671-014-0302-6.

Hilton, Lara, Susanne Hempel, Brett A. Ewing, Eric Apaydin, Lea Xenakis, Sydne Newberry, Ben Colaiaco, et al. 2017. "Mindfulness Meditation for Chronic Pain: Systematic Review and Meta-Analysis." *Annals of Behavioral Medicine* 51 (2): 199–213. https://doi.org/10.1007/s12160-016-9844-2.

Hofmann, Stefan G., and Angelina F. Gómez. 2017. "Mindfulness-Based Interventions for Anxiety and Depression." *Psychiatric Clinics* 40 (4): 739–749. https://doi.org/10.1016/j.psc.2017.08.008.

"How Does Mindfulness Training Affect Health? A Mindfulness Stress Buffering Account - J. David Creswell, Emily K. Lindsay, 2014." n.d. Accessed April 26, 2022. https://journals.sagepub.com/doi/abs/10.1177/0963721414547415?journalCode=cdpa.

Hoyler, Marguerite, Samuel R. G. Finlayson, Craig D. McClain, John G. Meara, and Lars Hagander. 2014. "Shortage of Doctors, Shortage of Data: A Review of the Global Surgery, Obstetrics, and Anesthesia Workforce Literature." *World Journal of Surgery* 38 (2): 269–280. https://doi.org/10.1007/s00268-013-2324-y.

Iglesias, Tim. 2019. "Mindfulness as Resistance." *Southwestern Law Review* 48: 381.

Kabat-Zinn, Jon. 2003. "Mindfulness-Based Interventions in Context: Past, Present, and Future." *Clinical Psychology: Science and Practice* 10 (2): 144–156. https://doi.org/10.1093/clipsy.bpg016.

———. 2005. *Wherever You Go, There You Are: Mindfulness Meditation in Everyday Life.* 10th anniversary ed. Hyperion.

Katterman, Shawn N., Brighid M. Kleinman, Megan M. Hood, Lisa M. Nackers, and Joyce A. Corsica. 2014. "Mindfulness Meditation as an Intervention for Binge Eating, Emotional Eating, and Weight Loss: A Systematic Review." *Eating Behaviors* 15 (2): 197–204. https://doi.org/10.1016/j.eatbeh.2014.01.005.

Khoury, Bassam, Manoj Sharma, Sarah E. Rush, and Claude Fournier. 2015. "Mindfulness-Based Stress Reduction for Healthy Individuals: A Meta-Analysis." *Journal of Psychosomatic Research* 78 (6): 519–528. https://doi.org/10.1016/j.jpsychores.2015.03.009.

Lynch, Thomas R., and Leslie L. Bronner. 2006. "Mindfulness and Dialectical Behavior Therapy (DBT): Application with Depressed Older Adults with Personality Disorders." In *Mindfulness-Based Treatment Approaches: Clinician's Guide to Evidence Base and Applications*, 217–236. San Diego, CA: Elsevier Academic Press. https://doi.org/10.1016/B978-012088519-0/50011-3.

McCarthy, Megan, Catherine Houghton, and Karen Matvienko-Sikar. 2021. "Women's Experiences and Perceptions of Anxiety and Stress during the Perinatal Period: A Systematic Review and Qualitative Evidence Synthesis." *BMC Pregnancy and Childbirth* 21 (1): 811. https://doi.org/10.1186/s12884-021-04271-w.

McKnight, Patrick E., and Todd B. Kashdan. 2009. "Purpose in Life as a System That Creates and Sustains Health and Well-Being: An Integrative, Testable Theory." *Review of General Psychology* 13 (3): 242–251. https://doi.org/10.1037/a0017152.

Nietzsche, Friedrich, Bernard William, Josephine J. Nauckhoff, and Adrian Del Caro. 2001. *The Gay Science*. Cambridge: Cambridge University Press.

Norris, Catherine J., Daniel Creem, Reuben Hendler, and Hedy Kober. 2018. "Brief Mindfulness Meditation Improves Attention in Novices: Evidence from ERPs and Moderation by Neuroticism." *Frontiers in Human Neuroscience* 12. https://www.frontiersin.org/article/10.3389/fnhum.2018.00315.

Nove, Andrea, Petra ten Hoope-Bender, Martin Boyce, Sarah Bar-Zeev, Luc de Bernis, Geeta Lal, Zoë Matthews, Million Mekuria, and Caroline S. E. Homer. 2021. "The State of the World's Midwifery 2021 Report: Findings to Drive Global Policy and Practice." *Human Resources for Health* 19 (1): 146. https://doi.org/10.1186/s12960-021-00694-w.

"Ockenden Review: Summary of Findings, Conclusions and Essential Actions." n.d. GOV.UK. Accessed May 3, 2022. https://www.gov.uk/government/publications/-final-report-of-the-ockenden-review/ockenden-review-summary-of-findings-conclusions-and-essential-actions.

Ong, Jason C., Rachel Manber, Zindel Segal, Yinglin Xia, Shauna Shapiro, and James K. Wyatt. 2014. "A Randomized Controlled Trial of Mindfulness Meditation for Chronic Insomnia." *Sleep* 37 (9): 1553–1563. https://doi.org/10.5665/sleep.4010.

Orme-Johnson, David W., and Vernon A. Barnes. 2014. "Effects of the Transcendental Meditation Technique on Trait Anxiety: A Meta-Analysis of Randomized Controlled Trials." *The Journal of Alternative and Complementary Medicine* 20 (5): 330–341. https://doi.org/10.1089/acm.2013.0204.

Parfit, Derek. 2011. *On What Matters: Volume Two*. Oxford: Oxford University Press.

Pickert, Kate. 2014. "The Art of Being Mindful. Finding Peace in a Stressed-out, Digitally Dependent Culture May Just Be a Matter of Thinking Differently." *Time* 183 (4): 40–46.

Purser, Ronald. 2019. "The Mindfulness Conspiracy." *The Guardian*, June 14, 2019, sec. Life and style. https://www.theguardian.com/lifeandstyle/2019/jun/14/the-mindfulness-conspiracy-capitalist-spirituality.

Purser, R. E., & Loy, D. R. (2013). Beyond McMindfulness. *Huffington Post, 1*(7), 13.

Stonehocker, Jody, Joyce Muruthi, and William F. Rayburn. 2017. "Is There a Shortage of Obstetrician-Gynecologists?" *Obstetrics and Gynecology Clinics of North America* 44 (1): 121–132. https://doi.org/10.1016/j.ogc.2016.11.006.

Trousselard, M., D. Steiler, D. Claverie, and F. Canini. 2014. "[The History of Mindfulness Put to the Test of Current Scientific Data: Unresolved Questions]." *L'Encephale* 40 (6): 474–480. https://doi.org/10.1016/j.encep.2014.08.006.

Tsai, Shao-Yang, Satish Jaiswal, Chi-Fu Chang, Wei-Kuang Liang, Neil G. Mug-gleton, and Chi-Hung Juan. 2018. "Meditation Effects on the Control of Involuntary Contingent Reorienting Revealed With Electroencephalographic and Behavioral Evidence." *Frontiers in Integrative Neuroscience* 12. https://www.frontiersin.org/article/10.3389/fnint.2018.00017.

Walsh, Roger, and Shauna L. Shapiro. 2006. "The Meeting of Meditative Disciplines and Western Psychology: A Mutually Enriching Dialogue." *The American Psychologist* 61 (3): 227–239.

Widdicombe, Lizzie. 2015. "The Higher Life." *The New Yorker*, June 7, 2015.

Zenner, Charlote, Solveig Herrnleben-Kurz, and Harald Walach. 2014. "Mindfulness-Based Interventions in Schools - A Systematic Review and Meta-Analysis." *Frontiers in Psychology* 30 (5): 603. https://doi.org/10.3389/fpsyg.2014.00603.

Žižek, Slavoj. 2001. *Enjoy Your Symptom! Jacques Lacan in Hollywood and Out*. New York: Routledge.

2

THE MINDFUL PRACTITIONER

Craig Hassed and Richard Chambers

Personal introduction

We, the authors of this chapter (CH & RC), have a longstanding personal and professional commitment to mindfulness and its myriad uses clinically and educationally. Having worked in clinical practice (CH for nearly 40 years as a doctor and RC for nearly 20 as a psychologist) and teaching and researching at Monash University in Australia (CH for over 30 years and RC for over 10) we have been involved in training many thousands of medical and allied health professionals at undergraduate and postgraduate levels, with the emphasis on enhancing clinical performance, wellbeing and mental health.

We both became interested in this line of work initially because of a personal need for self-care and personal development that arose as tertiary students and junior clinicians. Having discovered the immense value of living more mindfully, this naturally evolved into a professional interest as clinicians to share these insights and practices with clients. This, in turn, led to a commitment to help other professionals to bring mindfulness into their personal and professional lives through including it in tertiary education.

Much energy and attention are rightly directed to the therapeutic applications of mindfulness, many of which are relevant to the birthing sphere. It is equally relevant, however, for the health practitioner to be mindful in the process of performing their work. Why? Well, essentially, the ability to be present and self-aware is a prerequisite for virtually all other clinical competencies. For example, it is important for practitioners to take a proactive attitude to better managing workload, work stress and mental health for many reasons – not least of which is because a burned-out and impaired practitioner is less likely to care effectively for their clients/patients and is more likely to make clinical errors. Furthermore, a more present and attentive practitioner

DOI: 10.4324/9781003165200-2

tends to be more compassionate and communicates more effectively with colleagues and clients.

For these and other reasons which will be explored in this chapter, mindfulness can be seen as a kind of meta-skill that underpins other essential self-care and clinical skills. It is like the primary higher or executive function upon which other executive functions rely. In brief, it is very hard to get other things right if we can't get the attention bit right first. So, this chapter will explore the why and how of mindfulness and its applications by the practitioner in the process of doing their work.

Reducing burnout and improving practitioner mental health

In one of life's great ironies, healthcare professionals experience elevated rates of mental health issues compared to the rest of the population (Eaves & Payne, 2019; Harvey et al., 2021; Maharaj, Lees & Lal, 2018). Even students in courses such as medicine, nursing, midwifery (Oates et al., 2019) and allied health experience sharp rises in stress, anxiety and other forms of psychological distress as they progress through their studies, and once they start working this trend continues (Dyrbye, Thomas & Shanafelt, 2005). One in three doctors report experiencing burnout at any given time (De Hert, 2020), with similar trends also observed in nurses and allied health professionals (Friganović et al., 2019; Pradas-Hernández et al., 2018). Within the birthing sphere, 46% of obstetrics and gynaecology specialists report burnout (the highest rate amongst any medical specialisation) and a 2019 survey of midwives in Australia similarly found that almost half had considered leaving the profession (Harvey et al., 2019).

There are multiple factors contributing to this issue. These include shift work, which is widely recognised as being a major contributor to mental health issues, as well as the pressure of ever-increasing caseloads. Interfacing with other aspects of the medical system – such as navigating the tension between viewing childbirth as a normal human behaviour, versus considering it a 'medical emergency' – contribute to these background pressures, meaning that working in the birthing sphere can be additionally stressful. Add in the anxiety and distress of expectant parents before, during and after birth and the ever-present risk of litigation in many countries when things go wrong, and it becomes clear why this can be a very challenging sector to work in. Finally, the tendency of many birthing professionals to prioritise other people's needs and wellbeing over their own acts as an amplifier of the underlying stresses of the profession (Young, Smythe & McAra-Couper, 2015).

The implications of burnout amongst birthing professionals are complex and varied. It can lead to higher rates of absenteeism and greater staff turnover which are major problems for hospitals and health centres. More hidden are the impacts on performance, such as presenteeism – that is, being physically at work but performing at reduced capacity. A meta-analysis of physicians found that depressed doctors make almost twice as many medical errors (Pereira-Lima et al., 2019), and nurses with poor mental health report 71% more errors (Brandford & Reed, 2016). Finally, patients commonly report lower levels of satisfaction when their healthcare is provided by practitioners with burnout or other mental health problems (Panagioti et al., 2018). A systematic review of 58 studies on mindfulness and the compassion characteristics of healthcare professionals found that mindfulness was effective at improving self-compassion, burnout, depression, anxiety, stress and compassion fatigue (Conversano et al., 2020).

There is therefore a clear need for mindfulness in healthcare generally, and the birthing sphere in particular. In the next section, we outline how mindfulness may be employed in both bottom-up and top-down ways.

Bottom-up applications of mindfulness

The term "bottom-up" may evoke images of new-born infants, but here we refer to approaches taken by individuals (in contrast to "top-down" which refers to organisational approaches and policy decisions). Mindfulness provides a number of practical strategies that can be employed in a bottom-up way by healthcare professionals. First, mindfulness being primarily used as a practice aimed at increasing awareness helps people to start paying more attention to their moment-by-moment experience and their unrecognised stress, anxiety and depression. Noticing tension held in the body, low levels of energy or a racing mind that cannot focus properly on the present moment is a necessary first step to changing what is going on underneath. For some people, this immediately orients them toward healthier behaviours and ways of approaching life. Others may need to pause and reflect on what would recharge them, considering – or perhaps remembering – things that genuinely nourish their body, mind and soul. Individuals vary, but commonly these include finding meaning in what they do, quality sleep, time in nature, genuine connection with people they can be vulnerable and authentic with, healthy food, good hydration and physical exercise. It is also important to *do* these things mindfully, as there is a big difference between going hiking while stewing on problems at work versus actually being present with our surroundings. The former mentally fatigues us, whereas the latter refreshes us.

Mindfulness also provides an opportunity to observe the operation of the mind and recognise the mental habits underlying stress, anxiety and depression. Many people assume that stress is either endogenous *"it's just a chemical imbalance in the brain which I can't do anything about other than take medications"* or purely environmental *"I'm like this because of a busy job, difficult boss, and too much traffic on the roads – none of which I have any control over"*. But when we look closely, we can start noticing that sometimes we react to being stuck in traffic with frustration and resentment, while other times we just turn on music, keep our attention focused on driving and adopt an accepting attitude that the situation is what it is. Attitude has a massive effect: the former leads to stress, while the latter doesn't. Shifting attitude in a situation that we cannot change fosters an internal locus of control, and it is an empowering way of relating to stress. It means completely accepting something the way it is, not wishing it to be otherwise, and then engaging our attention with it. Once we notice that stress and anxiety are created by worrying and obsessing about the future, dwelling and ruminating on the past, or judging and reacting to what is happening in the present moment, we can start to work with these ubiquitous mental habits. With mindfulness, we simply bring the attention back to what is actually happening in that moment, that is, to the senses. In any moment that we do this, we are no longer feeding the negative thoughts that give rise to stress.

> Mindfulness tip – Start to notice moments where you are stressed. Learn to recognise signs of stress in the body – things like increased heart rate, shallow breathing and muscle tension. In these moments, try to notice what images, stories or thoughts are in the mind that might be driving this stress response. If possible, experiment with returning your attention to the present moment (e.g., by focusing on your breathing, feeling your feet making contact with the floor, or focusing on the task you are doing). Notice the effect this has on stress.

What makes this easier, of course, is a daily formal meditation practice. Meditation simply means 'mental training' and mindfulness meditation involves training the attention to stay present, while simultaneously cultivating qualities such as curiosity, acceptance and non-reactivity even in the presence of discomfort. For a woman in labour that means one thing, for a health practitioner under work pressure it means another. When this is systematically trained in a quiet space devoid of stress and distractions, the ability to remain present and nonreactive gets strengthened, as with anything we practice. We then find that we can stay more present and be less reactive even during challenging situations. Over time, the brain's stress circuitry gets triggered less often and with less amplitude. This is why many people are embracing mindfulness as a capacity that helps them maintain functioning at a high level, even in challenging environments. Bestselling author, Tim Ferris, interviewed elite performers in business, entrepreneurship and sport and found that 80% had a daily meditation practice (Ferris, 2017).

Top-down applications of mindfulness

In addition to these bottom-up approaches, it is also worth considering top-down ways mindfulness can be used to reduce burnout and improve practitioner mental health. It is not enough to just leave it up to individual practitioners to apply these principles – but for real change to happen, a systemic approach must be employed. This entails considerations such as setting up physical work environments and work practices to promote mindfulness, ensuring demands and expectations placed on practitioners allow for adequate work/life balance and wellbeing, and having clear guidelines around the use of digital technology to minimise its negative impacts on attention and performance. Furthermore, it is imperative that leaders themselves practice mindfulness to ensure those they lead function well and have good mental health. Research shows that mindful leaders are more likely to have transformational (rather than transactional or passive) leadership styles, and that this predicts employee engagement and organisational performance (Carleton, Barling & Trivisonno, 2018).

Work stress and coping with workload

The three elements of workplace stress described by Karasek and Theorell in 1990 are control, support and demands. Having little external locus of control at work is stressful but not as much as having no internal locus of control. Using mindfulness to switch to a greater internal locus of control by consciously choosing our attitude to the situation has been discussed above, but essentially, if we choose an open and accepting attitude to an uncomfortable situation then we engage with it more, feel empowered, we begin to learn from it, and we are less controlled by rumination and avoidance.

Fostering support within the workplace can be both formal (e.g., debriefing, counselling, leaders who listen to their workers' needs, work systems that support practitioner wellbeing) and informal (e.g. a supportive work culture, looking out for your colleagues, taking human moments). Mindfulness can certainly help people to give and receive formal feedback more consciously, but because of its ability to foster compassion (Brito-Pons, Campos & Cebolla, 2018) and pro-sociality (Donald et al., 2019), it is particularly helpful in helping to transform workplace culture. Providing both formal and informal support is important because without it practitioners won't look out for each other and will feel undermined and demotivated in times of high workload.

Demands can be both real and perceived. For real and excessive demands, especially when prolonged, the aim is either to increase our ability to meet those demands with appropriate training, or to moderate those demands by reducing workload or increasing staffing levels. As far as the perception of demands is concerned, when unmindful we are often consumed by rumination or worry exaggerating how major the demands actually are. Rumination and worry are sometimes described as the 'second arrow', the first arrow being the challenging situation we may be confronting but the second and more damaging one is our negative thinking about the situation leading to an inability to effectively engage with it. Rumination and worry are both forms of default mental activity – the distracted mode the brain goes into when we unhook from present-moment sensory input. Default thinking can cause distraction, make demands appear bigger than they are and undermine our ability and self-confidence with negative thought patterns about ourselves. This commonly leads to avoidance and procrastination which compounds a problem by wasting the time, energy and resources we had available to us to meet those demands in the first place. Being able to short circuit the tendency to be consumed by ruminative patterns of thinking by recognising it and practicing mindfulness engages our attention with the actual situation in front of us free of the amplifying effect of default mode.

From a practical point of view, managing high workload and conserving energy mindfully requires moment-by-moment attention. We often consume energy with the low level, internally generated stress and tension we carry through the workday. This significantly depletes energy. From a mindfulness perspective, when running a marathon, we give our attention to one 'step' (i.e. one job, one moment, one interaction) at a time rather than worrying about the 42,000 steps we might still need to take. If we can do this then we reduce the mental load and fatigue commonly associated with rumination and worry. Mindfulness means keeping simple moments, simple. The workday or night will contain some complex clinical moments but also many simple moments. For example, we may have finished dealing with a complex clinical situation and now you have a three-minute walk to another ward or birthing suite. If unmindful, we are likely to fill those three minutes with rumination, negative self-talk and overthinking. If mindful, however, then we can just give our attention to the present moment – simply feeling the body walking. If we do that then at the end of the walk we step into the next clinical situation with a calmer, more attentive state of mind rather than an overloaded and distracted one.

Like punctuating our day with lots of commas, we can also take time for frequent mini meditations throughout the workday. These could be anything from a few seconds to a couple of minutes according to what the situation allows. For example, you might have just finished recording some notes on a patient before eating some lunch, and so before rushing off it might be good to sit quietly and centre yourself in the present free of preoccupations about past or future. Then you move off, walk and eat your lunch mindfully – taste the food.

As far as the stress or fight-or-flight response is concerned, we do need it from time to time when confronting a significant present-moment threat. We activate it based on being mindful of the threat. This activation is adaptive and meant to be good for our health in dealing with a real threat. Unfortunately, when we aren't mindful, we far more commonly activate the response when we don't need it. This is not adaptive – it is called anxiety. It is a trick of the mind (the default circuits) in projecting something we anticipate in the future or relive from the past. It is a little like confusing a rope for a snake in low light. If we are mindful, we can, as it were, discern the difference between an actual snake that is about to bite us, compared to a rope that only appears like a snake. If we ground ourselves in present moment reality, we have the chance to deactivate the stress response when we don't need it. This – having a clear perception of the present – has massive implications for how we perform under pressure and the decisions we make.

Clinical performance and decision-making

When we switch off the unnecessary and unmindful activation of the stress response, the brain's stress centre (amygdala) quietens down and the executive functioning area of the brain that we rely on for performance and decision-making (prefrontal cortex) comes back online. This doesn't mean we immediately totally relax – the stress hormones adrenaline and cortisol will remain in our bloodstream for up to 90 minutes before they are fully metabolised – but at least we are no longer feeding the stress response.

The attitude to stress or anxiety when we notice it has a large effect on whether it escalates and we lose more focus, or it settles, and we are able to get back on-task. Acceptance, self-compassion and gentleness lead down one path, and reactivity, self-criticism and frustration lead down another. It's not so much that we are trying to control the response as learning to stand a step or two back from it and not be controlled by it. As neuroscientist Kelly McGonigal has shown (McGonigal, 2013), it is very helpful to simply recognise stress as fight/flight reactivity and see that it is the nervous system trying to keep us alive, rather than appraising stress as 'negative'. Her research found that relating to stress this way actually avoids many of the negative consequences, whereas appraising it negatively tends to exacerbate them.

Once our overall levels of arousal start to return to baseline, we can also regain some perspective. 'Amygdala hijack' is a term describing when the stress centre overwhelms the executive functioning areas (Goleman & Davidson, 2017). It is associated with performing poorly under pressure, freezing up, or making bad and/or impulsive decisions. It leads to an increased likelihood of misperceiving innocuous events and stimuli as threatening (mistaking the proverbial rope for a snake). But when we regain some control over our attention, we become able to see more clearly once again and therefore focus our attention on what we are able to control and learn to accept what we are not. Attention and attitude (e.g., acceptance) are therefore the two core qualities at the heart of mindfulness, and so improving trait mindfulness – our ability to regularly display mindful traits in daily life – makes it much easier to keep things in perspective.

Another problem when we are unmindful and on automatic pilot is that we are much more subject to various forms of unconscious bias which commonly lead to diagnostic and decision errors (Sibinga & Wu, 2010). For example, if a health professional steps into a clinical situation with an assumption about a person (e.g., they over-react to their pain) then it is easy to see and interpret the history and clinical signs to confirm what the health professional already thinks (confirmation bias), whether they do or not, and to ignore or resist other data that might suggest an alternate diagnosis (anchoring bias). This may cause a significant delay in responding to an actual but unexpected event like a birth complication such as obstructed labour. The point about health professionals practicing mindfulness is not that all of a sudden, they magically don't have cognitive biases, it's more a matter that the biases go from being unconscious to conscious. Assumptions are not automatically taken as facts. So, when we are about to step into a clinical situation, and the mind makes assumptions before even assessing it, the mindful clinician is more likely to recognise it, to self-correct and look more objectively at the data. The person may have over-reacted to pain in the past, but what is happening here and now? Be curious, look and see.

The other benefit of mindfulness from a decision-making perspective is the potential for preventing the black and white thinking that is commonly observed in hyperkinetic work environments, like hospitals, where the cognitive load is high (Hallowell, 2005). Such environments cause what is called 'attention deficit trait'. When the mental load is high the mind just wants to take the shortest route to an easy decision, generally the most habitual, simplest and least innovative one, but it may not be the one that is right for the situation.

Nobel Prize-winning economist, Daniel Kahneman, described two modes of decision-making in his book, *Thinking, Fast and Slow*: system 1 (i.e., fast, automatic, intuitive) and system 2 (i.e., slower, analytical, reasoned). The virtue of system 1 is that it is fast and efficient, but the downside is that it increases the likelihood we will make errors and fall prey to cognitive biases (such as negativity, anchoring, confirmation and stereotyping biases). The virtue of system 2 is that it helps to prevent errors and leads to more reasoned decisions, but downside is that it is slower and consumes more cognitive resources (and therefore energy!), and in everyday life we don't always have as much time as we might like to deliberate on decisions. Plus, we can all at times overthink decisions while we ignore the obvious. The point is, if we are mindful, we can tell more easily when we are in the wrong mode (e.g., being hasty when more care is needed, or overthinking an emergency situation rather than acting) and we can take steps to switch modes.

Therefore, many of the informal mindfulness strategies mentioned previously, like walking mindfully between clinical interactions, eating mindfully, doing one job at a time and being present when someone is speaking, can provide mental rest and reduce cognitive load. This is a great remedy for attention deficit trait, and it can help us to be more present when making important decisions by being aware of when we need to be in system 1 or system 2.

Clinical errors

Modern working environments like hospitals are becoming increasingly complex. As a result, many clinical errors occur through distraction, complex multitasking, overreliance on system 1 thinking, poor mental health and fatigue. Luckily, however, all of these may be partially or fully remediated through mindfulness.

Distraction

With the level of addiction that many people have to their smartphones, just the fact that it goes off in the pocket, even on silent, when someone was performing an attention-demanding task was enough to increase the error rate by 28% (Stothart, Mitchum, & Yehnert, 2015).

> Mindfulness tip – get unnecessary distractors out of the environment especially when doing something complex, risky or important.

Complex multitasking

This is trying to pay attention to two or more complex tasks at exactly the same time and is one of the most encultured but fraught and unmindful modern practices. So, for example, a charge midwife/nurse might be trying to respond to another midwife/nurse's questions while doing a drug round. The myth is that we both can and should do this to save time and be more productive, but the reality is quite different. Both tasks suffer, and in terms of errors, it can mean forgetting information, giving out the wrong medication, or giving an incorrect answer to the question. The human brain – including the female brain – does *not* pay attention to multiple complex things at the same time. When trying to complex multitask, the mind (and brain) has to rapidly switch attention between tasks which leads to missed information that we are not even aware we are missing (attentional blink), increased mental load, impaired memory, activation of the stress response and, importantly, a manyfold increased risk of errors depending on how complex the task is. Furthermore, the evidence clearly indicates that women are just as poor at multitasking as men (Hirsch, Koch, & Karbach, 2019).

> Mindfulness tip – Give attention to one thing at a time and only switch when you really need to. Efficient attention switching is necessary in complex and fast-moving clinical situations, but it is not multitasking. In multitasking the attention is scattered and often off target whereas in efficient attention switching the attention is like an agile but precise laser beam focused on one thing at a time.

Poor mental health

The twin problems that come with poor mental health for health professionals are the loss of wellbeing for the professional themselves, implications for the wellbeing of patients because the professional is far more likely (possibly six-fold) to make clinical and prescribing errors as a result (Fahrenkopf et al., 2008). The reasons include rumination – a form of being in default mode – which draws attention away from the task, as well as the impairment of memory and executive functioning that comes with depression. Luckily, mindfulness has been shown in extensive reviews of studies on healthcare professionals to be associated with significant improvements in mental health (Spinelli, Wisener & Khoury, 2019).

> Mindfulness tip – Practice prevention and self-care regularly, but if you notice yourself or a colleague in need of mental healthcare then seek help with a well-trained mental health professional, preferably one with mindfulness training.

Fatigue

Things have changed a lot since the days when overwork and fatigue were seen as badges of courage and commitment in healthcare. Luckily, those times have mostly passed, but fatigue and the negative impact that it has on vigilance, eye-hand coordination, cognitive functioning and errors are still too common.

Mindfulness tip – Use mindfulness to help you conserve energy and use it wisely. Know how to switch off and rest well when you have the chance. Also, be mindful and self-aware enough to notice when fatigue is significant at work in which case you will be able to increase vigilance when you need it the most.

Empathy, compassion and reducing vicarious stress

A key requirement in healthcare – and especially birthing – settings is the ability to connect empathically with expecting parents without experiencing vicarious stress and 'compassion fatigue'. Managing these competing demands can be extremely challenging and is a major source of stress for many in the birthing sphere. If practitioners err too much on the side of protecting their own mental health by distancing themselves emotionally from their patients, they risk miscommunication and disconnection which are key factors in the levels of satisfaction for those in their care (Doyle, Lennox & Bell, 2013) and has even been found to predict malpractice litigation (Roter, 2006). Depersonalisation, manifesting as negative, callous and cynical behaviours, is one of the hallmarks of burnout.

Unfortunately, the intense focus of healthcare education on the biomedical and technical aspects can marginalise and de-emphasise the human aspects (Bornstein, 2013; Brennan, 2021) and sometimes discourages expression of emotion from clinicians. Medical training in particular is notorious for teaching doctors to 'care less' about their patients, in favour of cultivating a professional distance. This confusion between objectivity and dehumanising the clinical interaction is often done to protect medical professionals from vicarious stress and trauma, which can ultimately lead to 'compassion fatigue' and burnout. However, such emotional distancing can lead to patients experiencing healthcare staff as cold and uncaring. Fortunately, there have been increasing efforts in recent years to address this imbalance and emphasise the importance of professional *and* humane relationships between clients/patients and clinical staff.

Mindfulness offers a more adaptive alternative. With practice, it is possible for healthcare and birthing professionals to maintain empathic connection with themselves – and, by extension, with their patients – while simultaneously maintaining professional boundaries and avoiding burnout. To understand how this is possible, we need to take a closer look at 'compassion fatigue' and how it is created. We intentionally keep referring to 'compassion fatigue' whereas in fact what some healthcare professionals actually experience is *empathy* fatigue, not compassion fatigue.

Empathy operates on multiple levels. *Cognitive* empathy refers to attempting to understand the lived experience of someone else (by 'stepping into their shoes'). *Emotional* empathy goes further by 'feeling into' their experience, via the activation of mirror neurons and a process known as empathic resonance. Someone in empathic resonance with the emotional (or physical) pain of someone else has the same pain areas activated in their brain as are active in the brain of the person actually experiencing the pain. Excessive empathic resonance over time is what can lead to negative affect, and ultimately vicarious stress and trauma. In contrast, when people experience 'empathic concern' – a combination of emotional empathy and a desire or action to alleviate the suffering of the other person, different brain areas are activated. This is what happens in true compassion. The result is a *decrease* in negative affect, and indeed increased levels of *positive* affect (Klimecki et al., 2014). Research shows that compassion for oneself and others predicts wellbeing over time (Neff, Rude & Kirkpatrick, 2007). This may be one of the main reasons that doctors who rate higher in mindfulness have not only better mental health, but also greater compassion, more emotional intelligence, better communication and more satisfied patients (Beach et al., 2013).

> Mindfulness tip – Wherever possible, attempt to balance both empathy (deeply connecting with other people on cognitive and/or emotional levels) and compassion (taking action or making wishes to alleviate the suffering of others).

Communication

In addition to the obvious benefits for healthcare and birthing professionals, compassion and empathic listening skills are also central to patient satisfaction and should be a central part of any training offered to healthcare and birthing professionals. This is especially important given the high levels of anxiety and distress experienced by expectant parents and during the birthing process.

A good starting point is basic mindful listening practice. If we pay close attention when we are communicating with others, it quickly becomes obvious that much of the time we are 'listening' to our thoughts and evaluations about what others are saying (default mode), rather than actually listening to the words that are being said. This is especially true in busy and stressful workplaces like birthing and healthcare settings. It is therefore obvious why simply learning to give patients our full attention can be a very powerful practice in and of itself.

We contend that once this basic listening is established, we can start to listen more deeply and start to pay attention to the nonverbal components of conversation which is the majority of what is being communicated. What's more, we can start to 'listen to understand', rather than waiting for our turn to respond, as author Steven Covey entreats us to do in his classic *The 7 habits of Highly Effective People*. We can even begin listening for deep connection via active, empathic and compassionate listening. In doing so, we start to connect with the deepest parts of people – with the actual living, breathing human being in front of us, rather than a 'patient' we have to get through a procedure and out the door.

> Mindfulness tip – Next time you are communicating with someone, notice the habitual tendency to 'listen' to your thoughts about what they are saying instead of what they are actually saying. Experiment with paying

full attention to the verbal and nonverbal aspects of what they are communicating and notice the effect this has on the interaction.

Mindfulness also allows us to become aware of our speech. Again, the first thing many people discover about their speech when they begin paying attention is just how *un*mindful it is. Oftentimes it is laden with judgements, unquestioned assumptions and biases. There is the habit of complaining and rambling, often with little or no awareness as to how we are being perceived. But once we notice these things we can move from 'unconscious incompetence' to 'conscious incompetence', tracking what we are saying and how we say it. Ultimately, we can start to cultivate 'conscious competence' by thinking before speaking and pausing regularly to reflect on whether what we have just said was received the way we intended it to.

> Mindfulness tip – Before speaking, pause for a moment and ask yourself what your intention is in this particular interaction. Are you providing information? Or trying to convince them of something? Or perhaps just gossiping? Pause at moments throughout the conversation to check back in with this question. And also experiment with checking whether your message is being received accurately or not.

Research has shown that communication between healthcare professionals and patients influences the quality of the relationship, which in turn predicts better treatment compliance and enhanced health/wellbeing outcomes (Street et al., 2009). Research also shows that the quality of the therapeutic alliance predicts patient satisfaction, rather than just the provision of information. A well-known and highly cited study by Levinson and colleagues (1997) contrasted the communication style of physicians who had malpractice suits brought against them in court with those who didn't. The study found that no-claims physicians did a better job of telling patients what they should expect from treatment at each visit, laughed and used humour more often, and periodically stopped to ensure their patients understood what was being said. The extra three minutes taken to do these things during each consultation resulted in a significantly decreased likelihood of having claims made against them. Communication and therapeutic alliance becomes particularly important in birthing settings, where the potential magnitude of complaints and/or malpractice claims is so high.

Improving teamwork and culture with mindfulness

The same communication principles outlined above can equally be applied to colleagues, managers, administrators and other stakeholders in birthing settings. Doing so can potentially improve team performance and even change organisational culture (Crowther et al., 2019).

As a starting point, birthing professionals can ensure they pay full attention to colleagues when speaking to them. There are countless other things it is possible to do and think about while supposedly listening to someone – uncompleted tasks, the conversation that was just had with a patient, concerns about high-risk patients – but all of these things serve to take us out of the present moment. There is a time and place for systematically working through these things, but this is not while talking to a colleague! As with all mindfulness practices, changing this ingrained habit takes awareness first and, when noticed, consistent effort, but over time becomes easier. Important times to practice mindful listening are during meetings and handovers, where important information is being communicated. However, making an effort to be fully present with colleagues even during informal 'water-cooler' moments has the potential to improve workplace culture by increasing the sense of connectedness between team members. And it's not just mindful listening that is important! Paying attention to our speech ensures we communicate ideas clearly, helps minimise the judgments and assumptions that we habitually tend to make (and give voice to), and ensures that we communicate in an authentic way – speak when we need to and keep our peace when we need to. The same principles also apply to electronic communication, ensuring that the way we use digital technology fosters a greater sense of connection.

Ultimately, as the mindfulness of individual team members starts to increase, a phenomenon known as "collective mindfulness" can start to emerge. Collective mindfulness means that members of a team or organisational unit are more likely to enculturate mindful work practices and culture, and to notice details or unique situations and act upon them (Sutcliffe & Vogus, 2014). This is particularly important in healthcare settings – and arguably even more so in birthing contexts, given the potential medical significance of irregularities to the birthing process. Furthermore, a study by Liu and colleagues (2020) found that team mindfulness positively moderated the relationship between individual mindfulness and work engagement. A team that cultivates both individual and collective mindfulness may therefore become a group of highly engaged individuals with excellent resilience, interpersonal skills, compassion and attentiveness to their work. Moreover, a maternity workforce that nurtures healthy resilience will flourish and be more sustainable without harming individual and collective wellbeing (Crowther, 2017).

Mindfulness for patients and their partners

So far in this chapter, we have explored some aspects of mindfulness that help to make a more mindful health practitioner, but what about the patient? It is beyond the scope of this chapter to give detailed instructions for all the clinical uses of mindfulness, and much of this will be covered in other chapters. What we will do in this section is give an overview of some of the clinical applications of mindfulness that are particularly relevant to birthing and about which practitioners should inform their patients. We will also provide some cautions about the use of mindfulness.

There are many different clinical applications of MBIs but there are three main applications of mindfulness in the birthing sphere that are worth emphasising here.

First, MBIs like mindfulness-based cognitive therapy (MBCT) can help greatly with mental health particularly in terms of stress, anxiety and depression. The period from pregnancy through to the early years post-birth can be enormously stressful and challenging. Having some simple and effective strategies to help women and their partners navigate those stresses and challenges can be enormously helpful and liberating. It is also worth remembering that significant emotional distress for a woman during pregnancy not only activates her stress system, but the mediators of her stress response cross the placenta and can negatively impact the physical, neurological and psychological development of the foetus. Therefore, caring for the next generation of children must start with the psychological care of women in the lead-up to pregnancy and thereafter.

Second, pain and other symptoms associated with pregnancy and childbirth can be anxiety-provoking. The distress is not just when such symptoms are actually present, but significant distress can be caused for weeks or months prior to childbirth in anticipation of discomfort. MBIs have been found to be extremely helpful for people coping with pain and other physical symptoms because it helps a person not only to minimise the distress associated with anticipation of discomfort, but because it can negate the amplifying effect of emotions like anxiety or fear on the experience of discomfort when it is present. Staying present, moment-by-moment and being less emotionally reactive to the discomfort can help enormously.

Third, it is important to consider the benefits of mindfulness for effective parenting. A distracted, unmindful parent cannot care as well or safely for a child as a present, engaged and attentive one. Being aware and present is a pre-requisite for both caring and compassion as well as helping to deal with the personal and vicarious stress that can be a part of being a parent. Adopting an accepting attitude is one of the hallmarks of mindfulness and there are very few areas of life where an accepting attitude is more relevant than in parenting – accepting of the disruption to one's previous life, accepting of going without sleep, accepting of uncomfortable emotions, accepting of our humanity and sometimes less than perfect parenting…. Learning to flow with events rather than resist them can have a massive effect on the amount of stress we experience during adversity. Another key capacity that mindfulness offers a parent is the ability to switch on, for example when awoken in the night, and switch off again, for example when back in bed. To do this we need to be in the present moment for this saves an enormous amount of burden in the form of the stress, energy and mental load in the form of rumination and worry.

A word of caution

A health professional may understand some of the principles of mindfulness, and even practice it personally, which is a good foundation upon which to provide advice to patients when mindfulness might be relevant and helpful for them. Referring women and their partners to ante-natal mindfulness classes (see Chapter 7) where the generic skills of mindfulness are contextualised for pregnancy, childbirth and parenting, such as the increasingly popular Calmbirth approach that teacher's mindfulness (see chapter 7) can be tremendously helpful. However, it must be noted that significant mental and physical health problems are not necessarily simple to deal with. First, mindfulness shouldn't be imposed on someone who is not interested, ready or motivated to learn about it. Second, although mindfulness may be very helpful, if it is being delivered by someone without a deep understanding of it and how to apply and teach it, nor the necessary health professional credentials, then it can be poorly taught or inappropriately applied leading to potential problems including frustration or exacerbation of anxiety. Therefore, for complex health problems, it is recommended to refer willing birthing women/persons and their partners to experienced practitioners of mindfulness. If a health professional wishes to deliver MBIs in practice then it is useful to get further training in how to teach it and in what contexts it can be most effectively and safely applied.

Final reflections and future directions

In this chapter, we have made the case that mindfulness is a core skill with many different and relevant applications for the maternity health practitioner and patients alike within the birthing sphere. Reading a book or using an app can be useful but, where possible, it is more useful and instructive to do a course running over a series of weeks to help establish the practice in daily life. Face-to-face courses allow for more direct interaction with an experience instructor, but online courses can also be very useful and accessible, such as the free introductory mindfulness-based online courses found on the Monash Mindfulness website (www.monash. edu/mindfulness). The point is to establish the practice as a normal part of life that flows into professional life as one becomes a mindful practitioner.

References

Beach, M.C., Roter, D., Korthuis, P.T., et al. "A Multicenter Study of Physician Mindfulness and Health Care Quality." *Annals of Family Medicine*, 11, no. 5 (2013): 421–428. https://doi.org/10.1370/afm.1507

Bornstein, D. "Medicine's Search for Meaning." *New York Times* (2013). https://opinionator.blogs.nytimes.com/2013/09/18/medicines-search-for-meaning/

Brandford, A.A., & Reed, D.B. "Depression in Registered Nurses: A State of the Science." *Workplace Health & Safety*, 64, no. 10 (2016): 488–511.

Brennan, M. "Are We Losing Our Humanity in Medicine's Quest for Pure Science?" *BMJ Opinion* (2021). https://blogs.bmj.com/bmj/2021/09/02/are-we-losing-our-humanity-in-medicines-quest-for-pure-science/

Brito-Pons, G., Campos, D. & Cebolla, A. "Implicit or Explicit Compassion? Effects of Compassion Cultivation Training and Comparison with Mindfulness-based Stress Reduction." *Mindfulness*, 9 (2018): 1494–1508. https://doi.org/10.1007/s12671-018-0898-z

Carleton, E.L., Barling, J., & Trivisonno, M. "Leaders' Trait Mindfulness and Transformational Leadership: The Mediating Roles of Leaders' Positive Affect and Leadership Self-efficacy." *Canadian Journal of Behavioural Science*, 50, no. 3 (2018): 185.

Conversano, C., Ciacchini, R., Orrù, G., et al. "Mindfulness, Compassion, and Self-Compassion Among Health Care Professionals: What's New? A Systematic Review." *Frontiers in Psychology*, 11 (2020): 1683.

Crowther, S. "Resilience and Sustainability amongst Maternity Care Providers." In G. Thomson & V. Schmied (Eds.), *Psychosocial Resilience and Risk in the Perinatal Period: Implications and Guidance for Professionals* (pp. 185–200). London: Taylor & Francis, 2017.

Crowther, S., Cooper, C., Meechan, F., & Ashkanasy, N.M. "The Role of Emotion, Empathy, and Compassion in Organisations." In S. Downe & S. Byrom (Eds.), *Squaring the Circle: Normal Birth Research, Theory and Practice in a Technological Age* (pp. 111–119). London: Pinter & Martin Limited, 2019.

De Hert, S. "Burnout in Healthcare Workers: Prevalence, Impact and Preventative Strategies." *Local and Regional Anesthesia*, 13 (2020): 171.

Donald, J.N., Sahdra, B.K., Van Zanden, B., Duineveld, J.J., Atkins, P., Marshall, S.L., & Ciarrochi, J. "Does your Mindfulness Benefit Others? A Systematic Review and Meta-analysis of the link Between Mindfulness and Prosocial Behaviour." *British Journal of Psychology (London, England: 1953)*, 110, no. 1 (2019): 101–125. https://doi.org/10.1111/bjop.12338

Doyle, C., Lennox, L., & Bell, D. "A Systematic Review of Evidence on the links Between Patient Experience and Clinical Safety and Effectiveness." *BMJ Open*, 3, no. 1 (2013): e001570.

Dyrbye, L.N., Thomas, M.R., & Shanafelt, T.D. Medical Student Distress: Causes, Consequences, and Proposed Solutions. *Mayo Clinic Proceedings*, 80, no. 12 (2005): 1613–1622. https://doi.org/10.4065/80.12.1613

Eaves, J.L., & Payne, N. "Resilience, Stress and Burnout in Student Midwives." *Nurse Education Today*, 79 (2019): 188–193. https://doi.org/10.1016/j.nedt.2019.05.012

Fahrenkopf, A.M., Sectish, T.C., Barger, L.K., et al. "Rates of Medication Errors among Depressed and Burnt-Out Residents: Prospective Cohort Study." *BMJ*, 336, no. 7642 (2008): 488–491. https://doi.org/10.1136/bmj.39469.763218.BE

Ferriss, T. *Tools of Titans: The Tactics, Routines, and Habits of Billionaires, Icons, and World-Class Performers.* New York: Houghton Mifflin, 2017.

Friganović, A., Selič, P., Ilić, B., & Sedić, B. "Stress and Burnout Syndrome and Their Associations with Coping and Job Satisfaction in Critical Care Nurses: A Literature Review." *Psychiatria Danubina*, 31, Suppl. 1 (2019): 21–31.

Goleman, D., & Davidson, R. *The Science of Meditation: How to Change Your Brain, Mind and Body.* London: Penguin UK, 2017.

Hallowell, E.M. "Overloaded Circuits: Why Smart People Underperform." *Harvard Business Review*, 83, no. 1 (2005): 54–62, 116.

Harvey, S.B., Epstein, R.M., Glozier, N., Petrie, K., Strudwick, J., Gayed, A., Dean, K., & Henderson, M. "Mental Illness and Suicide among Physicians." *Lancet (London, England)*, 398, no. 10303 (2021): 920–930. https://doi.org/10.1016/S0140-6736(21)01596-8

Harvey, S., Spurr, P., Sidebotham, M., & Fenwick, J. "Describing and Evaluating a Foundational Education/Training Program Preparing Nurses, Midwives and Other Helping Professionals as Supervisors of Clinical Supervision Using the Role Development Model." *Nurse Education in Practice*, 42 (2020): 102671.

Hirsch, P., Koch, I., & Karbach, J. "Putting a Stereotype to the Test: The Case of Gender Differences in Multitasking Costs in Task-Switching and Dual-Task Situations." *PLoS One*, 14, no. 8 (2019): e0220150. https://doi.org/10.1371/journal.pone.0220150

Karasek, R., & Theorell, T. *Healthy Work. Stress, Productivity, and the Reconstruction of Working Life.* New York: Basic Books, 1990.

Klimecki, O.M., Leiberg, S., Ricard, M., & Singer, T. "Differential Pattern of Functional Brain Plasticity after Compassion and Empathy Training." *Social Cognitive and Affective Neuroscience*, 9, no. 6 (2014): 873–879.

Levinson, W., Roter, D.L., Mullooly, J.P., Dull, V.T., & Frankel, R.M. "Physician-patient Communication: The Relationship with Malpractice Claims Among Primary Care Physicians and Surgeons." *Jama*, 277, no. 7 (1997): 553–559.

Liu, S., Xin, H., Shen, L., He, J., & Liu, J. "The Influence of Individual and Team Mindfulness on Work Engagement." *Frontiers in Psychology*, 10 (2020): 2928.

Maharaj, S., Lees, T., & Lal, S. "Prevalence and Risk Factors of Depression, Anxiety, and Stress in a Cohort of Australian Nurses." *International Journal of Environmental Research and Public Health*, 16, no. 1 (2018): 61. https://doi.org/10.3390/ijerph16010061

McGonigal, K. (2013, June). https://www.ted.com/talks/kelly_mcgonigal_how_to_make_stress_your_friend?

Neff, K.D., Rude, S.S., & Kirkpatrick, K.L. "An Examination of Self-compassion in Relation to Positive Psychological Functioning and Personality Traits." *Journal of Research in Personality*, 41, no. 4 (2007): 908–916.

Oates, J., Topping, A., Arias, T., Charles, P., Hunter, C., & Watts, K. "The Mental Health and Wellbeing of Midwifery Students: An Integrative Review." *Midwifery*, 72(2019): 80–89. https://doi.org/10.1016/j.midw.2019.02.007. Epub 2019 Feb 14. PMID: 30826662

Panagioti, M., Geraghty, K., Johnson, J., Zhou, A., Panagopoulou, E., Chew-Graham, C., Peters, D., Hodkinson, A., Riley, R., & Esmail, A. "Association between Physician Burnout and Patient Safety, Professionalism, and Patient Satisfaction: A Systematic Review and Meta-analysis." *JAMA Internal Medicine*, 178, no. 10 (2018): 1317–1331.

Pereira-Lima, K., Mata, D.A., Loureiro, S.R., Cripp, J.A., Bolsoni, L.M., & Sen, S. (2019). "Association between Physician Depressive Symptoms and Medical Errors. A Systematic Review and Meta-analysis." *JAMA Network Open*, 2019. https://doi.org/10.1001/jamanetworkopen.2019.16097

Pradas-Hernández, L., Ariza, T., Gómez-Urquiza, J.L., Albendín-García, L., De la Fuente, E.I., & Cañadas-De la Fuente, G.A. "Prevalence of Burnout in Paediatric Nurses: A Systematic Review and Meta-analysis." *PloS One*, 13, no. 4 (2018): e0195039. https://doi.org/10.1371/journal.pone.0195039

Roter, D. "The Patient-physician Relationship and its Implications for Malpractice Litigation." *Journal of Health Care Law and Policy*, 9 (2006): 304.

Sibinga, E.M., & Wu, A.W. "Clinician Mindfulness and Patient Safety." *JAMA*, 304, no. 22 (2010): 2532–2533.

Spinelli, C., Wisener, M., & Khoury, B. "Mindfulness Training for Healthcare Professionals and Trainees: A meta-analysis of Randomized Controlled Trials." *Journal or Psychosomatic Research*, 120 (2019): 29–38. https://doi.org/10.1016/j.psychores.2019.03.003

Stothart, C., Mitchum, A., & Yehnert, C. "The Attentional Cost of Receiving a Cell Phone Notification." *Journal of Experimental Psychology: Human Perception and Performance*, 41, no. 4 (2015): 893. https://doi.org/10.1037/xhp0000100

Street Jr, R.L., Makoul, G., Arora, N.K., & Epstein, R.M. "How Does Communication Heal? Pathways Linking Clinician–Patient Communication to Health Outcomes." *Patient Education and Counseling*, 74, no. 3 (2009): 295–301.

Sutcliffe, K.M., & Vogus, T.J. "Organizing for Mindfulness." In A. Ie, C.T. Ngnoumen, & E. Langer (Eds.), *The Wiley Blackwell Handbook of Mindfulness* (pp. 407–423).2014.

Young, C., Smythe, L., & McAra-Couper, J. "Burnout: Lessons from the Lived Experience of Case Loading Midwives." *International Journal of Childbirth*, 5, no. 3 (2015): 154–165.

3

MINDFULNESS AND COMPASSIONATE MIDWIFERY IN CHILDBIRTH TRAUMA

Diane Menage and Jenny Patterson

This chapter presents our separate but closely aligned PhD research findings. Both of us explored women's experiences of midwifery care, in the UK, albeit from opposite perspectives: Diane explored experiences where compassion featured, and Jenny explored the experiences that women described as traumatic. In this chapter, we bring these two perspectives together to explore how mindfulness in midwifery practice may enhance a compassionate approach and mitigate that which can be termed traumatic.

I, Jenny, am a midwifery lecturer at Edinburgh Napier University, Scotland, and have practiced as a midwife since 2007 both within the Scottish National Health Service and independently. I have a particular interest in trauma and Post Traumatic Stress Disorder (PTSD) associated with childbirth, either for child-bearing women and people, or the maternity care professionals, alongside the role maternity care professionals have within these experiences. I believe the conscious intention to focus on the individual that one is engaging with, their unique present needs, encompasses and requires a mindful approach. In other words, when interacting with women and birthing people, being attuned to what is important to an individual, is inherently mindful.

I, Diane, had a career in nursing before qualifying as a midwife in 2002. I have practiced midwifery in a variety of settings within the UK NHS and independent practice. I currently teach undergraduate and postgraduate midwifery students at De Montfort University in Leicester, UK. My interests include compassion, self-compassion, and leadership. I see an attentive, mindful approach as a skill that encompasses the fundamental skills of how to be with another person in a way that enhances listening, noticing, and connecting. When women and birthing people know they are being seen and listened to, they feel respected and share information more freely. This contributes to building trust and helps midwives understand the issues, providing care that is appropriate and improves safety (Lewis 2015).

DOI: 10.4324/9781003165200-3

The focus of this chapter

We strongly believe that individualised, attentive, reflective, and mindful care is at the heart of safe midwifery practice and that *mindful self-compassion* underpins this. When we veer from an attentive, mindful approach, we risk generalising care based on standardised procedures that may fail to acknowledge or address individual needs. As we shall show, missing individual needs may contribute to a poor perception of care or poor outcomes.

Midwifery care has many strands but for the purposes of this chapter, we will simplify this into two dimensions: practical and personal. Practical encompasses physical and clinical aspects of care, the practical skills a midwife uses to monitor, support, and facilitate the childbearing process. Personal refers specifically to human interaction with the woman or birthing person, their partner and family, as well as colleagues and the multidisciplinary team. Single-minded attention to practical tasks risks neglecting the personal dimension. When midwives, for example, pay attention to a monitor without attention to the person attached to the monitor; communicate clinical information to a colleague without heed to the woman or birthing person present; or focus on our tasks without heed to our human needs, we fail to be mindful of the personal dimension. Some may argue that practical care skills are paramount for safe midwifery, while the personal dimension, often referred to as soft skills, sometimes need to take a back seat. Here we will highlight why this is both incorrect and inherently dangerous. We will demonstrate that mindful compassion (towards self and other) within the personal dimension must be at the centre of every act of midwifery care.

First, we present Jenny's research findings about the experience of birth trauma and subsequent PTSD from the perspective of both women and midwives. This will set the scene for understanding the role of a mindful compassionate approach in midwifery care and what maternity care providers need in order to provide mindful compassionate care. We then present Diane's research findings about women's experiences of compassionate midwifery care and how this influenced their childbirth experiences. Our joint findings reflect the synergy between mindfulness and compassion and promotion of compassionate caregiving (Conversano et al. 2020). From this, we weave together our joint understanding of mindful, compassionate midwifery care as a powerful intervention that can improve childbirth experiences and outcomes for women and birthing people. Finally, we will postulate that this powerful intervention can transform the working lives of midwives, their interactions with one another and with the families they care for.

Jenny's research

Even though trauma was observed in association with childbirth from the 1970s (Robinson 2007), PTSD, first defined in 1980 (APA[1] 1980), was not clinically acknowledged to be associated with childbirth until 1994 (APA 1994). The existence of birth trauma and subsequent PTSD is now widely acknowledged (BTA 2021). PTSD is a condition that follows a clinically defined traumatic event that is one *during which the person either experiences or witnesses, actual or threatened, death or harm* (APA 2013). It is important to understand that the individual's perception of the event, their subjective experience is significant (Garthus-Niegel et al. 2013). It has been shown that up to 45% of women and birthing people may experience childbirth as a traumatic event that meets the above criterion (Alcorn et al. 2010), with around 4% of all women, birthing people and their partners developing full PTSD (Ayers et al. 2007; Yildiz, Ayers, and Phillips 2017; PTSD UK 2021). Many more than this develop partial symptoms (Zaers, Waschke, and Ehlert 2008; Polachek et al. 2012). As such UK organisations such as the *Birth Trauma Association (BTA)* (BTA 2021) and *Make Birth Better (MBB)* (MBB 2021), have become mainstream, widely referenced sources of information, education, and collaboration for families and maternity care staff.

Labour, birth, and the early postnatal period are the most common times for birth trauma to occur (Ford and Ayers 2011; Harris and Ayers 2012; Patterson, Hollins Martin, and Karatzias 2019). We also now know that the main source of trauma, the key 'hotspots' or strong memories that persist, most often relate to *how* something was done rather than *what* was done. In other words, the interpersonal aspects of the care provision, the personal dimension, have been shown to be core to birth trauma (Sorenson and Tschetter 2010; Reed, Sharman, and Inglis 2017) and the strongest predictors of PTSD post childbirth (Harris and Ayers 2012).

I interviewed women who had developed full PTSD following a recent birthing experience, and midwives who provide care during labour, birth, and the early postnatal period. The women were asked to "Please tell me about you experience of interacting with midwives and others during your childbirth journey". Midwives were asked to "Please tell me about your experience of interacting with women while providing their maternity care".

Both the women and the midwives spoke at length and with emotion about their experiences. Both related the deep joy they felt when human connection was present; when they were truly listened to or able to listen; when their human needs were recognised and responded to. When this happened, the women expressed strong positive memories and deep fondness for the midwife, often crying with joy. Similarly, the midwives expressed joy, privilege, and deep job satisfaction. Yet in contrast, negative and traumatic memories were more frequent, and all related to a lack of personal connection: feeling abandoned or abandoning; not being heard, not having time to listen; with some women feeling actively abused either physically or verbally (Patterson, Hollins Martin, and Karatzias 2019). We will unpack these from the perspective of being mindful to the personal dimension. In the following summary, all names associated with quotes are pseudonyms.

Among the themes I identified, 'Abandonment' was a strong and prevalent experience among both groups. Abandonment related to a sense of isolation with no one to turn to or that those present were disconnected and unaware of, or unable to respond, to need. Disconnection or lack of awareness contrasts with a mindful approach.

For the women, feeling abandoned contributed to fear, lack of control, and feeling unsafe, all key features of trauma (Ford and Ayers 2011; Patterson, Hollins Martin, and Karatzias 2019). Whilst this included not having anyone present with them for long periods, it most often related to just not being seen, not being visible to the midwife. For example, Catriona arrived at labour assessment in a wheelchair found by her companions to help get from the car park to the entrance. Catriona was looking forward to being 'enveloped in a warm motherly embrace' but instead found that the midwives initially ignored her and focused on the wheelchair stating, "What on earth are we going to do with that?". This is a clear example of attention being on the practical, while missing the personal. Some might consider this trivial, yet for Catriona, this was a key source of trauma and flashbacks that persisted for years. She suddenly found herself in a situation that felt unsafe, where no one saw her or recognised her needs. Sadly, this perception persisted with the midwives focused on their computer or notes with cursory acknowledgement of Catriona. She felt unable to trust the midwives, unable to relax or trust that she was in safe hands. For Julie, her midwife with whom she had built a connection and felt supported by, took a break. The replacement midwife was uncomfortable with Julie's vocalisations and insisted that she use the Entonox (gas and air). This was not just a verbal insistence, but a physical holding of the mask on Julie's face while telling her to 'be quiet'. Far from being mindful of the individual woman, this was physically abusive. Julie moved very quickly into a state of fear and panic and feeling unsafe, from which she never fully recovered. Another example is the experience of Marie who had a clearly disclosed and documented a history of sexual assault, who during an internal examination had her requests for this to stop ignored until her husband shouted at the midwife. These examples highlight a focus on either the midwife's own discomfort or a practical task, rather than the individual they are caring for.

From the perspective of the midwives, 'listening is the very first thing to do' (Alice) whilst abandoning women was described as the 'very worst thing' (Brenda, Kerry). The midwives' sense of abandoning women often related to the practical necessity of having to leave to collect equipment or drugs, which frequently led to being drawn into other tasks away from the woman and delaying their return. This created anxiety and distress for the midwives who were keen to be with and present to the women. The expressed distress related to abandoning was most acute directly following the birth of the baby and placenta when midwives were required to provide care for another labouring person. This forced separation created distress for the midwives who keenly wished to remain present for the woman in the first hours post birth, supporting transition, breastfeeding, and sharing their reflection on the birth. Doing 'the nice little bits together after' (Alice).

Another key theme that emerged was 'Torn in Two' (Patterson, Hollins Martin, and Karatzias 2019), where the midwives expressed distress at feeling torn between attending to demands of the system and the individual needs of the women. They often felt unable to provide the individual-focused care that they wished to and that they saw as essential for safety. The midwives described coping with this by disengaging from women. This disengagement limited the ability to be mindful or compassionate and created further tension for the midwives who felt unable to create a balance between the practical and personal dimensions of their role. This not only reduced their role satisfaction but contributed to distress and anxiety regarding their provision of safe care. Furthermore, being forced to abandon women and birthing people, as well as witnessing or contributing to the neglect of their individual needs or those of colleagues, leads to burnout, trauma, and PTSD for many maternity care professionals (Leinweber and Rowe 2010; Wright, Matthai, and Budhathoki 2018).

Diane's research

My research focused on the lived experience of compassionate midwifery care and revealed compassion as a powerful intervention which reduced women's suffering, helping them to feel safer and more able to cope (Ménage et al. 2020). The participant's experiences in my study spanned the childbirth sphere: pregnancy, labour, birth, and the early postnatal period (while there are regional variations, this was up to four weeks after the birth for the women in the study). Women's detailed narratives of midwives who they recognised as providing compassionate care, illustrated how during these experiences some midwives were able to connect and 'be with' them at times when they were frightened; distressed; in physical or emotional pain; or suffering in any other way. The phrase 'tuned-in' encapsulates this quality of 'being with'. While this was enhanced when midwives already knew the woman involved, it was also recognised in midwives that they had never met before. There was something about the way that the midwife was with the women that was almost immediately recognised, suggesting that it was not only the midwife who was 'tuned-in' to the woman, but the woman was also 'tuned-in' to the midwife. Marree's words below illustrate this instant recognition (all names are pseudonyms).

'I instantly got that feeling from, you know like just the attitude, her face….'
Maree

Compassion is a process that starts with the recognition of another's suffering and incorporates behaviour aimed at alleviating that suffering (Gilbert 2009). However, in my study on women's lived experience of compassion it was left to the women themselves to decide what they thought compassionate midwifery was, in what contexts they were aware of it, and how they experienced it. Women needed compassion when they felt frightened, vulnerable, and disempowered. Their sense of disempowerment was related to being in an unfamiliar setting, usually with unfamiliar people combined with the uncertain nature of birth and becoming a parent. Feelings of lack of control and lack of agency put women on high alert, assessing the behaviour of the midwife and identifying her behaviour as compassionate, or not. There are important links here with Jenny's study which suggested that when women have an unmet need for compassion, they felt increasingly disempowered and abandoned by those who they had expected compassion from. Yet, my study revealed that compassion from a midwife reduced these feelings. The essence of compassionate care at this time (when women felt frightened, vulnerable, and disempowered) was experienced through the midwife's quiet, calm attention to the woman and the ability to really see and hear her and what was going on for her. There was a sense that 'less was more' in that it often did not involve a lot of talking or activity but was more likely to be about a warmth and stillness. The importance of listening was emphasised:

> …she was listening more, she was listening first to what I had to say and she was kind of being observant to the situation …it was like paradise, it was like finally someone that I can you know talk to, and they can just listen without feeling, I don't know, that they have all the answers…
>
> *Katrin*

If there were words spoken, tone of voice, body language and touch were just as important.

> almost like a grounding, so just putting a hand on, settling you, a hand over my hand, a squeeze of a hand… there was just something very settling about it, and it was as simple as a hand on a hand, er, or moving my hair out of my face because they could see it was in my face, that nurturing sort of eh, was not intrusive and er for me it was really lovely…
>
> *Mary*

These findings concur with the literature on midwifery presence and attentiveness (Berg et al. 1996), and build on it by providing contextual details about how and why women experience this as compassion and what impact it had on them. While this attentiveness enabled midwives to notice what was really going on for women it was different to purely clinical observation. Whilst clinical observation may have also been involved, women did not seem to get a sense of the 'obstetric gaze' (Davis and Walker 2010) which seeks to observe, measure, and document women's bodies in relation to medical parameters. Midwifery attentiveness, experienced as compassion in this study, might be described as a holistic or humanistic gaze of the woman as a unique person in herself, in her body, and in the world.

The significance of the woman's experience of her midwife really *being with* her was striking in some of the interviews. At times when women were upset and emotionally distressed, it acted as compassionate 'first aid'. The concept of midwives holding space for women during birth was explored by Lemay and Hastie

(2018) who described it as a 'conscious presence' which allows the midwife to attune to the woman in the moment. They explain how this attunement is the key to holding or guarding space for a woman. Andrews (2017) contends that this is the ancient art of *being with woman* during her birth journey. However, in this study, women described midwives who were attuned and present, holding space and they experienced this as a compassionate and therapeutic response to their suffering during pregnancy, birth, and in the early postnatal period.

The findings of this study highlight women's need for midwives who are able to stay with them when they are upset, distressed, or in pain. However, staying with women when they are suffering can be difficult as it may trigger painful emotions for the midwife. As a result, midwives may use other tactics which divert the woman from her painful emotions or experiences. Midwives may *fill* the space, rather than hold the space (Andrews 2017) with talk or with administrative or technical tasks which can lead to the midwife being 'absently present' (Berg et al. 1996). Similarly, Hunter (2002) described a 'professionally detached stance' adopted by midwives who felt unable to cope, which is unlikely to meet women's needs.

Experiences of compassionate care were identified and understood, by women, as being authentic, real, and *ordinary*. The midwives involved did not have to 'put on' compassion like a mask or role. This is important because 'putting on' compassion is likely to be unsatisfactory for all parties. Women in the study could often see through such an approach and there is a body of research from outside maternity care that has shown in-authentic 'niceness' as tiring and a chore for those trying to sustain it. Hochschild's (1983) comparison of presenting the *professional face*, which involves 'surface acting' and the 'authentic face' which comes from human connection assists in an understanding of this phenomenon. According to Hochschild, the *professional face* is difficult to sustain, yet authentic connection, contrary to popular belief, causes less 'job strain' and is more sustainable. While this sort of connection can involve significant emotional labour, for midwives and birth workers, it is balanced with a reciprocity which provides emotionally rewarding relationships and a greater sense of job satisfaction (Hunter 2006).

Reflecting on our joint findings in relation to midwifery theory

There are theoretical approaches and an assessment scale relating to midwifery care that serve to deepen our understanding of the role of mindfulness within midwifery care. In relation to the practical and personal dimensions of care, the *Vigil of Care* and *Care as Gift* approaches outlined by (Fox 1999) and discussed by (Walsh 2011) stand out. A *Vigil of Care* approach is focused on monitoring wellbeing, performed by an expert who sees the 'patient' as an entity that needs to be measured, and administered to. It is a top-down system-centric approach that, from the perspective of safety, values the practical dimension over and above the personal dimension. This approach does not have individual human needs at the core. In contrast, the *Care as Gift* approach views safe and effective care to be that which connects directly to the individual, sees the person, and values a holistic level of care built on trust, love, and generosity. Sorenson (2003) developed a scale to measure the *Quality of Provider Interaction* (QPI). This scale runs from *disaffirming* (where the person receiving care is treated as an object and dehumanised) to *affirming* (where the person is seen as an individual, listened to, and involved in their care). This scale mirrors the continuum between *Vigil of Care* and *Care as Gift*. These theoretical perspectives can be seen to connect with the experiences not only of the women and birthing people, but of the midwives and other maternity care providers too. Further reflection on this is provided by the term Sanctuary Trauma first coined by Silver (1986):

> Likely to occur when a woman turns to others, from whom she expects comfort, during or after a traumatic experience, and is subsequently treated with harshness or indifference.
>
> *(p. 215)*

This quote specifically refers to women and while not all birthing people or midwives identify as women, the importance of this observation is the impact of interpersonal factors. In the context of childbirth, within a wider picture that includes objective factors such as obstetric interventions, and maternal and neonatal outcomes, interpersonal factors are the strongest predictor of PTSD post childbirth (Harris and Ayers 2012). During a traumatic birthing experience, it is highly likely that individuals will turn to those around them for support. Women and birthing people will turn to their care providers, while midwives will seek support from colleagues and managers. When this sought-after support is not forthcoming the distress is potentially compounded. This was reflected in Jenny's findings regarding the sense of abandonment/abandoning. For the midwives, abandoning women occurred due to a lack of attentiveness by management regarding the support midwives require to fulfil their role. Thus, importance of *'being with'* emerged strongly from within both sets of research and is reflected by overlapping themes (Figure 3.1).

Whereas Diane observed that women experienced compassion as a welcome *intervention* in that it was akin to an identifiable, therapeutic approach which transformed care by reducing their suffering. Most often this meant that their fear and anxiety were reduced. Consequently, they had more trust in their care. Interestingly, this trust was not exclusively trust in the 'compassionate midwife', it seemed to extend beyond this to increasing trust in their care as a whole and in their trust in themselves. In turn, this appeared to help women feel more able to cope. Compassionate midwifery has the potential to alleviate suffering around childbirth and conversely lack of compassion increases suffering. In some circumstances that may go on to manifest itself as trauma (Figure 3.2).

Our joint findings relating to midwives' distress at being 'Torn in Two and feeling unable to provide high-quality compassionate care reflect the inherent

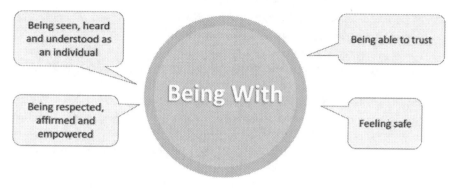

FIGURE 3.1 Being with.

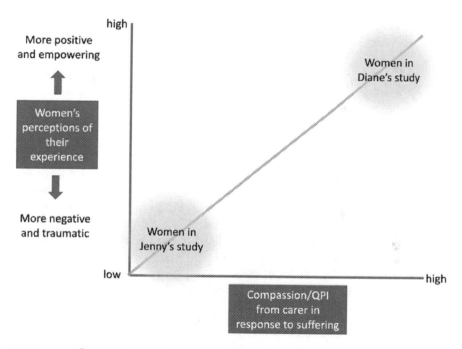

FIGURE 3.2 Compassionate midwifery and trauma.

tensions between a *Vigil of Care* and a *Care as gift* approach to midwifery care. Furthermore, the difference between these approaches is clearly represented in Diane's observation earlier regarding *midwifery attentiveness* experienced as compassion and generating trust, compared to an *obstetric gaze*, described by Davis and Walker (2010), that measures and documents. The danger within models of care that are not attuned to individual human needs is that when workloads are excessive, managing workflow becomes the priority and human needs are further sidelined. In these circumstances, people feel dehumanised and disaffirmed, which can create a toxic environment and as our findings show, can increase the risk of poor psychological outcomes such as distress, trauma, and PTSD. However, psychological outcomes are only part of the story.

Within maternity, the physical and physiological processes of labour are deeply entwined with the emotional and psychological states (Anderson 2002; Buckley 2015) and spiritual and cultural needs (Crowther, Stephen, and Hall 2020) of the woman or birthing person. When we re-examine our research findings together, we can see signs of trauma and fear appearing to disrupt the optimal hormonal processes. These hormonal processes are necessary to support the physical and emotional changes during labour and birth and yet these are integrated with the mind, body, and behaviour (Dixon, Skinner, and Foureur 2013). Therefore, fear and trauma may potentially impact negatively on physiological labour progress, necessitating clinical interventions and leading to poorer maternal and fetal outcomes. While this was not a direct aspect of Jenny's research, she observed that women described their labour stalling or stopping when they shifted from a supportive environment to one of trauma.

Developing a culture of mindful compassion in midwifery

The vast majority of midwives set out to provide high-quality, compassionate care to women, birthing people, and families and yet they are frustrated and upset that they cannot always achieve it (Mander and Patterson 2018). Women's stories about their compassionate midwife illuminate the position of the midwife as the person trying to juggle a number of conflicting demands, contradictions, and paradoxes regarding their role and expectations on them. Midwives have to find a way of balancing these things successfully to be able to sustain compassionate care. The model of *Compassionate Midwifery in Balance* (below) depicts the position of the midwife endeavouring to balance compassionate care. Note the precarious fulcrum or balance point. There is little margin for error (Figure 3.3).

The evidence from women is clear. Listening, noticing, and *being with* women and birthing people, is a fundamental way to show compassion, but finding ways to listen, notice and be with ourselves is just as important if, as midwives and birth workers, we are going to be able to achieve that all-important balance which enables compassionate care to flow.

Box 3.1 Stop and reflect

Stop and reflect

In what ways do you see yourself as trying to balance your work and your life? What sort of things knock you off balance?

How can you bring a mindful practice into your life and work to mitigate the possibility of being 'knocked off balance'?

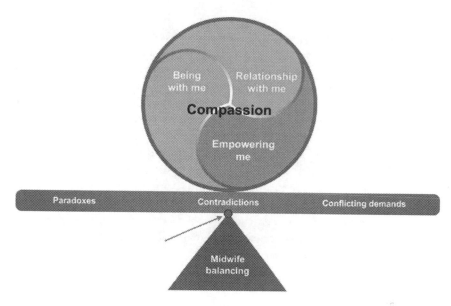

FIGURE 3.3 Compassionate midwifery in balance (Ménage et al. 2020).

Balance is important in everyone's life, and we will all have different ideas about what that means and how it feels when we do not feel balanced. There are a number of reasons why midwives and maternity workers may not be able to achieve balance in their professional roles and provide high-quality, compassionate care even when it is exactly what they want to do. Firstly, they may be suffering themselves. This could be to do with an impossible workload, a demand to continually multi-task and they may be working in a culture of fear and blame which raises their anxiety levels to a point where there are barriers to providing compassionate care. Fear induces a threat response which is effectively a block to compassion (Gilbert 2009) and as a result midwives may have *lost themselves* and become detached from their original reasons for becoming midwives. In a sense, they become abandoned from their own philosophy of care and develop a lack of mindfulness when they just follow the 'rules'. This happens all too often as midwives try to align with the prevailing work culture and feel worn down within an inflexible system (Hunter et al. 2019). It also separates midwives from the spiritual aspects of birthing and inhibits *spiritual midwifing*. Spiritual midwifing honours the relational, cultural, and environmental impacts on birth; it acknowledges our common humanity and what is meaningful and sacred at birth. This disconnect from the spiritual can negatively affect psychological, emotional, and physical wellbeing (Crowther et al. 2021). Mindfulness practices offer a way for midwives to take notice of what is happening in the moment and may also offer solutions. For example, by developing mindfulness techniques midwives may be more able to create a quiet, safe space for both themselves and those they are caring for at the time of birth and immediately afterwards.

Second, within midwifery education and practice, there has been a focus on learning medicalised care procedures and more recently on the importance of providing information to improve public health and aid informed choices around birth. Both certainly have an important place in midwifery care, but other aspects of care have been completely neglected. Historically, an attentive mindful approach has not been developed in midwives' nor obstetricians' education and training, with these interpersonal skills still not being given the importance they warrant. Models of midwifery care that are systems-centred rather than people-centred and excessive workload further exacerbate the problem (Kirkham 1999, 2020; Catling 2017; Hunter et al. 2019). In these working environments, maternity workers are expected to prioritise workflow rather than people. This leads to the crux of the issue. That is: how do midwives and other maternity care professionals maintain practice authentically, in the face of the pressures of modern maternity care settings and without being adequately prepared for this in their pre-registration education and training?

Finding a way of achieving balance and sustaining compassionate care is no easy task and yet the complex skills needed to be able to do this are not the skills that most people have been taught within their general education or in their professional preparation. Indeed, the focus is usually heavily weighted towards thinking and doing rather than noticing and being. Arguably, mindful self-compassion techniques provide one of the best techniques for developing skills which promote balance.

Compassion is associated with respectful, patient connection with another being as a means of noticing their suffering and being able to relieve it (Ménage et al. 2017, 2020). It requires *'radical listening and curiosity'* (Ménage 2017). But it is worth remembering that compassion must flow in three directions in order to be sustained:

Box 3.2 Compassion must flow in three directions

Self to other
Other to self
Self to self

Gilbert (2009)

Generally, in midwifery, when we think of compassion, we think of how we can provide compassionate care to those we care for. In other words, we think about compassion flowing from ourselves to others. Interestingly, those that we care for often show compassion and empathic concern for those who are caring compassionately for them (Ménage et al. 2020). This is compassion flowing from others to self and we may also experience this from compassionate work colleagues and others. However, when compassion can flow from self to self this is self-compassion, and it is every bit as powerful as compassion from another.

Indeed, it is perhaps the most useful and accessible form of compassion possible. But practising self-compassion takes just that: practice. However, Neff (2017) points out that mindfulness is crucial to the ability to give oneself compassion, hence the concept of *mindful self-compassion*. Mindfulness is the means of connecting to our common humanity in the present moment. It is this that gives us a real opportunity to notice our own suffering and respond with compassion.

Box 3.3 Stop and reflect

Stop and reflect

How do you show compassion to yourself?
Are you comfortable with the concept of self-compassion?
Can think of some examples of how you demonstrate compassion to yourself?

For some people, self-compassion sounds selfish or self-indulgent and for these reasons, it can feel uncomfortable. This is a common misconception and has nothing to do with these things. It is about treating yourself as if you were somebody that you cared about and had taken responsibility for. There is a very strong link between mindfulness and self-compassion which explains why the term *mindful self-compassion* is now well established. There is a body of research which has linked mindful self-compassion to a number of emotional and physical health benefits and to better interpersonal relationships (Neff 2011) and there are many courses teaching the techniques which develop this as an evidence-based tool for self-resilience. While we may understand the significance of connecting with the woman we are caring for, do we understand how important it is to connect to ourselves too?

Box 3.4 Stop and reflect

Stop and reflect

Under what circumstances do feel really connected to yourself in the present moment?

You may have been able to think of examples when you felt connected to yourself and experienced the here and now rather than thinking about other people, issues, and plans. For some, it might be when you relax in a hot bath at the end of the day or when you go for a walk or when you do something creative. Or you did not fully understand what connecting to yourself entails? That would not be unusual at all.

Mindfulness is a practice in which we can develop the skills to connect with ourselves. Not with our thoughts or our actions, but the essence of ourselves. There are many techniques and most use a focus on the body's rhythms to come into the present moment. The breath is one of the most common rhythms to notice and follow. Curiosity is developed in this very simple method of just following the 'in' and the 'out' breath. It sounds easy and yet it is not because the mind is usually running around at speed planning and analysing what needs to happen next and why. This is the nature of the human mind and we have been practising this all our lives. For this reason, mindfulness can seem very difficult at first and it is a mistake to think that the aim is to *get good at it* anyway. Thoughts will of course come into the mind the moment that we do not want them to. Many people find this the main problem with mindfulness, but it should not be. Practising mindful self-compassion using the techniques developed by Gilbert (2009), Neff (2011), Kabat-Zinn (2016) and Puddicombe (2016) shows us that thoughts and distractions are normal and unavoidable. Finding ways to stand back and observe them rather than follow them slavishly is the way to stay in the moment and connect with oneself in an authentic and therapeutic way. Introducing this technique to midwives from the very start of their education would ensure that midwives have the opportunity to develop mindful self-compassion as a tool for their careers and for life. Diane has been introducing student midwives to compassionate mindfulness over the last three years. Appendix 1 describes her experience of this.

Summary

This chapter explores how mindful midwifery care, or a lack of this, significantly influences how women and birthing people perceive their childbirth experience. This perception is far from trivial. This is not about whether one has a good feeling or not about one's birthing experience, rather it is about the reality of trauma and PTSD. Yet, when the perception is one of compassionate care this reduces fear, increases safety, and thus reduces trauma. At the heart of the issue lie the interpersonal interactions, either between women/birthing people and their midwives, or between midwives and other maternity care providers. The so-called soft skills required to optimise these interactions are not yet fully recognised as essential skills to be embedded in midwifery or obstetric education. We argue that the skills of compassion (for self or others), and mindfulness are integral to safe maternity care and contribute to improved psychological and physical outcomes for women, birthing people, and their families. We have provided some reflective activities to promote a compassionate and mindful approach (Figure 3.4).

Take home messages

- Interpersonal factors are significant contributors to trauma and PTSD.
- Models of midwifery care that fail to address the human needs of women and birthing people contribute to harmful environments in which poor psychological or physical outcomes are more likely.

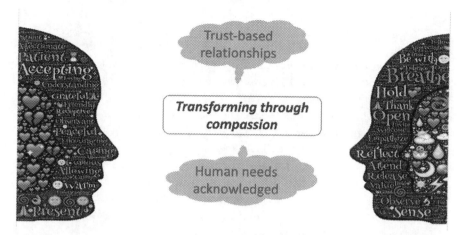

FIGURE 3.4 Transforming through compassion.

- Models of midwifery care that fail to address the human needs of midwives and other maternity care providers contribute to harmful environments that cause psychological or physical harm to staff. This in turn contributes to poor quality care.
- Compassionate midwifery care is a powerful intervention to reduce fear and increase safety.
- Compassionate, mindful skills can enhance the interactions between women/birthing people and their care providers, and between maternity care providers themselves.
- Learning mindful self-compassion techniques has proven benefits and can be learned. They should be embedded within midwifery and obstetric education.

Box 3.5 Appendix 1: Diane's experience of introducing mindful self-compassion techniques to student midwives

I walked into the classroom and prepared to start my lecture for a cohort of third-year midwifery students. I always try to take a moment to really look at them and connect. How are you I asked? They seemed particularly tense and distracted. One or two spoke up. They were 'tired' stressed-out' 'overloaded with work' they said. 'Our dissertations are due in on Friday and we still have this module to do as well as clinical exams!' On the spur of the moment, I decided to try something different that I had been finding invaluable. I told them that I wanted them to be brave and just try something. It would only take five minutes of their time but would they agree to try it, they nodded agreement. I said the following slowly and calmly:

OK just get comfortable in your seat, feet on the floor and hands on your lap [they shuffled about a bit and looked a bit puzzled but they did as I suggested] *Take a deep breath, in…..and out. Again, slowly in….. and out and with the next breath gently close your eyes. Now just breath in your normal way but follow the breath and notice the pattern of the in and out breath. Your mind will wander but when it does just let it go come back to a focus on your breath.*

Now bring to mind a person (or animal that you care deeply about) think of them now and imagine that you can see them in front of you. Say to them silently: may you be well, may you be happy, may you be peaceful and at ease. Now bring to mind everyone in this classroom. Wish them well by saying to them silently: may you be well, may you be happy, may you be peaceful and at ease. Now bring to mind yourself. Focus on just you and nobody else. Say to yourself silently: may you be well, may you be happy, may you be peaceful and at ease.

Now turn your attention to your breath again. Notice your in breath and your out breath and follow each in turn. Now be aware of your self as you sit on your chair in this room and be aware of your feet on the floor and hands on your lap and when you are ready open your eyes.

I looked at all the faces looking back at me and the tension had visibly lifted. How was that for you? Their responses varied. Many of them said it was amazing and they felt better already. Others noted that it had eased their anxiety and relaxed them. One or two were not sure but certainly felt no worse. Somebody said that the hard part was wishing themselves well. This is common I reassured them. We are not used to showing ourselves authentic compassion. But with practice, it gets easier.

It had only taken a few minutes but the students were more focused and engaged with the lecture than they had been for a while. That was the start of offering mindfulness and mindful self-compassion sessions at the beginning of some my classes. I have now tried this with first-, second-, and third-year students and always find that the students get something from it. I also provide them with information on how they can find out more about different mindfulness and self-compassion techniques and I put recordings of short mindfulness meditations on their module platforms for them to utilize as well as signpost them to other resources. Feedback from students continues to demonstrate that these short sessions are much appreciated by many of the students and I find that if I don't offer these for a while the students will ask me for them. As I continue to develop my own practice in mindful self-compassion I find more ways to share this with both students and colleagues.

Note

1 APA: American Psychiatric Association who publish the Diagnostic and Statistical Manual of Mental Disorders.

References

Alcorn, Kristie L., O'Donovan, Analise, Patrick, Jeff C., Creedy, Debra, and Devilly, Grant J. 2010. "A Prospective Longitudinal Study of the Prevalence of Post-Traumatic Stress Disorder Resulting from Childbirth Events." *Psychological Medicine*, 40: 1849–1859.

Andrews, Erica. 2017. "Holding Space: With Women in the Labyrinth." *Midwifery Today*, 121: 9–11.

Anderson, Tricia. 2002. "Out of the Laboratory: Back to the Darkened Room." *MIDIRS Midwifery Digest*, 12: 65–69.

APA. 1980. *Diagnostic and Statistical Manual of Mental Disorders, 3rd edition*. Washington, D.C.: American Psychiatric Association.

APA. 1994. *Diagnostic and Statistical Manual of Mental Disorders, 4th edition*. Washington, D.C.: American Psychiatric Association.

APA. 2013. *Diagnostic and Statistical Manual of Mental Disorders, 5th edition*. Washington, D.C.: American Psychiatric Association.

Ayers Susan, McKenzie-McHarg Kirstie, Eagle Andrew. 2007. "Cognitive Behaviour Therapy for Postnatal Post-Traumatic Stress Disorder: Case Studies." *The Journal of Psychosomatic Obstetrics & Gynecology*, 28(3): 177–184. doi: 10.1080/01674820601142957. PMID: 17577761.

Berg, Marie, Lundgren, Ingela, Hermansson, Evelyn, and Wahlberg, Vivian. 1996. "Women's Experience of the Encounter with the Midwife during Childbirth." *Midwifery*, 12(1): 11–15.

BTA. 2021. The Birth Trauma Association (BTA). https://www.birthtraumaassociation. org.uk

Buckley, Sarah J. 2015. *Hormonal Physiology of Childbearing: Evidence and Implications for Women, Babies, and Maternity Care*. Washington, D.C.: Childbirth Connections Programs, National Partnership for Women & Families. https://www.nationalpartnership.org/our-work/resources/health-care/maternity/hormonal-physiology-of-childbearing.pdf

Catling, Christine. 2017. "The Culture of Midwifery in Australia." *Women and Birth: Journal of the Australian College of Midwives*, 30: 21–22. https://doi.org/10.1016/j.wombi.2017.08.055

Conversano, Ciro, Ciacchini, Rebecca, Orrù, Graziella, Di Giuseppe, Mariagrazia, Gemignani, Angelo, and Poli, Andrea. 2020. "Mindfulness, Compassion, and Self-Compassion among Health Care Professionals: What's New? A Systematic Review." *Frontiers in Psychology*, 11: 1683.

Crowther, Susan, Stephen, Audrey, and Hall, Jenny. 2020. "Association of Psychosocial–Spiritual Experiences Around Childbirth and Subsequent Perinatal Mental Health Outcomes: An Integrated Review." *Journal of Reproductive and Infant Psychology*, 38(1): 60–85.

Crowther, Susan A., Hall, Jenny, Balabanoff, Doreen, Baranowska, Barbara, Kay, Lesley, Ménage, Diane, and Fry, Jane. 2021. "Spirituality and Childbirth: An International Virtual Co-Operative Inquiry." *Women and Birth*, 34(2): e135–e145.

Davis, Deborah L, and Walker, Kim. 2010. "Case-Loading Midwifery in New Zealand: Making Space for Childbirth." *Midwifery*, 26(6): 603–608.

Dixon, Lesley, Skinner, Joan, and Foureur, Maralyn. 2013. "The Emotional and Hormonal Pathways of Labour and Birth: Integrating Mind, Body and Behaviour." *New Zealand College of Midwives Journal*, 48: 15–23.

Ford, Elizabeth, and Ayers, Susan. 2011. "Support during Birth Interacts with Prior Trauma and Birth Intervention to Predict Postnatal Post-Traumatic Stress Symptoms." *Psychology & Health*, 26: 1553–1570.

Fox, Nick J. 1999. *Beyond Health: Postmodernism and Embodiment*. London: Free Association Books.

Garthus-Niegel, Susan, Soest, Tilmann, Vollrath, Margarete E, and Eberhard-Gran, Malin. 2013. "The Impact of Subjective Birth Experiences on Post-Traumatic Stress Symptoms: A Longitudinal Study." *Archives of Women's Mental Health*, 16: 1–10.

Gilbert, Paul. 2009. *The Compassionate Mind*. London: Constable and Robinson.

Harris, Rachel, and Ayers, Susan. 2012. "What Makes Labour and Birth Traumatic? A Survey of Intrapartum 'Hotspots'." *Psychology & Health*, 27: 1166–1177.

Hochschild, Arlie, R. 1983. *The Managed Heart. Commercialization of Human Feeling.* Berkeley: University of California Press.

Hunter, Billie. 2002. *Emotion Work in Midwifery: An Ethnographic Study of the Emotion Work Undertaken by a Sample of Student and Qualified Midwives in Wales.* PhD thesis or dissertation. Ethos, British Library: University of Wales, Swansea.

Hunter, Billie. 2006. "The Importance of Reciprocity in Relationships between Community-Based Midwives and Mothers." *Midwifery*, 22(4): 308–322.

Hunter, Billie, Fenwick, Jennifer, Sidebotham, Mary, and Henley, Josie. 2019. "Midwives in the United Kingdom: Levels of Burnout, Depression, Anxiety and Stress and Associated Predictors." *Midwifery*, 79: 1–12. https://doi.org/10.1016/j.midw.2019.08.008

Kabat-Zinn, Jon. 2016. *Mindfulness for Beginners*. Louisville, CO: Sounds True Inc.

Kirkham, Mavis. 1999. "The Culture of Midwifery in the National Health Service in England." *Journal of Advanced Nursing*, 30(3): 732–739. https://doi.org/10.1046/j.1365-2648.1999.01139.x

Kirkham, Mavis. 2020. "Sustained by Joy: The Potential for Flow Experience for Midwives and Mothers and the Blocking of that Flow." In *Sustainability, Midwifery, and Birth (Second Ed.),* edited by Lorna Davies, Rea Daellenbach, and Mary Kensington, 99–115. Abingdon: Routledge. https://doi.org/10.4324/9780429290558

Leinweber, Julia, and Rowe, Heather J. 2010. "The Costs of 'Being With The Woman': Secondary Traumatic Stress in Midwifery." *Midwifery*, 26: 76–87.

Lemay, Céline, and Hastie, Carolyn. 2018. "Holding Sacred Space in Labour and Birth." In *Spirituality and Childbirth: Meaning and Caring at the Start of Life*, edited by Susan Crowther and Jenny Hall, 112–114. Abingdon: Routledge.

Lewis, Marie. 2015. *Exploration of the Concept of Trust within the Midwife-Mother Relationship*. PhD thesis or dissertation: Swansea University.

Mander, Rosemary, and Patterson, Jenny. 2018. "The BPG Survey: The Results." In *Untangling the Maternity Crisis* edited by Nadine Edwards, Rosemary Mander, and Jo Murphy-Lawless, 11–20. Abingdon: Routledge.

MBB. 2021. "Make Birth Better." Accessed Feb 10, 2022. https://www.makebirthbetter.org

Ménage, Diane. 2017. "Empathic Midwifery: Radical Listening, Curiosity and Imagination." *All4maternity*, July 1, 2017. https://www.all4maternity.com/viewpoint-empathic-midwifery-radical-listening-curiosity-imagination/

Ménage, Diane, Bailey, Elaine, Lees, Susan, and Coad, Jane. 2017. "A Concept Analysis of Compassionate Midwifery." *Journal of Advanced Nursing*, 73(3): 558–573.

Ménage, Diane, Bailey, Elizabeth, Lees, Susan, and Coad, Jane. 2020. "Women's Lived Experience of Compassionate Midwifery: Human and Professional." *Midwifery*, 85(1): 102662.

Neff, Kristin D. 2011. *Self-compassion*. New York: William Morrow.

Neff, Kristen D. 2017. *Self-Compassion: The Proven Power of Being Kind to Yourself.* New York: Harper Collins. 100–104.

Patterson, Jenny, Hollins Martin, Caroline J., and Karatzias, Thanos. 2019. "Disempowered Midwives and Traumatised Women: Exploring the Parallel Processes of Care Provider Interaction that Contribute to Women Developing Post Traumatic Stress Disorder (PTSD) Post Childbirth." *Midwifery*, 76: 21–35.

Polachek, Inbal S., Harari, Liat H., Baum, Micha, and Strous, Rael D. 2012. "Postpartum Post-Traumatic Stress Disorder Symptoms: The Uninvited Birth Companion." *The Israel Medical Association Journal*, 14: 347–353.

PTSD UK. 2021. Post Natal PTSD in Birthing Partners. Accessed Feb 10, 2022. https://www.ptsduk.org/what-is-ptsd/causes-of-ptsd/post-natal-ptsd-in-birthing-partners/

Puddicombe, Andy. 2016. *The Headspace Guide to Meditation and Mindfulness.* London: Hodder & Stoughton.

Reed, Rachel, Sharman, Rachael, and Inglis, Christian. 2017. "Women's Descriptions of Childbirth Trauma Relating to Care Provider Actions and Interactions." *BMC Pregnancy and Childbirth*, 17: 21. https://doi.org/10.1186/s12884-016-1197-0

Robinson, Jean. 2007. "Post Traumatic Stress Disorder." *AIMS Journal*, 19: 5–8.

Silver, Steven M. 1986. "An Inpatient Programme for Post-Traumatic Stress Disorder: Context as treatment." In *Trauma and its Wake Vol II*, edited by Charles R. Figley, 213–231. Levittown: Bruner/Maxel.

Sorenson, Dianna S. 2003. "Healing Traumatizing Provider Interactions among Women through Short-Term Group Therapy." *Archives of Psychiatric Nursing*, 17: 259–269.

Sorenson, Dianna S., and Tschetter, Lois. 2010. "Prevalence of Negative Birth Perception, Disaffirmation, Perinatal Trauma Symptoms, and Depression Among Postpartum Women." *Perspectives in Psychiatric Care*, 46: 14–25.

Walsh, Dennis. 2011. "Nesting and Matrescence" In *Theory for Midwifery Practice 2nd edition*, edited by Rosamund Bryar and Marlene Sinclair, 178–192. Basingstoke: Palgrave Macmillan.

Wright, Erin M, Matthai, Maude T, and Budhathoki, Chakra. 2018. "Midwifery Professional Stress and Its Sources: A Mixed-Methods Study." *Journal of Midwifery & Women's Health,* 63(6): 660–667.

Yildiz, Pelin D., Ayers, Susan, and Phillips, Louise. 2017. "The Prevalence of Posttraumatic Stress Disorder in Pregnancy and After Birth: A Systematic Review and Meta-analysis." *Journal of Affective Disorders*, 208: 634–645.

Zaers, Stefanie, Waschke, Melanie, and Ehlert, Ulrike. 2008. "Depressive Symptoms and Symptoms of Post-traumatic Stress Disorder in Women After Childbirth." *Journal of Psychosomatic Obstetrics & Gynecology*, 29: 61–71.

4

POIPOIA TE WAIRUA O TE MĀMĀ

A Māori perspective on mindfulness and the birth sphere

Miriama Ketu-McKenzie

'Ko au te awa, ko te awa ko au'
I am the river and the river is me.

These words belong to a renowned whakatauki (Māori proverb) from the Whanganui region of Aotearoa New Zealand.[1] They were chosen as an opening for this chapter for two reasons: First, the elegance with which they capture the way in which Māori traditionally viewed the relationship between the natural world and themselves. Second, because they present a window through which links between te ao Māori[2] and current conceptualisations of mindfulness, can be made explicit.

This chapter explores several of the points at which concepts in mindfulness and concepts in te ao Māori, converge. It discusses the relevance of mindfulness practice for wāhine Māori (Māori women) and is written from the perspective of a Māori female Clinical Psychologist of Ngāti Raukawa (ki te tonga) and Ngāti Tūwharetoa[3] descent – who was first introduced to formal mindfulness practice in 2012.

Back then, the term 'mindfulness' was virtually unheard of in the Clinical Psychology training circles to which I belonged. As a student who was drawn to the profession following the loss of a cousin to suicide, I was learning that to heal problems of the mind, the content of one's individual thoughts needed to be analysed, faults in logic needed to be corrected and any corresponding un-healthy behaviours needed to be broken down and understood in terms of their reinforcing and contingent forces. Problems of the body were conceptualised in a similar way. I was taught that physical problems were typically caused by one or more faults in a particular part of the body, and that in much the same way as a mechanic analysed a car for issues, diagnosed the problem, fixed/replaced the faulty parts, then put the machine back together, the body and mind were seen

DOI: 10.4324/9781003165200-4

as needing specialist 'external mechanics' (i.e. psychologists, nutritionists, endocrinologists) to analyse and then fix their respective problems.

For those who hold to traditional Māori conceptions of wellbeing, the idea of viewing health as synonymous with the absence of pathological symptoms can seem reductionistic and overly functionalist. That is because Māori conceptions of health emphasise the importance of balance across multiple domains (e.g. the mind, the body, the spirit and relationships). Renowned Māori psychiatrist Dr Mason Durie best captures this discrepancy by noting that, where modern medicine tends to take a *centripetal* approach to wellbeing, focusing on analysing the individual components of a person, many Māori take a *centrifugal* approach to health, contextualising their wellbeing within a wider system of interconnectedness to, and interdependence upon, relationships with whānau (family), whenua (land), wairua (spirit) and tīpuna (ancestors). Following a hui attended by Māori elders in Hamilton 1982, Dr Durie integrated the above concepts into the model now known as 'Te Whare Tapa Whā'. His model compares health to the four walls of a whare (house), with psychological health, physical health, family health and spiritual health representing one wall each. The model implies that health is the result of interactions between each wall and that imbalance in any one area, affects the stability and integrity of the whole structure (see Figure 4.1).

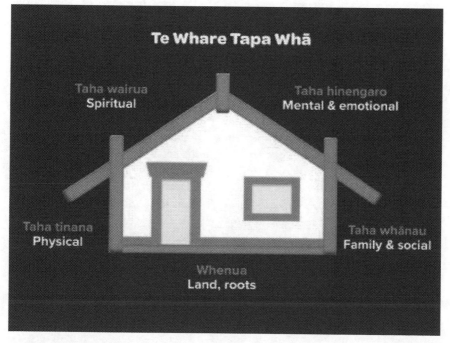

FIGURE 4.1 Te Whare Tapa Whā.
Source: Reprinted with permission from the Mental Health Foundation, NZ.

As the daughter of a Māori man and a Pākeha[4] woman, who was raised with close connections to our marae (traditional Māori fortified village) and to our wider whānau, I grew up exposed to both of those approaches to health. Nevertheless, I found it difficult in the early years of my clinical training to reconcile the mechanistic approach of Cognitive Behavioural Therapy (CBT) with the realities of working with Māori, who sought more holistic formulations of their problems than CBT alone could offer. On a personal level, therapies like CBT left me unable to explain why the family members on my European side were in largely good health and living well into their 90s even 100s, while at the same time many members of my Māori whānau were struggling with mental health issues and dying young, often of preventable chronic diseases.

While I was preparing my PhD research, my 62-year-old Māori father was diagnosed with end-stage renal failure and a year later his younger brother died suddenly of a stroke at age 56 – at a time when the life expectancy for Pākeha males was 80 years. Those events, combined with knowledge that my dad and his brother were raised in less than ideal home environments, compelled me to consider the relationship between mind and body in more detail. I eventually found myself studying the stress response system, where I learned that the Māori perspective of viewing mind and body as integrated and interrelated, was closely aligned with biological knowledge of how the hypothalamic-pituitary-adrenal axis (or HPA axis) works.

The HPA axis is a major neuro-endocrine system that connects perceptions held in the brain to physical responses in the body. This system is activated whenever the brain perceives a challenge or a threat, and under such conditions, coordinates a whole-body response that mobilises the body to run from or fight the threat at hand. To achieve this complex action, the hypothalamus in the brain instructs the pituitary gland to release adrenocorticotropic hormone (ACTH), which in turn triggers the release of cortisol from the adrenal gland. This cascade of events enables the rapid release of glucose into the bloodstream, while at the same time suppressing immune function so that the body is immediately able to run or to fight. This system works well when the perceived stressors are intermittent and rapid (i.e. when exposed to the threat of an animal predator that can be outrun or fought off). However, under conditions of chronic stress exposure (such as poverty or domestic abuse), or exposure to stress in childhood (when the threat is inescapable) the stress response system can effectively 'wear out', leaving the individual immune-compromised and vulnerable to mood disorders, cardiovascular disease and metabolic disease. This is a concept known as 'allostatic overload'.[5]

Understanding allostatic overload and the HPA axis helped me to integrate my two different worldviews because the science supported the Māori view in which the mind and body were closely interconnected parts of a greater whole. From that point on in my research, I started to see the differences in health outcomes between my two families not as differences of race or genetic predisposition necessarily, but as differences in exposure to stress across their lifetimes, starting in early life.

Early life stress

I first encountered the consequences of early life stress in the 1998 'ACE study' article published by Robert Anda and Vincent Felitti. Their research with over 13,000 Americans provided evidence of a clear, dose–response relationship between the number of adverse experiences endured in childhood (such as physical abuse, loss of a family member, witnessing violence against their mother) and the leading causes of premature death in the United States, including ischemic heart disease, cancer and chronic lung disease. Put simply, their research showed that the higher the number of adverse experiences one faced in early life, the more likely they were to develop cancer, heart disease, chronic lung disease, liver disease and skeletal fractures as adults. Consistent with this, the higher the number of adverse experiences one endured in childhood, the more likely they were as adults to smoke cigarettes, drink excessive amounts of alcohol, use drugs, become depressed and suicidal.

To account for their findings, Felitti and Anda proposed that adverse childhood experiences (or ACEs) disrupted neurological development, thereby impairing social, cognitive and emotional functioning. Those impairments then contributed to the adoption of health risk behaviours (such as excessive drinking, smoking), which in turn led to the development of chronic diseases and ultimately, to early death. A graphic of this model can be seen in the pyramid shown on the left in Figure 4.2. In essence, the ACE model proposes that early life stress accelerates the progression of disease across the lifetime, contributing

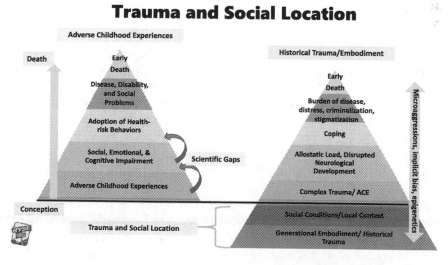

FIGURE 4.2 Extended ACE pyramid. Reprinted with permission from RYSE California.

to premature death. It is likely that the HPA axis plays a pivotal role in this progression, for it is responsible for the regulation of stress across multiple body systems.

At a personal level, this knowledge helped me to make sense of the differences in life expectancy observed between my two families. When applied to Aotearoa New Zealand as a whole, however, the ACE model offers a framework for understanding differences in premature deaths between Māori and Pākeha in general. For although life expectancy rates for both groups have improved over the past 150 years, Māori today are still expected to live an average of seven years less than their Pākeha neighbours, and it is anticipated that many of their deaths will be preceded by preventable, chronic diseases. Consistent with the ACE model outlined above, Māori are also more likely than Pākeha to smoke cigarettes and drink hazardous amounts of alcohol. However, by neither blaming nor dismissing the role that lifestyle choices plays, the ACE model provides a way of understanding health disparities between Māori and Pākeha that takes into account differences in exposure to stress and subsequent changes to the HPA axis. For when we consider that exposure to early life stress in the form of childhood physical abuse, sexual abuse, and witnessing inter-parental violence is also known to be significantly higher for Māori than it is for non-Māori in Aotearoa New Zealand, one could argue that the high adoption of health risk behaviours and reduced life expectancy rates in Māori are perhaps better understood as correlates of stress exposure rather than simply poor lifestyle choices. Notably, the same pathway from early life stress to chronic disease and early death outlined here is also seen in other populations who share similar histories to Māori.

Extending the ACE pyramid

Reports of frequent exposure to early life stress, as well as high rates of addiction, mental illness, chronic disease and premature death can be found in indigenous minorities across the globe, including those in Australia, Canada and Hawaii. In recognition of this, RYSE Center in California in 2017 proposed an extension to the original ACE pyramid, positing *historical trauma* and *social conditions* as precursors to adverse experiences in childhood. A graphic of this 'extended ACE pyramid' is shown in the pyramid on the right side of Figure 4.2. By adding extra layers, the extended ACE pyramid accounts for ways in which historical trauma (such as colonisation) might contribute to the high frequency of exposure to adverse childhood events among such populations, by impacting the social conditions into which an indigenous child is born, altering the intrauterine environment and altering gene expression through epigenetics.

Essentially, the extended ACE pyramid proposes that historical trauma negatively alters the social conditions of indigenous people (e.g. through the removal of land, the suppression of cultural rituals and changes in gender roles, forced labour, inadequate housing, mass death), which directly impacts the health of those bringing indigenous children into the world, and increases the likelihood that their children will be exposed to adverse experiences that could disrupt their neurological development – leading them to adopt unhealthy coping strategies that contribute to the development of disease and early death.

While it is beyond the scope of this chapter to provide a detailed overview of the neurobiological sequelae activated when young brains and bodies are exposed to stress, it is sufficient to note that the broad pathways outlined in both the ACE pyramid and the 'extended ACE pyramid' are supported by neuroscientific evidence which shows that exposure to chronic stress in utero and/or within the first 1,000 days of life can result in excessive activation of the developing HPA axis – with life-long implications for the mind and the body. Put simply, the research suggests that a mother who is pregnant and faced with unrelenting stress is likely to have a chronically activated HPA axis. Such an HPA axis is likely to regularly release excessive amounts of cortisol into the bloodstream, which can negatively impact a baby's development, contributing to low birth weight and the formation of a hyper-reactive HPA axis. Such intra-uterine exposure can increase the risk of developing Type-2 diabetes in adulthood due to HPA axis-related changes in glucose regulation that were programmed at birth. In addition, exposure to stress (such as maternal separation or neglect) in the perinatal and infancy periods of development, can also influence the reactivity of the HPA axis such that those exposed to early life stress outside of the womb, are also more vulnerable to developing chronic health problems when exposed to stress later in life. Although there remain gaps in our knowledge of how the timing, frequency, duration and severity of certain stressors affect each of the stress response pathways differently, the research is unequivocal in the fact that stress exposure in utero and the months following the birth can have extremely adverse effects on a growing HPA axis and executive functioning, and that those effects are cumulative over time – resulting in a stress response system that is unable to adequately respond to other life threats (such as cancer and infection) and is thus, more vulnerable to developing chronic disease.

A third area in which maternal health can influence a developing baby is in the area of epigenetics – the study of how life experiences interact with gene expression. Recent research by Professor Peter Gluckman and Dr Tatjana Buklijas has shown that our life experiences have the power to both suppress certain genes and activate others. The implication here, is that, the strands of DNA passed down by mothers across generations, might change in response to their life experiences – such that mothers who have experienced overwhelming life events (like the grievous loss of many of their people during the process of colonisation) can through ongoing intergenerational effects, pass the remnants of their grief onto their grandchildren and great-grandchildren. To understand how this applies to Māori in Aotearoa New Zealand specifically, an understanding of historical trauma, subsequent changes to social conditions, and the impacts of those on the health of wāhine Māori is required.

Historical trauma

Researcher and lawyer Ani Mikaere has argued that prior to the arrival of Europeans in Aotearoa New Zealand, wāhine were highly valued in Māori society. Their prestige was embedded in the myths and legends Māori shared across generations, many of which portrayed wāhine as powerful goddesses who were to be revered and respected for the unique gifts with which they were endowed. Consistent with this, Mikaere asserts that in pre-colonial Māori society, the place of wāhine was on par with that of tāne Māori (Māori men). This was because every person in the tribe was considered part of the collective whole, and therefore, both wāhine and tāne played a part in ensuring that the collective was protected. That protection extended to conception and birth, where wāhine in particular were viewed as essential to the survival of the collective because they provided the whakapapa links that joined Māori to their ancestors – the very first of whom was a woman.

In fact, Māori were so concerned about protecting their future progeny that they created *tikanga* (rules) to guide the tasks a wāhine could or could not carry out while of child-bearing age. An example of this can be seen in the fact that the privileged role of kaikaranga (the person who calls people onto the marae) was only ever bestowed upon wāhine for whom the years of bearing children had passed. This was to protect the fertile womb (and a developing baby) from any harm that could come to them through the spiritual realm. The reason they were so fiercely protected was because Māori believed that if any spiritual harm came through the wāhine to the womb, then that harm could be passed down through future generations of Māori. As mentioned earlier, because Māori considered spiritual health to be as important as physical health, ensuring the physical, mental and spiritual health of future generations was of paramount importance.

Their instinct to protect their child bearers was warranted, for within 100 years of colonial contact, more than half of the Māori population was eradicated – decreasing from over 100,000 to less than 42,000, and it was wāhine Māori who bore the burden of this loss with 25% of Māori girls dying within their first year of life (compared with 10% Pākeha girls) and 50% dying before age seven (compared with 15% of Pākeha girls) – largely of communicable diseases to which they had never before been exposed and had no immunity for. A consequence of this was that few survived to child-bearing age, thereby limiting population growth.

Loss of health and life on this scale marked a distinct change for Māori, for when Pākeha first began settling in Aotearoa in the early 1800s, Māori were described by Pākeha observers as being in excellent health. Estimates suggest that the average life expectancy from birth for Māori at that time was approximately 30 years – the same life expectancy rate for Pākeha. However, by 1893, the impacts of colonisation had led to the average life expectancy from birth for a wāhine Māori decreasing to 23 years, while the average life expectancy from birth for a Pakeha woman in Aotearoa increased to 55 years – the greatest life expectancy for European women anywhere in the world. By the mid-20th century, the discrepancy in life expectancy between Māori and Pākeha had become so great, that the life expectancy for a Māori person in 1945 was less than that of Pākeha living in 1876.

In addition to the great number of Māori lives lost during colonisation, during the years 1860–1939 specifically, the percentage of Māori-owned land in Aotearoa decreased from approximately 80% to 9%, and the social structures that comprised Māoridom (e.g. Māori language, Māori spiritual practices, Māori rituals, values and beliefs), were all but lost. Those who survived the colonisation process were effectively acculturated into Pākeha systems of living. In practice, this meant that many Māori were forced off land which had once provided them with kai (food) and protection and into areas where they had to earn money in order to survive. Those changes altered the social fabric of the tribe, resulting in many whānau moving away from the village-like structure of the Pā, which inexorably changed the structure of the family – for colonial housing and land divisions did not accommodate for large numbers of extended whānau.

As a consequence of this, living conditions for Māori during the 1890s and the quality of their housing was sub-standard when compared with Pākeha. This was in part because Māori had little in the way of material wealth once they lost access to their tribal lands, and in part because they struggled to adjust to the expectations that an individualistic society placed on their collectivistic way of life. As such, their dwellings were overcrowded, hygiene was poor, access to medicine was difficult and Māori were generally treated as second-class citizens in their own land. There was an added insult for wāhine Māori in particular, who upon marriage, became *'chattels'* of their husbands, and were considered to have *'less worth than a man's horse'* once English law and Christian values dominated their society. It is those combined events – the radical changes to the fabric of tribal society, the decline in the status of women, the large-scale loss of life, the material poverty and the stress of adjusting to a new system of living in which Māori were largely powerless – that together constitute the term 'historical trauma', and which are considered here to have altered the expression of genes transmitted across generations.

Social conditions

Recalling the extended ACE pyramid, the historical trauma that Māori endured resulted in the survivors living in social conditions that were at times extremely stressful and hazardous to their health – this was especially true for wāhine, the child-bearers. Although it would be remiss to deny that health and social conditions for Māori have greatly improved since 1900, inequities that favour Pākeha lives over Māori remain in most every area today. Recent reports from the 2018 census in Aotearoa New Zealand show that less than half of all Māori live in homes that they own (compared with 72% Pākeha); 25% of Māori still live in overcrowded conditions (compared with 5% of Pakeha); nationally, the median net worth for Māori is just \$23,000 (compared with \$114,000 for Pākeha) and fewer than 22% of Māori can speak their own language.

Consistent with the theory that poor social conditions can affect the intra-uterine environment, comparisons with non-Māori women show that wāhine Māori are more likely to report feeling stressed, depressed and anxious through-out their pregnancies and are significantly more likely to drink heavily during the first trimester of their pregnancy. Wāhine Māori are also more likely than non-Māori to smoke throughout their pregnancies and they are more likely to experience complications during childbirth. Although these statistics do not ac-count for the individual causes of stress among wāhine Māori, the available ev-idence suggests that Māori women are more likely to experience stress in the form of intimate partner violence, than their non-Māori counterparts and they are also more likely to have been abused physically, sexually and emotionally in childhood than non-Māori. For all of the above reasons, they're also more likely to be living in poverty and unable to access support from extended whānau.

Given the evidence presented in the original ACE model which suggests that stress accelerates the pathway to chronic disease and premature death, it may come as no surprise to learn that Māori mortality rates of cardiovascular and cerebrovascular disease are twice as high as they are for Pākeha, Māori mortal-ity rates for cancer are 1.5 times greater, Māori mortality rates for diabetes are 3.5 times greater and Māori mortality rates for chronic obstructive pulmonary disorder are 3 times greater. When one considers that the life expectancy rates between Māori and Pākeha were on a par when they first encountered one an-other, it would be wrong to assume that the health disparities observed between them today were solely attributable to bad genes. A more likely proposal is that they are the consequence of disparities in exposure to stressors that started with the arrival of colonisation, have been transmitted intergenerationally, and are continuing to affect Māori across the lifetime, starting from birth. The message of hope within this is that there is also preliminary evidence showing that the reactivity of a stress response system that was exposed to early life stress can be altered with mindfulness practice. This is because mindfulness practice helps to regulate the HPA axis, thus promoting more healthful adaptations to stress.

Enter mindfulness

As a PhD candidate in 2012, I happened upon a mindfulness symposium at a New Zealand Psychological Society conference and encountered my first 'mindfulness of breath' exercise. I decided then that I would study the benefits of mindfulness as an intervention for Māori, for during that brief practice, I recognised that the quality of presence I had felt during the exercise was both familiar – because I had felt it before at both our marae and in church as a child – and alien because I was experiencing it while sitting in an office-type space, surrounded by people I didn't know, and without any of the traditional signifiers of spiritual practice that I had come to associate with such a strong *feeling* of connection.

After consulting with several Māori elders and investigating the intersect between concepts within mindfulness and Māori notions of health, the following five points were considered to support the hypothesis that mindfulness might be a 'good fit' with Māori worldviews:

First, mindfulness draws on 2500 years of Eastern philosophy which views the mind, the body, the spirit and relationships with others, as interdependent and interconnected. To that end, health is considered to be the consequence of integrating those various elements, and can be attained by increasing awareness of how each influences the other, and not attaching to whatever is present in any given moment. The holistic nature of this approach has much in common with traditional Māori views of health (recall Figure 1 and Te Whare Tapa Whā), as compared with the bio-medical model.

Second, formal mindfulness is a spiritual practice, and in te ao Māori spiritual health is considered as vital to wellbeing as physical health.

Third, Mindfulness Based Stress Reduction (MBSR) is a group-based therapy, which makes it ideal for those whose values are highly collectivistic.

Fourth, there is overlap between the functions of mindfulness meditation (e.g. to increase focus and to become intentional about one's way of being in the world), and the function of certain practices and rituals within te ao Māori, such as performing karakia (ritual chants) as a way to set an intention for a specific hui (meeting).

Fifth, mindfulness as a way of being, promotes awareness of how one influences and is influenced by their relationships with others, their relationship to their tīnana (body), their relationship to the earth and so on – all of which are concepts that overlap with traditional Māori ways of living (recall the whakatauki at the start of this article).

For all of those reasons, I undertook a research project which first evaluated the degree of dysregulation in the cortisol levels of a group of wāhine Māori who had experienced high amounts of stress in childhood, and then assessed the benefits of exposing those wāhine Māori to an eight-week mindfulness-based stress reduction course. Following consultation with several Māori elders, ethical approval and informed consent procedures, eight wahine Maori were recruited into the study from Te Wai Pounamu (the South Island). As was predicted, during the baseline testing period almost all of the wāhine showed chronic patterns of cortisol dysregulation – with some showing chronically low cortisol output and others presenting with chronically high levels, which was assumed to be a correlate of early life stress. Multiple samples were taken at various times throughout the day in order to capture the cortisol awakening response, the overall daily output of cortisol, and cortisol responses to an acute stressor. Moreover, tests evaluating levels of depression, anxiety, perceived stress, symptoms of trauma, eating behaviour and mindfulness were conducted across the eight-week period.

The results showed across-the-board improvements in the majority of the tests, and importantly, those improvements appeared to correlate with increases in mindful awareness. Among the most interesting of the findings, however, was what the wāhine themselves said about how mindfulness fits with Māori ways of seeing the world:

> *'What I know about our worldview is that everything's for a purpose and I think a lot of what's in the mindfulness stuff, keeping yourself clear, being aware of what's happening and what it is and why, where it comes from and what your reaction is, there's definitely a link.'*
>
> *Ani*

> *'When I think of different Ringatu[6], those karakia go forever, miles and miles and miles, early hours of the morning, on particular days, you know, but what are you doing at those times? You're not just spitting out words, you actually are in a state of meditation.'*
>
> *Ripeka*

As well as what they said about completing an 8-week MBSR course – to which they had previously had no exposure:

> *'I'm a bit surprised actually, at how deep if you like, you can get, how deep the reach can be.'*
>
> *Kiri*

> *'I've enjoyed the connection with other Māori women, women I've never met before, and the ones I have met, I've gotten to know them better…there's a special bond now that we've got.'*
>
> *Arohia*

Taken together, the case for promotion of mindfulness practice within te ao Māori seems evident. However, nowhere is the need for mindfulness-based interventions more clearly seen than in the birthsphere – where Māori minds, bodies and stress response systems are formed.

In te aō Māori, the individual person is considered to be just one link in a chain that extends all the way back to the beginning of time, and all the way forwards to future generations. Consistent with early tikanga, it could be argued that for Māori to safeguard future generations from harm, the best place to start is within the stress response systems of the people who will bear the children, namely the wāhine. In an age where gaining access to our traditional practices is difficult, mindfulness offers a unique opportunity for both western medicine and indigenous views to find a meeting point, and for Māori to gain relief from the consequences of chronic and early life stress exposure. Mindfulness is well aligned with traditional views of health and wellbeing because it is a psychosocial-spiritual-physiological practice that works by increasing attentional awareness. As such, mindfulness may well be a practice that other indigenous peoples working to correct colonial injustices, can use to help re-populate, reclaim and re-connect to their whakapapa (heritage) within the childbirth sphere. For Māori, because mindfulness promotes a non-religious spirituality that involves training oneself to be connected to what is within you, what is around you, what is above you and what is underneath you, it can be argued that regular mindfulness practice mimics the function of traditional Māori practices by increasing awareness of and respect for the relationship between ourselves and the world around us. In keeping with the traditional imperative to protect future progeny, if our goal is to positively influence the minds, spirits, bodies and relationships of future generations of mokopuna (grandchildren), what practice could be more important?

Notes

1 Aotearoa is the Māori name for New Zealand in te reo Māori (Māori language). In contemporary New Zealand society the two names are either used together – 'Aotearoa New Zealand' or separately depending on context and speaker(s)/author(s).
2 Te ao Māori refers to the Māori world view which acknowledges the interconnectedness and interrelationship of all living and non-living things.
3 During introductions, Māori identify themselves by naming the various tribes to which they affiliate. Doing so links them back to their ancestors and helps their listener to locate the parts of the country to which they are attached. The tribal lands of Ngāti Raukawa ki te tonga and Ngāti Tūwharetoa are located in the lower half of the North Island of Aotearoa New Zealand.
4 Pākehā refers to non-Māori who are primarily of European descent.
5 Allostatic load refers to the cumulative burden that stress places on the body. Allostatic overload occurs when one's environmental challenges overwhelm the individual system's ability to cope.
6 Ringatu refers to a Māori religion founded by Te Kooti Arikirangi te Turuki. Many of its followers memorise karakia (ritual scriptures, chants and prayers) which they then repeat to invoke spiritual guidance.

Bibliography

Anderson, I., Crengle, S., Kamaka, M. L., Chen. T-H., Palafox, N., & Jackson-Pulver, L. (2006). Indigenous health in Australia, New Zealand and the Pacific. *Lancet*, 367, 1775–1785.
Barlow, C. (1991). *Tikanga Whakaaro: Key concepts in Māori culture*. Melbourne: Oxford University Press.
Brunton, P. J., Sullivan, K. M., Kerrigan, D., Russell, J. A., Seckl, J. R., & Drake, A. J. (2013). Sex-specific effects of prenatal stress on glucose homoeostasis and peripheral metabolism in rats. *Journal of Endocrinology*, 217, 161–173.
Crowther, S., Stephen, A., & Hall, J. (2020). Association of psychosocial–spiritual experiences around childbirth and subsequent perinatal mental health outcomes: An integrated review. *Journal of Reproductive and Infant Psychology*, 38(1), 60–85.

Durie, M. (1994). *Whaiora: Māori Health Development*. Auckland: Oxford University Press.

Durie, M. (2011). Indigenizing mental health services: New Zealand experience. *Transcultural Psychiatry*, 48(1–2), 24–36.

Felitti, V. J., Anda, R. F., Nordenberg, D., Williamson, D. F., Spitz, A. M., Edwards, V., Koss, M. P., & Marks, J. S. (1998). Relationship of childhood abuse and household dysfunction to many of the leading causes of death in adults. The Adverse Childhood Experiences (ACE) study. *American Journal of Preventive Medicine*, 14(4), 245–58.

Friedman, H. S. (2002). *Health Psychology: Second Edition*. Upper Saddle River, NJ: Pearson Education, Inc.

Glover, M., & Kira, A. (2011). Why Māori women continue to smoke while pregnant. *The New Zealand Medical Journal*, 124(1339), 22–31.

Gluckman, P. Hanson, M., Buklijas, T., Low, F. M & Beedle, A. S. (2009). Epigenetic mechanisms that underpin metabolic and cardiovascular diseases. *Nature Reviews Endocrinology*, 5, 401–408.

Hirini, P., Flett, R., Long, N., & Millar, M. (2005). Frequency of traumatic events, physical and psychological health among Māori. *New Zealand Journal of Psychology*, 34(1), 20–27.

Ketheesan, S., Rinaudo, M., Berger, M., Wenitong, M., Juster, R. P., McEwen, B. S., & Sarnyai, Z. (2020). Stress, allostatic load, and mental health in indigenous Australians. *Stress*, 23(5), 509–518.

Kim, P. J. (2019). Social determinants of health inequities in indigenous Canadians through a life course approach to colonialism and the residential school system. *Health Equity*, 3(1), 378–381.

Low, F., Gluckman, P., & Poulton, R. (2021). Intergenerational disadvantage: Why maternal mental health matters. *Koi Tū: Evidence Brief*, 1–12.

Marie, D., Fergusson, D. M., & Boden, J. M. (2009). Ethnic Identity and exposure to maltreatment in childhood: Evidence from a New Zealand Birth Cohort. *Social Policy Journal of New Zealand*, 36, 154–171.

McCown, D., Reibel, D., & Micozzi, M. S. (2011). *Teaching Mindfulness: A Practical Guide for Clinicians and Educators*. New York: Springer.

McEwen, B. (2017). Neurobiological and systemic effects of chronic stress. *Chronic Stress*, 1, 1–17.

Mead, H. (2003). *Tikanga Māori: Living by Māori values*. Wellington: Huia Publishers.

Mikaere, A. (2019). Colonisation and the imposition of patriarchy. In Mikaere, A. (Ed.), *Mana Wāhine Reader: A Collection of Writings 1999–2019*, Volume II (pp. 4–19). Waikato: Te Kotahi Research Institute.

Ministry for Culture and Heritage (2021). *Māori Land Loss, 1860–2000*. Wellington, accessed 4 April 2022, https://nzhistory.govt.nz/media/interactive/maori-land-1860-2000

Ministry of Health (2021). *Mortality Web Tool*. Wellington: New Zealand, accessed 4 April 2022, https://www.health.govt.nz/publication/mortality-web-tool

Ministry of Social Development (2016). *The Social Report 2016 – Te Pūrongo oranga tangata*. Wellington, accessed 4 April, 2022, https://socialreport.msd.govt.nz/health/life-expectancy-at-birth-html

Nicholas, J. L., & Marsden, S. (1817). *Narrative of a Voyage to New Zealand, Performed in the Years 1814 and 1815*. London: Black & Son.

Sheng, J. A., Bales, N. J., Myers, S. A., Bautista, A. I., Roue-infar, M., Hale, T. M., & Handa, R. J. (2021). The Hypothalamic-Adrenal-Axis: Development, Programming actions of hormones, and Maternal-Fetal Interactions. *Frontiers in Behavioural Neuroscience*, 14, 1–21.

Stats, N. Z. (2018). *Te Pā Harakeke: Māori Housing and wellbeing 2021.* Wellington, accessed 4 April 2022, https://www.stats.govt.nz/reports/te-pa-harakeke-maori-housing-and-wellbeing-2021

Pool, I. (2019). Death and life expectancy – Effects of colonisation on Māori, Te Ara – The Encyclopaedia of New Zealand. [Online]. Available at http://www.TeAra.govt.nz/en/death-rates-and-life-expectancy/page-4

Rossen, F., Newcombe, D., Parag, V., Underwood, L., Marsh, S., Berry, S., Grant, C., Morton, S., & Bullen, C. (2018). Alcohol consumption in New Zealand women before and during pregnancy: findings from the Growing up in New Zealand study. *The New Zealand Medical Journal*, 131(1479), 24–34.

Schrader, B. (2013). Māori Housing – te noho whare – Whare and health, Te ara – the Encyclopaedia of New Zealand. [Online]. Available at http://TeAra.nz/en/maori-housing-te-noho-whare/page-2

Signal, T. L., Paine, S. J., Sweeney, B., Muller, D., Priston, M., Lee, K., Huthwaite, M. (2017). The prevalence of symptoms of depression and anxiety, and the level of stress and worry in New Zealand Māori and non-Māori women in late pregnancy. *Australian and New Zealand Journal of Psychiatry*, 51(2), 168–176.

Stephens, M. A. C., & Wand, G. (2012). Stress and the HPA axis. *Alcohol Research*, 34(4), 468–483.

Vargas, J., Junco, M., Gomez, C., & Lajud, N. (2016). Early life stress increases metabolic risk, HPA axis reactivity and depressive-like behavior when combined with postweaning social isolation in rats. *PLoS One*, 11(9). [Online]. Available at doi: 10.1371/journal.pone.0162665. eCollection 2016.

Walsh, M., & Grey, C. (2019). The contribution of avoidable mortality to the life expectancy gap in Māori and Pacific populations in New Zealand – a decomposition analysis. *The New Zealand Medical Journal*, 132(1492), 46–60.

5

MINDFUL INQUIRY INTO LIFEWORLDS AND DEATHWORLDS

An unmarried mother and a gay father

Valerie Malhotra Bentz

The four cornerstones of Mindful Inquiry (Bentz and Shapiro 1998) are linked together. Jeremy Shapiro and I discovered the inherent congruence between Mindfulness and three powerful traditions in social sciences: phenomenology, critical theory and hermeneutics. There are two sides to phenomenology: Husserlian and Schützian. The first requires that we look at the existentials of direct experience: lived time, space, embodiment and emotions (van Manen 1997). The second, Schützian lifeworld phenomenology, asks us to unpack the way the experience exists in particular situations. All situations exist within a hermeneutic context which may vary, and which allows for alternative and multiple meanings. Likewise, all experiences exist within systems of power explicated within the framework of critical theory—economic, political and social. Buddhist philosophies of mindfulness require attention to all of these levels for the principles of compassion and the unfolding connection to the wonder of being (Figure 5.1).

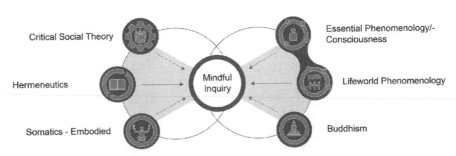

FIGURE 5.1 Relationships of aspects of mindful inquiry to the practice and each other.

Source: Original artwork by Anna Haefele.

DOI: 10.4324/9781003165200-5

The Buddhist way of being of compassion was for most of human history the norm:

> When we observe societies around the world outside of industrialized nations, especially those who have no established hierarchies, we notice an approach to moral development that is not top-down but one that is more bottom-up, emerging from ancient evolved practices of a life lived in companionship (Narvaez, 2014). These small-band hunter-gatherer societies (SBHG) are the kind of society in which our genus is presumed to have spent 99% of its history and, while under some stress, still exist all over the world (Lee and Daly 2005).
>
> *(Narvaez 2020, 2)*

What we have come to call *Deathworlds* (physical, social or psychological places where life is not supported or in some places can no longer survive) have been increasing on planet earth.

Along with this rather recent shift in human history, our birthing and child-rearing practices have led to the adoption of a worldview where individualism, greed and selfishness prevail (Four Arrows).[1] As Narvaez (2020) so aptly describes:

> Baselines have shifted (Narvaez, 2016a; Narvaez & Witherington, 2018). An accurate deep history view of *homo sapiens* shows us that we have wandered off the species-normal pathway of raising good, virtuous, connected human beings (Christen et al., 2017; Narvaez, 2013, 2014, 2015, 2016b, 2016c, 2018). Industrialized child raising practices break the continuum of bondedness to the living web, establishing a sense of disconnection deep within the child's psyche that lasts a lifetime without intervention. As a result, industrialized societies tend to raise humans poorly and then try to fix the dysregulated results with all sorts of sanctions and manipulations.
>
> *(2)*

Transformative Phenomenology (Rehorick and Bentz 2008, 2017) is a way of researching lived experience beginning with one's own. In keeping with the focus on the importance of examining one's own experience—research from within (Bentz 2018)—I will use examples from my own experiences of pregnancy and childbirth in the context of critical theory, phenomenology and hermeneutics (an overview of these practices is shown in Figure 5.2).

The deathworldly past of Milwaukee: a look at my pregnancy and birth experience through critical theory and phenomenology

I highlight here in brief form my lived experiences, combining critical theory, Husserlian phenomenology and Schützian Lifeworld phenomenology. The birth

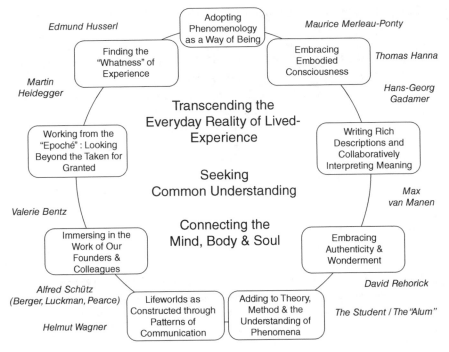

FIGURE 5.2 Ten qualities of transformative phenomenologists with influential philosophers and practitioners.

Source: Copyright (2020) by Valerie Bentz and James Marlatt, used with permission, original
artwork.

of my daughter was my second pregnancy, the first ending in a horrific, then-
illegal abortion. Both pregnancies were situations of fear, anxiety, social isolation
and being out of touch with my body.

Critical theory: the context

I was born and raised a fourth-generation German Lutheran in Milwaukee, Wis-
consin. I was barely aware that the land and the neighborhood I grew up in once
belonged to Indigenous groups, mostly the Potawatomi people. Their Algonquian
word for Milwaukee was *Millioke*, meaning "good and pleasant land." *Potawatomi*
means "keepers of the sacred fire" but the Potawatomi people call themselves
Neshnabek meaning "the true people." In the colonial wars between the French and
the English for Indigenous land, Potawatomi braves first fought with the French,
then later with the United States forces against the English. The United States won,
and by 1850, most of the Potawatomi, along with related peoples including the
Ojibwe (Chippewa) and the Minomenee, lost their land through a series of "treaties."

The Deathworld aspects of living as colonizers on top of the genocidal
wars against Indigenous peoples and taking their lands still echo and resonate
in our communities. Indigenous communities handled pregnancy, birth and

child-rearing in rich contexts of care (Narvaez 2020). In addition, the settlers, such as my great-grandparents, fled from desperate situations. Fortunately for me, there were strong remnants of maternalistic ways in my German family.

Around the time Indigenous groups became largely landless, my maternal great-grandmother, Mrs. Teich, became one of many German immigrants, who, fleeing oppression in Germany, settled in Milwaukee, which became the most German city in the nation. She was a founder of Bethlehem Lutheran church and school, where I was the fourth generation to attend. She lost her husband at a young age due to a work-related accident. At that time, there were no child labor laws, nor government aid to widows and families. My great-grandmother worked as a maid to raise her three daughters and started the first Lutheran Kinderheim home for orphans in her cottage on 26th street. My grandmother, Ida, had to leave school after the third grade to help earn money for the family as a washer girl.

Having already lost her father to an accident, Ida lost her husband, Emil Bentz, as a young man while he was working for the Milwaukee Rial. The effects of workplace hazards were not limited to my maternal line—my paternal grandfather, John Sajeck, lost his arm working in a factory. There was no worker's compensation. He was a mean and bitter man who mercilessly beat my father with a belt. My father had to quit high school to work in a factory to help support his mother and five siblings, although he later quit factory work and joined the police force.

I was born in Mt. Sinai hospital (Jewish based) in the midst of World War II. My father was dedicated and loving, although he was not demonstrative with hugging and having fun. My mother was a loving mother who breastfed me. She chose to remain bed-ridden for weeks prior to my birth instead of choosing abortion, though she was given the option as I was laying in her womb lopsided. My parents did not get along well, so the home was filled with discord and arguments. Ma would go into rages, and my older sister was as much a tormentor to me as a mentor. My place of peace and comfort was always at my grandmother Bentz' cottage on the next block.

The neighborhood was tight-knit and nurturing for me as a child, centering on Bethlehem Lutheran church and school with lots of activities and celebrations. Yet it was surrounded by trauma as the city adjusted to the migration of Black Americans to the North after the Civil War and immigrants from the European continent following the destruction of two world wars. Each culture established its own neighborhood. The industrial revolution also brought with it the pollution of the "good and pleasant land." The rivers leading to Lake Michigan were choked with industrial waste when I was growing up. The air was cloudy in winter partly from all the coal being burned in furnaces.

Echoes of Racism and Sexism: Rape, Abortion, Agony, Fear and the Birth of My Daughter

My older sister brought shock, shame and disgrace to our family by giving birth out of wedlock to a baby fathered by a Black friend from Harlem who she met while she was a graduate student at Columbia University. She said she had looked for an illegal abortionist but was too frightened to go through with it. The long-term outcomes of her unmindful birth of my nephew Chris and her emotional neglect of him as an infant still negatively affect his offspring. My own shame over this event in our family led me to become an activist on behalf of racial equality. I also had my own unwanted pregnancy, but that story concluded differently.

While home from college after my junior year, I was offered a ride home from a YMCA dance where I went with a high school friend by a charming immigrant from India, Raj. On a pretext, he asked that we stop at his apartment where he gave me a drink with a drug in it and raped me. I did not tell anyone about this and was in a state of panic and anxiety. The next morning, he came to the front door with flowers and gifts. My mixed emotions and feelings of guilt for what had happened led me to continue seeing him through the summer. He left for India and I found myself pregnant. My friend's mother knew a doctor who gave abortions. I had an excruciatingly painful abortion without anesthesia.

Second pregnancy

I went back to college, graduated and Raj returned from India, continuing to court me with poems and love letters. After graduation, I returned to Milwaukee and became pregnant for the second time. My love and attachment to Raj was born as much of guilt and shame as it was a feeling of intense unreality. My emotional state was undergirded by fear and anxiety, and I was out of touch with my body.

The lifeworld/deathworld of the unmarried mother

Alfred Schütz' lifework centers on providing a framework for us to understand how Lifeworlds are experienced and understood from within in everyday life. The situation of being an unwed mother carries a history of "stocks of knowledge," "typifications" and "relevances" (Schütz 1970).

There are Deathworldly aspects within Lifeworlds that mitigate against peaceful and hopeful experiences. In the absence of a community of care, the emotional climate of a pregnancy and birth can be filled with fear, anxiety and shame (Bentz 1989; Hamington 2004).

At the beginning of my second pregnancy, I was working at the Milwaukee County Department of Public Welfare (DPW) as a foster home licenser. In the same office, there was an Unmarried Mother (UM) unit. The workers would happily return from a day visiting pregnant or new mothers bragging about how many Termination of Parental Rights (TPRs) they had gotten that day. At that time, I knew that we were short of foster homes for newborns, some of whom were staying in the hospital for up to six months before they could be placed in foster homes! Yet the prospective and current mothers were shown a movie where the baby was given away to eager parents in a lovely home. When I started to show, I knew I could not continue employment at Milwaukee DPW. I found it ironic that I was about to be one of those typified by my co-workers as a UM and in need of counseling to *do the right thing* and terminate parental rights.

Early in my pregnancy, I had a mindful moment. My decision not to seek an abortion was made in consultation with a good high school friend, Dorothy Schmidt. We were at Lake Michigan beach that summer when I must have been two to three months pregnant. I realized that I had a strong love for the little one inside me and that regardless of the challenges, I would become a mother. My older sister invited me to come to Ottawa, where her husband was teaching, and have the baby there.

The treatment I received at Ottawa Civic Hospital where I gave birth was horrendous. I went early in the morning in active and excruciatingly painful labor because I had lost my water. I was put in a separate section of the ward reserved for unmarried mothers. A UM tag was put at the top of the bedstand. As I screamed in pain, nurses scolded me to shut up as I was disturbing others. Finally, a doctor came and held my legs together giving me a spinal shot for pain. After a seemingly long while another doctor came and did a forceps delivery. I was not schooled in nursing and was told that most mothers were giving their babies formula, so that is what I did.

Stocks of knowledge

The stocks of knowledge in the everyday lifeworld of a young woman of Lutheran heritage in Milwaukee becoming pregnant out of wedlock were devastatingly powerful and Deathworldly. Enormous pressure and shame were put on the women and their families in these situations. Ann Alexander (unpublished protocols, January 11–April 25, 2021) used Schüztian concepts to elucidate her experience of facing the shame and typifications of being an unmarried mother in the 1960s. She was given no alternative but to relinquish her baby. However, decades later, her son found her and she became a "birth mother," a much more positive, lifeworldly designation.

Hermeneutics of mindful pregnancy and childbirth

A hermeneutic approach to birth is a calling to mindful pregnancy and birth. Theodore Droysen's four levels of hermeneutics is a powerful approach with which to begin. These levels are described as the pragmatic level, the psychological level, the social and cultural level, and the moral and ethical level (Bentz 2010).

The pragmatic level involves whether the conditions of the pregnancy and the lifeworld of the mother and infant in community are conducive to providing care and nurturance which will allow for the child to develop a kind and ethical nature and moral imagination (Bentz 1989; Narvaez 2014). It explores whether there will be resources available for providing for the baby and child's well-being in harmony with the larger lifeworld, including nature.

The psychological motivations similarly should be free of ego attachment. The desire to have a child to fulfill an empty inner self, or to continue one's own individual genes and eggs, or for a woman to snag a man or obtain a welfare check, would be ruled out of a mindful pregnancy. Mental illness and undue stress would preclude getting pregnant. Similarly, a family or culture that puts pressure on women to bear children so that they could be grandparents or produce more Mormons or Catholics or Muslims would be a faulty egoic reason. Only love would be a proper psychological motivation at any level.

Social and cultural motivations would have to take into account conditions. Times of war, upheaval, poverty, and drug and addiction-infused environments should discourage pregnancies. In a high degree of prescience, anthropologist Margaret Mead argued that just as there are marriage licenses, there should be parent licenses. The criteria would include both parents being able to show means of support to provide for the child in case of divorce or death of one of the parents. Mindfulness training would be an excellent added criterion.

The ethical and moral level requires conditions in which the social and physical environment would foster a neurobiology conducive to positive moral development. The four levels also apply to who should be involved in making the decisions about whether a pregnancy and birth are to occur: the potential parents? Family? Tribe? Community? Nation? Global Society? At the present state of world climate crises, all levels have a stake in every pregnancy and every birth.

Gadamer's three levels of hermeneutics

Gadamer's three levels of hermeneutics could also be fruitfully and insightfully applied to pregnancy and childbirth. In his first level, one would assess the overall situation in which the pregnancy and birth would occur. At the second level, one would examine it more particularly and personally. Thirdly, one would closely relate to it in the most immediate situation (Bentz and Rehorick 2008).

Heidegger's hermeneutic ontology and pregnancy and birth

Heidegger's (2001, 2013) ontology should particularly be applied and reversed in order to promote Lifeworlds over Deathworlds. Heidegger rightly asserted that humans can only be authentic when they acknowledge their morality fully. This hermeneutic ontology should be pushed forward into an analysis of human societies to take responsibility for providing mindful pregnancies and births.

Take, for instance, Heidegger's (2001, 2013) wonderful image of the seeker of truth going on a forest path into a clearing and there waiting where perhaps the gods may arrive. The gods in his image would be the light of insight. This clearing would be a space for a prospective mother to be, such as Mary was in the story of the annunciation of her pregnancy with Jesus, or my own as I was on the beach with a friend knowing that my pregnancy with Pam was a gift from the gods. Similarly, William Hart had such an inspired feeling about his adopted son, upon first seeing him in an incubator. (See next section.)

Buddhism and mindful pregnancy and birth

Since Buddhism is the source of the concept of mindfulness, it is a powerful way to look at pregnancy and birth. Compassion for all beings is a basic principle of Buddhism (Pei 2018). We should be aware of the suffering of beings and seek to end the suffering. Suffering begins with attachment and the very attachment to a sense of needing or having to give birth is one such example. With any attachment comes others that fall in their wake.

Buddhism would ask us to be aware of addictions as they may affect our decisions. More obviously, persons who have addictions to drugs, alcohol, sex, power, money or gambling should by no means get pregnant. Whole communities pay the price for births occurring under these mindless conditions, and the costs in pain and suffering to the infants themselves are well recognized.

The pregnant father: the experiences of William Hart, a gay man

Can a man experience being pregnant? Scholar and phenomenologist David Rehorick's account of his day-to-day sharing of bodily experiences of his wife's pregnancy would attest to this as very possible (Rehorick and Nugent 2008). He recounts symptoms of sympathetic pregnancy (couvade syndrome), such as swelling, backaches and headaches, and describes his lived experience of these events as he explored their origin. Men's experiences of fatherhood are not limited to couvade symptoms.

As I was contemplating writing this chapter, I was teaching a course called Writing Phenomenology where doctoral students write about a meaningful experience of their choice using Husserlian essential and Schützian lifeworld phenomenological techniques. William Hart chose to write about the experiences of becoming and being a father as a gay man. With Will's permission, I below quote some of his protocols which he wrote and shared over a period of several months.

William did not experience a nurturing mother or father as a child. His biological mother was incarcerated. He was raised by his father and a rejecting stepmother who favored her two biological sons. He and his older brother were sent to stay with his aunt (who happily was loving and nurturing to him) while his father went on vacation with his wife and two younger sons. Upon returning, his father interrupted a game of house William was playing with his cousin, and in his desire to avoid his father's criticism, William discarded a much-cherished doll, Riley. It was the process of reflecting on this experience that revealed to William the importance to him of fatherhood as a personal goal:

In a sad attempt to be accepted by my father, I tossed the doll into a toybox that was in the living room and said something about only playing because my cousin wanted to play. My aunt knew I was hurt and said something in defense of me to my father, but I don't recall what it was exactly. I do recall a sickening feeling as I saw Riley laying on a heap of toys, her glasses sitting crooked on her face. On our way back to my father's house, while he and my brother talked in the front seats, I couldn't stop thinking about Riley. How could I have abandoned her like that? Thrown her away like my mother had thrown away the opportunity to be with us instead of in prison. Pushed her aside like my father had done to us? Was I more like my father than I cared to admit because I let someone convince me to neglect something I loved and "just leave it at my Aunt's house?" Like most kids, I finally moved on and started thinking about something else but not before I promised myself that I would not be a father like the one I have. It wasn't a question of if I would be a father, but that I would be a great father that my kids could count on. I would have kids one day and I would love hard and hold them each day and tell them each day that they are perfect, and beautiful, and smart. I would make sure I could take care of them financially and find someone who shared the same passion for kids that I did. My kids would get to experience what this world has to offer, and our home would be the place where they felt loved and could breathe. That was the day that being a father became the foundation for how I would move through the stages of my life in order to reach the goal stage of fatherhood.

(William Hart, 2021)

Will came out as gay at age 16. He wrote about choosing his marriage partner with an eye to how they could become good parents together. He mindfully geared his life toward healthy eating, recreation and fitness. He and his partner moved to a community with outdoor activities, good schools, and other resources for parents and children. He describes his transcendence to fatherhood as a progression through various phases of life, at first distant from fatherhood, and finally in the center of it:

As an adult, even before I started the process of adoption, I took steps that I thought would help me become a parent. After I completed my undergraduate degree, I began working for Home Depot's corporate office because they have an amazing onsite childcare center. I made decisions that met my immediate needs, but also would set me up to be able to be a father, even though there was no plan to start a family at that time.

In order to discuss my transcendence to fatherhood, I will be using Michael Mamas model of The Three Realms of Existence. In his work he describes three "interconnected realms: The Physical, the Psychoenergetic, and the Transcendental (Mamas, 2005) and Merleau-Ponty's embodied consciousness.

The Physical realm makes up the physical structures of our bodies and also deeper levels including "cellular structure, molecules, and atoms" (Mamas, 2005). As I began the transcendence, I was unaware of the changes that were happening within my physical realm. I knew I wanted to be an active father so I physically changed by working out, engaging in more physical activities (I get to tell my kid that I went skydiving), and even physically changed my environment by moving into a home that was in a great school district and provided the space necessary to raise a family. I also changed my diet because I wanted to be able to instill healthy eating habits into my child. While most of these were decisions that I made to better myself, unconsciously I knew that I wanted to be a very specific type of father even though these decisions were made years before I actually became a father.

Deeper, my Psychoenergetic realm which "includes our thoughts, psychology, and emotions" (Mamas, 2005) was also changing. I expanded my knowledge of different methods to becoming a father and learned as much as I could about "non-traditional" families. I focused my emotional maturity on being able to show love, empathy, gratitude, and to understand the importance of patience and understanding. I thought of myself as a future father and therefore made decisions that aligned with what I wanted that role to look like for me. I prepared myself to be a present parent who could handle the emotional and psychological needs of a child. I think I was more attracted to men that I thought would be great parents. Potential fathers who complimented my strengths and excelled at the things I was weak in.

Finally, within the Transcendental Realm which Mamas describes as the level in which we "merge with the oneness of all things, while simultaneously maintaining our individuality" (2005). After meeting the man that I absolutely knew I wanted to build a family with and taking the conscious steps to prepare for adoption, we got the call. It was late in the evening on an October night when we first met our son. He was in the surgical NICU at a hospital not far from our home and was only a few weeks old, but his birth mother had already made the decision to give him a better chance with a different family. Born at 28 weeks and weighing in at 2lb 8oz, we didn't know exactly what to expect when we got to the hospital. We must have parked as far from the surgical NICU as possible because it felt like we had to clear many security checkpoints. At each checkpoint, we thought that this would be the one where the information wasn't correct, and we wouldn't get to see him. But we cleared each one. Every step I took, I knew was bringing me one step closer to this little guy I had been planning my whole life to take care of.

Finally, we got to the double doors that lead to the Surgical NICU where he was waiting. When the doors opened a nurse was waiting for us. I remember her saying, "You must be the fathers." We washed our hands and looked around the dark room and immediately spotted our son's space.

We knew it was his because there was an incubator and nothing else. No decorations or stuffed animals, just machines beeping around him, tubes going into the glass box that was keeping him safe and alive, and a generic "John Doe" type name listed on the whiteboard. Even though there was nothing legally final when we walked up to the incubator, the minute I saw him I knew he was meant to be mine. Tiny but beautiful and exactly what I had imagined my son would look like. Stronger than anyone I know and in this tiny, dark corner of the hospital, he lit up the room. In that moment, I felt how connected I was with everything around me. How all these little things had to take place for me to be sharing a space with someone I loved in the second that I found out about him. I felt a oneness that I can't really explain but I have often referred to it as my parental instincts kicking in. I could physically and mentally feel a change in me. I looked different. I knew that I would do anything to protect this child and that I needed to hold him and be near him as much as he needed to be held in order to regulate his body temperature, breathing, etc.

Cook-Greuter writes that the post conventional and transcendent tiers of development start "to question the unconsciously held beliefs, norms, and assumptions about reality" (2000). I questioned what it meant to be a father. Was I a father now because it was stated, because there was a baby that I was responsible for, or was it something deeper? Was it a connection with another life-form isolated from any biological or physical connection? I wondered if the connection may feel different if he was my biological son but at the same time understood that this experience and connection was for us. It may have felt different for others, but this was the connection that we had, and it was strong and perfect. There was a calmness and understanding that I can't describe but I knew that I was aligned with the universe and that any energy I had used on things that now seemed trivial would go into taking care of my son. I knew I wanted the world to be a better place and that just by being in it, he had already done his part to make it so. I felt that I was now who I had transcended to be for several years. I was someone's dad and not just anyone, but this baby who needed to hear that he is wanted, how brave and strong he was to get through his first surgery just 4 hours after he was born, and how he had changed my world and my connection with it, just by sharing the space I was in. There were a million things that could have happened that would have changed both our trajectories, but this union was also a union with the environments and spaces that we occupied. Mamas refers to this understanding of true consciousness as the "Unified Field" (2005).

According to Merleau-Ponty, there is no hard separation between bodily conduct and intelligent conduct. In habits, the body adapts to the intended meaning, thus giving itself a form of embodied consciousness (Merleau-Ponty, 1964). My body physically adapted to my new role as a father. As a pretty modest adult, I didn't think twice about sitting shirtless in this hospital room so that I could provide skin to skin contact to help my son. My body and consciousness were aligned that my role was to take care of this baby any way that I could. Interestingly enough, when my second son was born, the experience was quite different as he was born via surrogacy and is the biological son of my husband. His birth was planned, and we were a part of it from the very first moment. Our surrogate lived in Orlando and we had to rush to get there because our son was born about 35 minutes after we arrived, I felt amazement when I saw him that he was biologically linked to my husband, I felt gratefulness to the staff and of course to the surrogate for carrying our son while he grew, but I didn't feel the transcendence into fatherhood again. There was a calmness. I remember that after the baby was born, they let my husband cut the umbilical cord and then a nurse said, "Let's give him to 'mama' so she can see him and hold him." This could have easily upset the surrogate, my husband, or myself because she wasn't his mother. Biologically, his mother is a woman living in a completely different part of the US. For the amount of money we had spent and the amount of time we put into making sure everyone was aware of what was going on, a mistake like this could have easily been avoided. But we didn't care. We had made it in time to meet our son, he was in this world and healthy. We knew we were the fathers and this nurse who probably said something out of habit was just another being on a path of her own that was now interwoven with ours. We were not concerned and actually only heard it when we watched the video of the birth several days later. I will say that calmness quickly went away when the hospital produced a birth certificate with the surrogate's name on it which could have been a huge legal headache for us and did keep us in Orlando for a few extra days. As a parent, that document stated that our child belonged to someone that he didn't and as his parents, we immediately went into defense mode in order to fix an error that should never happen.

But the transcendence I felt with my first son had already happened. I was a father when my second son was born and while I felt many different emotions, especially the love at first sight feeling, I was already aware of the connectedness of the systems that led us to that delivery room on the other side of the country with our families patiently waiting to find out the sex of our newest child and that the baby was here and okay. The calmness that I had felt in that NICU 4 years earlier was still a part of who I was but had settled into a part of me that now felt comfortable. My awareness of each step we took to get from Phoenix to Orlando and how it closed the proximity of us, and our baby was something that I experienced from the moment we got the call that she was headed to the hospital.

The calmness and reflection I felt the day we walked into the surgical NICU and met our oldest son cannot be equated to another event in my life, thus far.

(William Hart, unpublished protocols, January 11–April 25, 2021)

William Hart's Schützian lifeworld protocols

Schütz puppets from transcending to fatherhood

In a conversation with my husband, we discussed our experiences of transcending to fatherhood. While we experienced it together as co-parents of our children, what we found was that our experiences had similarities that could be defined as typifications. There were various typifications shared by us including active fathers, prepared fathers, nurturers and learners. We also referred to ourselves as family guys, non-traditional family creators and individuals forging a new path within a heteronormative unit. The categories below typify the typifications that we had of ourselves. Schütz puppets, or *homunculae*, are developed to identify an essential reference schema of the phenomenological experience. Below are three of these essential references that get at the root of our experiences (William Hart, 2021).

Guardians of our environment

One of the main aspects of our transition to fatherhood was to create an environment where our children could be nourished, feel safe and understand love. Our home was critical to provide a space that would sustain our family unit and was central to our ability to not only pass the necessary home studies required for adoption, but to be a space that worked for us where we could provide opportunities for our kids but also have access to space that helped us be the best fathers possible. By being protective of our home and filling it with items that were safe, useful and aesthetically pleasing, we were ensuring that our space could work for us in the present and future. We are protective of our home and created a space that allowed us to parent the way that we wanted to. We chose a home in a neighborhood with ample green space, parks and that the home itself offered indoor and outdoor spaces that we could use to actively engage with our kids. We chose a one-story house because we didn't want the separation of levels to create distance and we chose several advanced security features in order to protect our family and the space that we wanted our family to feel safe in. This essential reference encompasses everything that took place prior to starting the process of becoming eligible adoptive parents (William Hart, 2021).

Pioneers of fatherhood

While gay parenting is not a new concept and we are by no means pioneers as LGBTQ fathers, we both identified a lifeworld with beliefs that we would be the first gay parents that a lot of people would encounter. This schema is based on the message of scarcity of active gay parents and came from stocks of knowledge that emerged during our experience of beginning the adoption process where we heard a lot of times that we were the first "gay couple" that a person had worked with. So, we both felt a pressure to be ideal candidates as to forge the path for other gay men and women who were interested in parenting. This is also referred to as "the best little boy in the world" phenomenon.

The second schema that we wanted to demonstrate through being fathers was one in which there is an acknowledgment of plenty of other families like us and the need for structures to successfully embrace LGBTQ parents. This schema is in alignment with studies on the massive number of children currently seeking homes in the United States. While the first schema reflects a limited number of LGBTQ parents seeking adoption, the second schema shows an abundance of children looking for families. Creating a shift from a limited number of LGBTQ parents applying for adoption starts with acknowledging the system creates disconnect and a feeling of otherness that could be stopping potential families before they make it to the formal adoption process. This essential reference encompasses the period of time between starting and completing the process of being eligible to adopt (William Hart, unpublished protocols, January 11–April 25, 2021).

Hopeful fathers

The third Schütz puppet that I identified from our conversations is the paradox of the hopeful father. This typification represents the irony that adoptive parents face, in that we had to go through a thorough process to become eligible to be parents and get ready to take care of a child, while the birth parents have the opportunity to show up at any time until the adoption is finalized and do minimal work to be reunited with a child that we love. Though processes exist that can expedite the process of termination of parental rights, a lot of them rely on the birthparent and any sign of possible reunification is shown preferential treatment. This showcases how adoptive parents are stretching themselves to meet the demands of adoption agencies while witnessing the preferential treatment of birth parents, even when it is not in the best interest of the child. While we loved Deacon from the moment we saw him, it would be almost a full year before his adoption was completed and we could exhale with the knowledge that we would not receive a phone call at any moment that the birthmother had decided she wanted to parent our child. This essential reference encompasses the period of time between Deacon being matched with us and the finalization of our adoption in August of 2015, 11 months after Deacon was born and we were matched with him.

As a researcher interviewing my husband on his experience transcending to fatherhood, I experienced amazement in learning about how similar and different our experiences were. I noticed during our conversations the waves of emotion that mirrored his from frustration to excitement, hope and a sense of completion. It was a powerful experience to have this conversation with him and placing ourselves back in the memories of our process helped us appreciate that we had the strength of each other to get through it and that, in the end, we got the most precious gift out of it. While we sometimes reflect on the experience and are in amazement that we were able to get through everything, it never felt like we were on the wrong path, just that we were on the right path that would lead us to Deacon and that we would do everything possible to meet a child that didn't even exist when we started the process. Yet, somehow, we knew him and loved him from the first day that we walked into the adoption office to sign up for classes to become eligible to adopt (William Hart, 2021).

Summary and conclusions

This chapter has discussed mindful pregnancy, childbirth and mother/fathering from two perspectives. One, Bentz, experienced becoming an unmarried mother and therefore a social pariah in a situation of shame and pain, overall not mindful. Nevertheless, I mindfully chose to give birth based on a deep feeling of transcendent love for my daughter while in my womb. I examined my experience based on the cornerstones of mindful inquiry: phenomenology, hermeneutics, critical theory and Buddhism. By contrast, William Hart's phenomenologically based descriptions of his becoming a father as a gay man were deeply mindful. His experience of transcendent love for his adopted sons was like mine, a deep feeling of meaningful purpose. Yet similar to me, he has had to exist in a social situation that overall is still not fully accepting of gay parenting.

The Deathworldly background for my birth experience is traceable to the genocidal removal of the Indigenous people from where I grew up, as well as the situations of oppression and poverty from which my German ancestors fled to Milwaukee. These presuppositions of the Dominant World view of individualistic competition with little support for parents from a caring community similarly affect the context in which William Hart as a married gay man faces. The work to restore our connections to each other, and other lifeforms of Narvaez and Four Arrows is crucial to restoring an overall mindful approach to pregnancy, birth and mother/fathering. A restoration of caring communities and relationships is vital for us all.

Note

1 See Appendix A, Table A1.

Bibliography

Bentz, Valerie. 1989. *Becoming Mature, Childhood Ghosts and Spirits in Adult Life.* New York: Aldine de Gruyter.
Bentz, Valerie 2003. The Body's Memory, The Body's Wisdom. in Itkomen, Matti and Buckhaus, Gary (eds) 158–185, Lived Images: Mediations in Experience, Liwords and I-hood. Jyvaskyla, Finland, University of Jyvaskyla Press

Bentz, Valerie. 2010. "Hermeneutics and Somatics Presentation." Posted July 19, 2010. https://valeriebentz.com/article/hermeneutics-somatics_07-19-2010/.

Bentz, Valerie. 2018. "Knowing as Being: Somatic Phenomenology as Contemplative Practice." In *Contemplative Social Research: Caring for Self, Being, and Lifeworld*, edited by Valerie Bentz and Vincenzo Giorgino, 50–79. Santa Barbara: Fielding University Press.

Bentz, Valerie, and Krzysztof Konecki. 2021. "Are Strangers More Likely to See Deathworlds in Lifeworlds?" Paper presented at *Schütz Circle Virtual Conference, Online*, June 5, 2021.

Bentz, Valerie and Jim Marlatt. 2021. Deathworlds to Lifeworlds: Collaboration with Strangers for Personal, Social, and Ecological Transformation. Berlin: De Gruyter.

Bentz, Valerie, Jim Marlatt and Carol Estrada. 2021. *Transformative Phenomenology: A Handbook*. Santa Barbara: Fielding University Press.

Bentz, Valerie and David Rehorick. 2008. "Transformative Phenomenology: A Scholarly scaffold for practitioners." In *Transformative Phenomenology*, edited by David Rehorick and Valerie Bentz, 3–32. New York: Lexington Press.

Bentz, Valerie, David Rehorick, James Marlatt, Ayumi Nishii, and Carol Estrada. 2018. "Transformative Phenomenology as an Antidote to Technological Deathworlds." *Schützian Research* 10: 189–220. https://doi.org/10.5840/schutz20181011.

Bentz, Valerie, and Jeremy Shapiro. 1998. *Mindful Inquiry in Social Research*. Thousand Oaks: Sage.

Cook-Greuter, Susanne. 2000. "Mature Ego Development: A Gateway to Ego Transcedence?" *Journal of Adult Development* 7, no. 4: 227–40. https://doi.org/10.1023/A:1009511411421

Four Arrows (Jacobs, Don). 2020. *The Red Road*. Charlotte: Information Age Publishing.

Hamington, Maurice. 2004. *Embodied Care: Jane Addams, Maurice Merleau-Ponty, and Feminist Ethics*. Urbana: University of Illinois Press.

Hart, William 2021. Unpublished protocols. Fielding Graduate University.

Heidegger, Martin, Zollikon Seminars: Protocols - Conversations-Letters, ed. Medard Boss, Evanston Ill. Northwestern University Press.

Mamas, Michael. 2005. "The Three Realms of Existence – A Model That Can Change Your Life." Accessed on June 13, 2020. http://www.rationalspirituality.org/michael-mamas-wisdom/articles/three-realms/.

Merleau-Ponty, Maurice. 1964. *Signs*. Translated by Richard McCleary. Evanston: Northwestern University Press.

Narvaez, Darcia. 2014. *Neurobiology and the Development of Human Morality: Evolution, Culture and Wisdom*. New York: Norton.

Narvaez, Darcia. 2020. "Moral Education in a Time of Human Ecological Devastation." *Journal of Moral Education* 50, no. 1: 55–67. https://doi.org/10.1080/03057240.2020.1781067

Pei, Marissa. 2018. *Eight Ways to Happiness: From Wherever You Are*. New York: Morgan James.

Rehorick, David and Linda Nugent. 2008. "Male Experiences of Pregnancy: Bridging Phenomenological and Empirical Insights." In *Transformative Phenomenology*, edited by David Rehorick and Valerie Bentz, 33–50. New York: Lexington Press.

Rehorick, David and Valerie Malhotra Bentz. 2017. "The Emergence of Transformative Phenomenology: Two Decades of Teaching and Learning at Fielding." In *Expressions of Phenomenological Research: Consciousness and Lifeworld Studies*, edited by David Rehorick and Valerie Malhotra Bentz, 18–44. Santa Barbara, CA: Fielding University Press.

Schütz, Alfred. 1970. *Alfred Schütz on Phenomenology and Social Relations*. Edited by Helmut Wagner. Chicago: University of Chicago Press.

van Manen, Max. 1997. *Researching Lived Experience*. Walnut Creek: Left Coast Press.

Appendix A

TABLE A1 Characteristics of Indigenous versus Dominant Worldview

Common Dominant Worldview Manifestations	*Common Indigenous Worldview Manifestations*
Living without a strong social purpose	Socially purposeful life
Primarily selfish goals for personal gain	Emphasis on generosity and future
Lacking empathy	generations
Disregarding holistic interconnectedness	Empathetic
Minimal contact with others	Continually honoring holistic
Blindness to hegemony	interconnectedness
Mainstream acceptance of injustice	High interpersonal engagement, touching
Fighting is the highest expression of	Hegemonic awareness and resistance to it
courage	Collective and organized resistance to
Learning as didactic	injustice
Dishonesty and deception are acceptable	Generosity is the highest expression of
Humor as entertainment	courage
Conflict mitigated via revenge and	Learning as experiential and collaborative
punishment	Dishonesty and deception are unacceptable
Learning is broadly contextualized	Humor as essential tool for coping
Self-knowledge less important	Conflict resolution as a return to
Individualism not connected to group	community
	Place-based learning and responsibility are
	key
	Self-knowledge is the most important
	Autonomy connected to group

Source: Adapted from Four Arrows (2020).
Learn to stay feeling relationally connected to others rather than detached, superior or inferior
Establish practices that keep ecological attachment alive (e.g., walking in parks without headset,
acknowledging other than humans as living companions; Kurth et al. 2020)
Learn to attend to consequences, short and long term, of personal and group decisions, always with
the web of life

6

FERTILITY AND MINDFULNESS

Janetti Marotta

More than 80 million people globally are affected by infertility. According to the Centers for Disease Control and Prevention (CDC) about 12% or 1 out of 8 women aged 15–44 in the United States have difficulty getting pregnant or carrying a pregnancy to term, regardless of marital status. According to a 2012 United Nations report, childless rates were found to be as high as 23% in Singapore and 19% in the United States with Austria, the United Kingdom, Finland, Bahrain, and Canada falling between the two.

Since the first successful in vitro fertilization (IVF) in 1978, by 2016 some 6.5 million babies have been born using IVF. Despite the plethora of modern advancements in fertility treatment, availability is dependent on where you live and financial considerations. Moreover, fertility treatment is not without emotional costs. Countless studies have found depression and anxiety to be highly prevalent among those dealing with infertility (Golombok 1992; Matsubayashi et al. 2001) and among those seeking treatment (Beutel et al. 1999).

As a clinical psychologist who has personally experienced infertility and specialized in this area since 1990, I have found mindfulness to be the perfect antidote to work with the overwhelming challenges of infertility. Unlike many other challenges we face in life, making more effort doesn't necessarily lead to success with infertility, and attempts to gain control over a situation inherently outside control, only amplifies a sense of insecurity and inadequacy. In the process, the qualities most needed to rise to the challenge dampen, i.e., patience, acceptance, and non-striving. Mindfulness offers a way through this paradox because it meets the present moment as it is, whether pleasant or unpleasant, without clinging to it or pushing it away.

Stemming from my infertility experience, I became a long-time practitioner of meditation and mindfulness and authored a book that applies the teachings and practices of mindfulness to the array of hardships infertility presents. In this

DOI: 10.4324/9781003165200-6

chapter, entitled *Mindfulness and Infertility*, highlights from my book, *A Fertile Path: Guiding the Journey with Mindfulness and Compassion*, are presented. Following the Introduction, this chapter includes the following:

- Research on Infertility and the Efficacy of Psychosocial Interventions
- Research on Mindfulness and the Efficacy of a Mindfulness-Based Approach
- The Benefits of Mindfulness for Infertility
- The Paradox of Infertility
- The Paradox of Mindfulness
- The Antidote of Mindfulness
- The Application of Mindfulness Principles and Practices

My story

My infertility history began in 1988, the year my husband, Steve, and I were married. After six years of repeated miscarriage, IVF, several IVF cycles with donor eggs (Donor IVF), and adoption, it was through traditional surrogacy, in which our surrogate's own eggs were fertilized through IUI with sperm from my husband, that we were blessed with our daughter, Cheyenne.

During this long-term struggle, my sense of self dwindled at the core. Infertility became a personal crisis because every area of life was impacted and my normal coping mechanism of control—trying harder to succeed—didn't work. I tried countless means available to treat my physical, emotional, and spiritual well-being. I engaged in individual, couples, and family therapy. I tried acupuncture, a prescribed acupuncture "exorcism," and medicinal teas. I went on several Vision Quests,[1] or Rites of Passage inspired by the spiritual practice among Native American Indians that uses wilderness to seek vision. Eventually, I became a Vision Quest guide and attended a Buddhist zendo.

Lastly, I immersed myself on an East/West spiritual path that led me on a pilgrimage to India. I became able to release my guilt, more fully grieve for our lost babies, and believe if I stayed opened to possibility, I would have a child. It was not about finding my way *out* of infertility but *through* infertility. It was by staying on the path—engaging in the process, not fixating on the goal. It is said we only change when we have more to lose than by not changing. It was at this juncture, that I put my own recovery above everything else. Crisis became opportunity as I grew in ways otherwise beyond my reach. Through awareness and the cultivation of mindfulness-roused qualities, I became able to *let things be*. With each emotional ebb and flow, each contraction and expansion, my ability to stay open and accepting became my own birthing experience.

Research on infertility and the efficacy of psychosocial interventions

The life crisis of infertility has been found to be so stressful that levels of depression and anxiety for women with the diagnosis of infertility are equal to patients with the diagnoses of cancer, HIV, and heart disease (Domar, Zuttermeister, and Friedman 1993). In a study that interviewed women before their first fertility clinic visit, 40.2% met criteria for a psychiatric disorder, as compared with an average occurrence of 3% (Chen et al. 2004). A 2014 review concluded that the prevalence of psychiatric problems among infertile couples is estimated to be 25% to 60%, with depression and anxiety being significantly higher in infertile couples than in fertile controls and the general population (De Berardis et al. 2014). In another study, infertility is reported to be the most stressful experience in many women's lives (Freeman et al. 1985).

While a successful IVF has enabled couples to have children without being otherwise able, there is not only a financial price but an emotional price as well. A review of the literature (Eugster and Vingerhoets 1999) determines that without question, IVF is physically and emotionally stressful for both women and partners, with anxiety and depression as the most common reactions to treatment. Studies report a 23% to 65% IVF clinic dropout rate, thus on average 50% of patients terminate treatment in a typical IVF clinic.

Research indicates the primary cause of fertility treatment dropout is not finances, diagnosis, or prognosis, but stress (Domar 2004). A review of the literature on patients dropping out of treatment concludes that psychological issues (most commonly treatment postponement, relational and personal factors, and psychological burden) are the greatest factors (Gameiro, Boivin, and Verhaak 2012). Women were found to be more depressed and anxious before beginning treatment, end treatment after a single IVF cycle (Smeenk, Verhaak, Stolwijk et al. 2004) and the most distressed patients do not seek psychological support at all (Boivin, Scanlan, and Walker 1999).

Substantial research demonstrates that psychosocial interventions to reduce the anxiety and depression related to infertility and its treatment are effective (Verhaak et al. 2007). The relationship between psychological interventions on pregnancy rate is also a subject of investigation. In an epidemiological study, women's high stress was determined to reduce the likelihood of conceiving by 40% (Akhter et al. 2016). A meta-analysis of 39 qualified studies found not only decreased symptoms of psychological distress for the intervention groups, but also that women in the intervention groups were twice as likely to become pregnant than those in the control groups (Frederiksen et al. 2015).

However, in another meta-analysis (Verkuijlen, Verhaak, Nelen et al. 2016), a substantial number of studies were eliminated from review because they lacked sufficient quality. Though psychological interventions were found to be associated with less psychological distress and higher pregnancy rates, only seven remained out of an initial 39. While the relationship between the effectiveness of psychological interventions on pregnancy rate may lead to significantly higher pregnancy rates, it is still somewhat debatable (Rooney and Domar 2018).

A series of articles introduced the importance of a more comprehensive model of mental health integration into infertility practice (Schlaff and Braverman 2015). In one article a collaborative model is strongly advised as symptoms of anxiety and/or depression are stressful for the patient and challenging for staff;

distressed patients are more likely to drop out of treatment; and psychological distress may be correlated with lower pregnancy rates (Domar 2015). An article by Boivin and Gameiro (2015) reinforces how an integrated approach could reduce treatment burden stemming from several sources, i.e., patient, clinic, and treatment.

Research on mindfulness and the efficacy of a mindfulness-based approach

The practice of mindfulness dates back more than 2,500 years ago to the time of Buddha and has now found its way into mainstream medicine. Mindfulness-Based Stress Reduction (MBSR) an eight-week program established by Jon Kabat-Zinn in 1989, has an established track record for treating chronic pain, numerous medical conditions, and a range of stress-related disorders. MBSR has been instrumental in spurring the extensive amount of research on mindfulness as a form of clinical intervention.

MBSR has also been influential in the development of other mindfulness-based programs including Mindfulness-Based Cognitive Therapy (MBCT), Dialectical Behavior Therapy (DBT), and Acceptance and Commitment Therapy (ACT) and as well the advancement of mindfulness to address specific populations, such as Mindfulness-Based Relapse Prevention (MBRP), Mindfulness-Based Therapy for Insomnia (MBT-I), and Mindfulness-Based Childbirth and Parenting (MBCP).

Mindfulness-based interventions have been determined to be effective for coping with emotional distress and a wide scope of medical and psychiatric conditions (Baer 2003; Davis and Hayes 2011; Hofmann, Sawyer, Witt, and Oh 2010; Teasdale, Segal, Williams, et al. 2000). In a review of empirical studies on the effects of mindfulness on psychological health (Keng, Smoski, and Robins 2011), studies demonstrate the beneficial effects of mindfulness on physical and mental health, behavioral regulation, increased subjective well-being, relationships, skill development, and brain and immune system functioning.

Mindfulness has also been applied to infertility. The ten-week Mindfulness-Based Program for Infertility (MBPI) determined that MBPI is an effective psychological intervention for women experiencing infertility. Treatment participants revealed a significant decrease in depressive symptoms, internal and external shame, entrapment, and defeat, along with a significant improvement in mindfulness skills and self-efficacy in ability to deal with infertility (Galhardo, Cunha, and Pinto-Gouveia 2013). In a seven-year follow-up study of MBPI, there were long-term effects of MBPI on mindfulness and experiential avoidance and therapeutic maintenance gains regarding depression and anxiety symptoms, independent of reproductive outcome (Galhardo, Cunha, and Pinto-Gouveia 2019).

A study on mindfulness-based cognitive infertility stress therapy (MBCIST) noted improvement on psychological well-being of infertile women, including self-acceptance, positive relations with others, autonomy, environmental mastery, purpose in life, and personal growth (Fard, Kalantarkousheh, and Far- amarzi 2018). Results from a mindfulness-based group counseling intervention in women undergoing IVF reported a decrease in depressive symptoms by in- creasing mental concentration from practicing mindfulness (Kalhori, Masoumi, Shamsaei, et al. 2020). Mindfulness-based interventions on pregnancy outcome have also been investigated. In a study that randomized first-time IVF patients into a mindfulness-based program versus a control, patients in the interven- tion group demonstrated a significant increase in mindfulness, self-compassion, meaning-based coping skills, and as well higher pregnancy rates (Li, Long, Lin et al. 2016).

A recent 2020 review by Patel, Sharma, and Kumar examined the effective- ness of mindfulness-based interventions (MBI) on the emotional well-being and pregnancy outcomes in infertility. MBIs were found to lead to significant reduc- tions in anxiety, depression, stress, and anger; improvement in well-being and enhanced self-efficacy; kinder responding and a more accepting manner; and decreased rumination, thought suppression, and other negative thinking styles. The authors note several studies on the impact of stress on conception signifying a plausible relationship between the relaxation response and fertility. MBIs are known to improve quality of sleep, regulation of cortisol levels, activities of the hypothalamic pituitary adrenal axis (HPA), and immune functions, all of which are known to play an important role in infertility. In conclusion, MBIs lead to reduced psychological distress and enhanced conception rates in infertility.

However, it does appear that more high-quality research on the impact of a mindfulness-based approach on pregnancy outcome is still needed to definitively support the hypothesis that stress impacts fertility.

The benefits of mindfulness for infertility

We are pre-disposed to perceive reality through a lens of judgment—to catego- rize into good or bad, like or dislike, success or failure. "Mindfulness involves opening to the present moment just as it is, without trying to hold on to what you like about it or get rid of what you don't like" (Marotta 2013, 4). Mindfulness teaches us how to accept reality for what it is and promotes the resilience neces- sary to deal with life challenges—such as the challenge of infertility.

Mindfulness lies at the heart of Buddhist psychology which centers on how you *get stuck* and how you *break free*. From the perspective of Buddhist psy- chology, cognitive, emotional, and behavioral patterns that cause suffering are rooted in clinging to what we want (grasping), pushing away what we don't want (aversion), and denying what is happening (ignorance). Mindfulness teaches us to notice these inherent tendencies so it's possible to loosen the grip of suffering. The practice develops insight because it teaches three factors necessary to be in harmony with—what the Buddha refers to as the *Three Characteristics of Existence*: life has suffering or dissatisfaction, everything changes, and there is an ever- fluctuating flow of experience.

That is to say, we're dissatisfied when our lives aren't how we want them to be, we struggle against change, and we fight to hold on to a permanent sense of self. Basically, we can't control life, we have difficulty with this lack of control, and we take this inability personally

(Marotta 2013, 2)

Through mindfulness, it is possible to notice when there is judgment or resistance to what is occurring. In other words, to observe when not being in harmony with the truth that "life has suffering." Mindfulness cultivates acceptance, meaning *being with* what's happening. Acceptance is the ability to *turn toward* that which is resisted. The situation, in this case, infertility, is not the problem; it's the *relationship* to it, the resistance that's the problem, i.e., the wish it wasn't happening, the self-blame, the regret of not seeking treatment sooner...the list goes on. It's not about changing, getting rid of, or judging thoughts, emotions, physical sensations, or experience. Rather, it's opening to it with acceptance.

By applying neutral attention, comes the ability to notice resistance to the law of impermanence—to observe fighting against the reality that "everything changes." All too common is the fear that infertility will go on forever, that the child will never come. Mindfulness cultivates patience, the understanding that some situations unfold in their own time.

When life is personalized as though it's happening to *me, mine, and I*, this is the ego—assumptions and beliefs about who you are. Mindfulness teaches there is no permanent self or ego—rather, there is egolessness, an "ever-fluctuating flow of experience"—the third characteristic of existence. Instead of saying: "I am infertile," it is reframed to: "This is infertility." Infertility is explored and understood from an impersonal perspective, one that is not clouded with unruly thoughts and overwhelming emotions.

Mindfulness trains to notice when in conflict with the three truths of reality—life has suffering or dissatisfaction, everything changes or is impermanent, and there is no solid self or ego rather there is egolessness, an ever-fluctuating flow of experience. Buddhist psychology adheres to the belief that acceptance to the three truths of reality brings suffering to an end.

The paradox of infertility

Infertility is a medical condition with psychosocial facets. Because our cultural conditioning links manliness with virility and womanhood with motherhood, infertility is viewed as a personal failure which challenges identity at its core (Deveraux and Hammerman 1998, 63–68).

For many, the fear of obtaining the diagnosis of infertility and receiving its treatment, results in consequential delays or evasion. Conversely, pursuing fertility treatment can set an addictive course when probabilities of success shrink over time. Too often, countless IVF cycles continue to be pursued when the likelihood of success is determined to be extremely low. Ironically, those very qualities most needed at this unpredictable and challenging time, such as non-judging, non-striving, and trust, are least accessible.

Repeated unsuccessful attempts to bear a child often have an adverse effect on primary relationships. The stress of infertility tends to magnify existing issues and dynamics. Differences between partners previously experienced as complimentary become controversial, splitting partners into opposing sides. Common side effects include not feeling understood or acknowledged, over-reacting or under-reacting, and experiencing loneliness or isolation (Deveraux and Hammerman 1998, 62–71) I have observed that as infertility extends over time, couples have less to give one another, when what they need is more and more.

Those who have never experienced infertility, tend to minimize, misunderstand, or empathize with the overwhelming impact of infertility and its treatment. Comments that are meant to be helpful from family, friends, and the general public are experienced as insensitive and uncaring. Despite an increasing need for support and understanding, there is the urge to withdraw further and further away from help. Navigating the demands of fertility treatment and unsuccessful outcomes impact the ability to manage the tasks and restrictions of work life. Careers are threatened at a time when needed as a source of self-esteem and income. However, when demands of the job are so wide and stakes of treatment so high, how is it possible to be effective and efficient on the job and relaxed as possible for treatment? There is a need to slow down, when expected to try harder.

The pressure to conceive is often experienced as a *race against the biological clock*. When hearing fertility "dips" at 35 years old and "dives" when turning 40, each day feels ever more crucial, as the chance of conception diminishes with age. Being 40 years old and every year after, feels like "old age." In the fertility world, age is measured by ovarian reserve which, at best, perishes somewhere in the 40s. As treatment is entered and extended, difficult decisions must be made under time pressures with life-long consequences. There is the need to be patient while needing to move forward quickly and slow down when expected to move faster and try harder.

Advanced Reproductive Technology (ART) presents multiple treatment options in creating a family, and each option has different issues and implications that need to be understood and decided upon such as IVF, Egg/Sperm/Embryo Donation, and Surrogacy. While it is important to be rationally minded, it is equally important to be intuitively driven. It is not only about knowing ART but knowing who you are. It is about knowing many things, but also one thing.

Infertility is often characterized as loss of control. The coping mechanism of control is counterproductive, as trying harder does not necessarily thwart greater failure. Paradoxically, within each attempt, each wish and desire, is the need to *let go*. While it is important to take control over those situations which can be controlled, the ability to relinquish control can only be found within oneself.

The paradox of mindfulness

In contrast to Western psychology, Buddhist psychology finds wisdom in paradox. The basic teaching of *turning toward* discomfort rather than away from it, is the basic principle. For this very reason, mindfulness uses paradox to meet life's challenges and becomes the ideal medicine to treat the paradoxical land-mines infertility presents.

> More than a stress reduction technique, mindfulness is a *way of life*—a method of meeting what Taoists call 'the ten thousand joys and the ten thousand sorrows' inherent in the human experience. Mindfulness cultivates the qualities most needed, such as acceptance, patience, and trust, and transforms the most insurmountable obstacles and plights to challenges and opportunities for growth. Mindfulness does not change or take away the situation, in this case infertility, but provides the vehicle to *become* the change itself. With awareness as the midwife, mindfulness teaches to relax, release, and let go: to breathe through every contraction of holding tight to what is wanted or trying to get rid of what is not wanted and open to the unfolding process of life. Through repeated practice, you learn resistance is how you get stuck, acceptance is how you break free.
>
> *(Marotta 2018, 4)*

The central quality mindfulness cultivates is acceptance, a state of open receptivity. Acceptance is a practice of getting curious, discovering what causes disease and discontent. It's the essential paradox of turning things around, moving toward that which is resisted. Mindfulness demonstrates the harder you try, the more stuck you become. It teaches to release the tight grip of wants and not wants, to open to it all, and let things be. The coping mechanism shifts from control—trying to change what is, to acceptance—being with what is and working from here.

The way change occurs is a fundamental difference between Western and Buddhist psychology. The paradoxical approach of mindfulness uses acceptance as an essential agent of change and believes change innately arises through insight and awareness. Here we meet another mindfulness paradox: when not trying to change, change naturally occurs.

> Mindfulness challenges assumptions about <u>who</u> you are and <u>why</u> you are doing <u>what</u> you are doing. It is not about following the prescription that leads from point A to point B; rather it is answering the invitation to *drop into your heart*—to come full circle on the wheel of paradox that starts with loving yourself just as you are and ends with loving yourself just as you are. Through this gateway, you give birth to yourself.
>
> *(Marotta 2018, 6)*

The antidote of mindfulness

The distinction between the instinctual reactivity from infertility distress and the way mindfulness responds to these difficulties is multi-faceted. The comparison below summarizes key aspects of mindfulness and highlights its potential for healing.

Coping Mechanism of Control vs. Awareness. Using the coping mechanism of control only exacerbates the loss of control endemic to infertility. Mindfulness uses present-moment non-judgmental awareness to *be with* what is happening. The focus is not to change what is happening but to change the *relationship* to what is happening.

Focus on Past and Future vs. Present. Infertility keeps the focus on past and future, overshadowing other aspects of life. Mindfulness anchors attention to the present moment. This shifts attention from what's wrong to what's *not wrong*.

Attention is Personalized vs. Neutral Attention. The inability to become pregnant or carry a pregnancy is typically experienced as a personal failure. Mindfulness does not personalize experience—attention is neutral.

Original Sin vs. Original Goodness. The tendency to personalize infertility is composed of personal narratives that all too often lead to feelings of unworthiness and the need to fix one's "broken sense of self." Mindfulness is based on the concept of *original goodness*—we are whole and complete already, <u>with</u> our various inadequacies and insecurities. Mindfulness does not encourage attempts to self-correct, but rather to become aware.

Reactive vs Responsive. The stress from infertility keeps the body on *low-grade alert* and emotions on automatic reactivity mode. Mindfulness teaches to pause—to breathe, disengage with neutral attention, and choose how to respond.

Outside In vs Inside Out. When using the coping mechanism of control, attention is focused on the goal—seeking outside success and validation to be okay. Mindfulness focuses on the process—how to work with what is happening and how to cultivate mindfulness qualities, i.e., acceptance, non-striving, patience, trust, and compassion.

Approach is Linear vs. Paradoxical. The normal reaction to difficulty, particularly with infertility, is to turn away, run, or avoid. Mindfulness is based on the wisdom of paradox—to *turn toward* that which you resist. "The wonderful paradox about the truth of suffering is that the more we open to it and understand it, the lighter and freer our mind becomes" (Goldstein 1993, 11–12). Happiness arises when you reduce the clinging to what you want, avoidance to what you don't want, and denial to see what is true.

The application of mindfulness principles and practices

The way into mindfulness is through the formal practice of meditation. Meditation is a training ground to bring awareness to what is occurring in the present moment without judgment. The practice translates into bringing this mindful attention into everyday life. Often, when learning meditation at Insight Meditation Centers, Vipassana meditation is taught. Vipassana is a traditional Buddhist practice for enhancing mindfulness. In Pali, an ancient language of Buddhism, Vipassana means "seeing things as they really are." Thus, Vipassana is often referred to as Insight Meditation. The sequence of practices at these centers teaches mindfulness of the breath, body, emotions, and thoughts. Each is used as an object of *attention*, while employing the *intention* to maintain focus on the object.

In meditation on the breath, observation is on breath sensations in the body, i.e., the rise and fall of the in-breath and out-breath, the rhythm, depth, and duration of the breath, the unique quality of each breath. In meditation on the body, attention is on body sensations, i.e., tightness, numbness, heat, cold, tingling. Instruction is to *turn toward* body sensations, breathing into and out from sensations so sensations can soften, fade, or simply be. Meditation on emotions focuses on the physical manifestations of emotions, i.e., to notice how sadness is felt as a heavy heart. Instruction is to *turn toward* distressing emotions with the quality of openness, making room for emotions to disperse or be as they are. Meditation on thoughts teaches us to see thoughts as "mental formations" like clouds forming and moving in the sky. The training is to not cling to or identify with thoughts, but simply to witness them coming and going.

To begin meditation, a relaxed, alert posture is established with eyes closed. Gently, awareness is brought to the object of attention. Whenever the mind wanders, as it naturally does, instruction is to return to the object of attention. It's not important how many times the mind wanders. It's the "coming back" that matters—the return to the present moment. The practice cultivates such qualities as patience, non-judgment, acceptance, compassion, and trust—essential qualities that develop the strength and resilience needed when confronted with infertility.

The intention of mindfulness meditation is not to change, get rid of, or judge thoughts, emotions, body sensations, or experience, but to open to it with acceptance—to not to change what is happening, but to change the *relationship* to what is happening. It is to notice resistance, i.e., impatience, boredom, sleepiness, judging, and to meet what's happening with acceptance, i.e., curiosity, engagement, and non-judgment.

The formal practice of meditation fosters the informal practice of bringing mindful awareness into everyday life. There are practices that teach how to apply mindfulness of the breath, body, emotions, and thoughts to work with life's difficulties, in this case, infertility. There are practices that use the breath and body to anchor and ground attention and practices to work with emotions and thoughts skillfully.

Mindfulness of the breath

It is estimated that 46.9% of the time the mind wanders, and what is known about a wandering mind is that it's an unhappy mind. Thus, almost half the time we're practicing mindlessness—a sort of virtual reality of past or future thinking that distracts from what is actually happening. Bringing attention to the breath redirects the mind from troublesome thoughts and associated emotions. Long, slow abdominal breaths also stimulate the relaxation response, helpful to lessen the physiological effects brought on by stress, including the stress from infertility.

A beginning informal mindfulness practice on the breath is to place breath reminders in notable places such as glass beads or colored adhesive dots. This may be, for example, on your laptop, cell phone, or bathroom mirror. When noticing a breath reminder, take 2–3 slow, deep breaths from the belly to stimulate the relaxation response and anchor attention to the present moment.

Mindfulness of the body

Considered an "embodied practice," mindfulness brings awareness to the body's response to thoughts, emotions, and experiences. Thoughts and emotions are connected to one another and manifested in the body. Too often, disturbing thoughts become wrapped in uncontrollable emotions which morph into alarming stories. These narratives are not only false but don't even exist in current time. However, the body is a reliable source that "speaks the truth" and is grounded only in the present moment. By noticing places of tension or tightness, and breathing into and out from these areas, body sensations have space to loosen, dissipate, or simply be. Mindfulness teaches to relax the body, and in doing so, the mind is still.

An informal mindfulness of the body practice is the PAUSE practice. This 2–3-minute practice grounds attention in the body. To begin, take 2–3 abdominal breaths and then return to natural breathing.

1 Notice thoughts. Without trying to interpret or analyze thoughts, simply acknowledge the dominate thought, i.e., "I'm afraid I'll never get pregnant."
2 Notice emotions. Without clinging to emotions, trying to avoid them or identify with them, simply acknowledge and label the dominate emotion. Rather than saying, for example, "I feel anxious," say "This is anxiety."
3 Notice body sensations. Place most of the time on the body, noticing points of tension, tightness, jitteriness…. Use the breath and body movement to release tension and find calm, i.e., move shoulders up and down, stretch, bend, breathe deeply. To end, bring this more relaxed, balanced attention with you.

Mindfulness of emotions

As the practice of mindfulness is rooted in non-judgmental present moment awareness, emotions, like thoughts, are not viewed as negative or positive. Rather, emotions are seen as destructive if resisted, i.e., judged, averted, fixated upon, or controlled. The basic tenet of mindfulness is to *turn toward* that which you resist.

In particular, the teaching is to *turn toward* distressing emotions with the quality of openness: a state of unlimited, wide acceptance. When emotions are neither held on tight or run away from, space is created for emotions to simply be.

To informally work with emotions, notice how you're *relating* to emotions: judging, evaluating, trying to fix yourself, personalizing. Ask yourself: "What am I doing that's wholesome?" "What am I doing that's unwholesome?" When overwhelmed by emotions, notice if you are hardening around them or shutting down. If so, can you soften to them and open up? For example, when experiencing sadness, bring attention to the felt sensations of sadness, i.e., heavy heart, shallow breathing, low energy. Breathe into these sensations, giving them room to soften, dissipate, or just simply be.

Mindfulness of thoughts

Judgmental thoughts fuel negative emotions as thoughts create stories that aren't even true. Thoughts become our personal narrative.

> Buddhist psychology starts from the perspective that it is primarily the beliefs we have, and how tightly we hold on to them, that accounts for our mental suffering. Rather than trying to get rid of thoughts, it's learning how to see thoughts skillfully.
>
> *(Kornfield 2008, 146–147)*

1 Thoughts are *mental formations*: By witnessing thoughts from a neutral perspective, it is possible to disentangle from thoughts and see them as "mental formations"—random events like clouds in the sky, forming, dispersing, and disappearing from sight.
2 Thoughts are *events* not facts: There is nothing defining about thoughts; nothing to identify with. Acknowledge the thought without repressing, judging, or identifying with it. Loosen identification with the thought by saying: "I am not my thought."

To informally *work with* thoughts with mindfulness, focus on the *relationship* to thoughts. Ask two fundamental questions: "What am I resisting?" "How can I open up?" Instead of judging thoughts as positive, negative, or inappropriate, make room for whatever thought arises without holding tightly to it by obsessing or ruminating (clinging), running from it by avoiding (aversion), or denying it altogether (delusion). Rather than identifying with the thought, stand back and observe it from a neutral perspective, as non-personal.

Conclusion

The central teachings and practices from *A Fertile Path* formed the focus of this chapter. Given this, I'd like to end with the same final thought expressed in this book.

Infertility is a catastrophe in every sense of the word. Yet, it is the very struggle of infertility, its diminishing of your reserves in every domain that can ultimately replenish and further you. It requires you to look for happiness not on the outside but on the inside. The continual contractions–through withdrawal, resentment, fear, and panic–make you thirst for expansion: trust, acceptance, peace, and finally liberation. Everyone seeks happiness, and it is at this very moment when happiness seems lost that the human spirit will fight hardest to find it where it lives. The final paradox is that infertility is inevitably a birthing process. The labor is difficult, frightening, and we resist, but the process carried through brings forth a new spirit in all who are open to it.

(Marotta 2018, 175)

Note

1 Vision Quests are an ancient type of rite of passage most commonly practiced among some Native American cultures as a supernatural experience to seek vision, advice, or protection. Presently, Vision Quests have been adapted by various wilderness programs to bring people into a deep connection with the natural world. For many, they are transformative journeys that act as a catalyst for generating change, finding meaning, and strengthening one's personal spirituality.

References

Akhter, Shekufe; Marcus, Michele; Kerber, Rich; Kong, Maiying; and Kira C. Taylor 2016. "The Impact of Periconceptional Maternal Stress on Fecundability." *Annals of Epidemiology* 26, no. 10: 710–716 e717. https://doi:10.1016.

Baer, Ruth A. 2003. "Mindfulness Training as a Clinical Intervention: A Conceptual and Empirical Review." *Clinical Psychology: Science and Practice* 10, no. 2: 125–143. https://doi.org/10.1093.

Beutel, M.; Kupfer, J.; Kirchmeyer, P.; Kehde, S.; Kohn, F.M.; Schroeder-Printzen, I.; Gips, H.; Herrero, H.J.; and W. Weidner. 1999. "Treatment-related stresses and depression in couples undergoing assisted reproductive treatment by IVF or ICSI." *Andrologia* 31: 27–35.

Boivin, Jacky and Sofia Gameiro. 2015. "Evolution of Psychology and Counseling in Infertility." *Fertility and Sterility* 104, no. 2: 251–259. https://doi: 10.1016.

Boivin, Jacky; Scanlan, L.C.; and S.M. Walker. 1999. "Why Are Infertile Patients Not Using Psychosocial Counselling?" *Human Reproduction* 14, no. 5: 1384–1439. https://doi.org/10.1093.

Chen, Ting-Hsiu; Chang, Sheng-Ping; Tsai, Chia-Fen; and Kai-Dih Juang. 2004. "Prevalence of Depressive and Anxiety Disorders in an Assisted Reproductive Technique Clinic." *Human Reproduction* 19, no. 10: 2313–2318. https://doi.org/10.1093.

Davis, Daphne M. and Jeffrey A. Hayes. 2011. "What are the Benefits of Mindfulness? A Practice Review of Psychotherapy-Related Research." *Psychotherapy (Chic)* 48, no. 2: 198–208. https://doi.org/10.1037/a0022062.

De Berardis D.; Mazza M.; Marini S.; et al. 2014. "Psychopathology, Emotional Aspects and Psychological Counselling in Infertility: A Review." *Clinical Therapeutics* 165, no.3: 163–169. https://doi.org/10.7417/CT.2014.

Deveraux, Lara L. and Ann J. Hammerman. 1998. *Infertility and Identity: New Strategies for Treatment*. San Francisco: Jossey-Bass Publishers.

Domar, Alice. 2004. "Impact of Psychological Factors on Dropout Rates in Insured Infertility Patients." *Fertility and Sterility* 81, no. 2: 271–273. https://doi.org/10.1016/j.fertnstert.2003.08.01.

Domar, Alice. 2015. "Creating a Collaborative Model of Mental Health Counseling for the Future." *Fertility and Sterility* 104, no. 2: 277–280.

Domar, Alice D.; Zuttermeister, P.C.; and R. Friedman. 1993. "The Psychological Impact of Infertility: A Comparison to Patients with Other Medical Conditions." *Journal of Psychosomatic Obstetrics & Gynecology* 14: 45–52.

Eugster, A. and A.J. Vingerhoets. 1999. "Psychological Aspects of In Vitro Fertilization: A Review." *Social Science & Medicine* 48, no. 5: 575–589.

Fard, Tahere Rahmani; Kalantarkousheh, Mohammad; and Mahbobeh Faramarzi. 2018. "Effect of Mindfulness-Based Cognitive Infertility Stress Therapy on Psychological Well-Being of Women with Infertility." *Middle East Fertility Society Journal* 23, no. 4: 476–481. https://doi.org/10.1016/j.mefs.2018.06.001.

Frederiksen, Yoon; Farver-Vestergaard, Ingeborg; Skovgard, Ninna Gronhoj; Ingerslev, Hans Jakob; and Robert Zachariae. 2015. "Efficacy of Psychosocial Interventions for Psychological and Pregnancy Outcomes in Infertile Women and Men: A Systematic Review and Meta-Analysis." *BMJ Open* 5, no.1: e006592. https://doi.org/10.1136/bmjopen-2014-006592.

Freeman Ellen W.; Boxer, Andrea S.; Rickels, Karl; Tureck, Richard; and Luigi Mastrionni. 1985. "Psychological Evaluation and Support in a Program of In Vitro Fertilization and Embryo Transfer." *Fertility and Sterility* 43, no. 1: 48–53. https://doi: 10.1016/s0015-0282(16)48316-0.

Galhardo, Ana; Cunha, Marina; and José Pinto-Gouveia. 2013. "Mindfulness-Based Program for Infertility: Efficacy Study." *Fertility and Sterility* 100, no. 4: 1059–1067. https://doi.org/10.1016/j.fertnstert.2013.05.036.

Galhardo, Ana.; Cunha, Marina. and José Pinto-Gouveia. 2019. "A 7-year Follow-Up Study of the Mindfulness-Based Program for Infertility: Are there Long-Term Effects?" *Clinical Psychology and Psychotherapy* 26, no. 4: 409–417. https://doi: 10.1002/cpp.2362.

Gameiro, Sofia; Boivin, Jacky; and Chris Verhaak. 2012. "Why do Patients Discontinue Fertility Treatment? A Systematic Review of Reasons and Predictors of Discontinuation in Fertility Treatment." *Human Reproductive Update* 18, no. 6: 652–269. https://doi.org/10.1093/humupd/dms031.

Goldstein, Joseph. 1993. *Insight Meditation: The Practice of Freedom*. Boston: Shambhala.

Golombok, Susan. 1992. "Psychological functioning in infertility patients." *Human Reproduction* 7: 208–212.

Hofmann, Stefan, G.; Sawyer, Alice T.; Witt, Ashley A.; and Diana Oh. 2010. "The Effect of Mindfulness-Based Therapy on Anxiety and Depression: A Meta-Analytic Review." *Journal of Consulting and Clinical Psychology* 78: 169–183. https://doi: 10.1037/a0018555.

Kalhori, Fatemeh; Masoumi, Sevedeh Zahra; Shamsaei, Farshid; Mohammadi, Younes; and Mahnaz Yavangi. 2020. "Effect of Mindfulness-Based Group Counseling on Depression in Infertile Women: Randomized Clinical Trial Study." *International Journal of Fertility and Sterility* 14, no. 1: 10–16. https://doi: 10.22074/ijfs.2020.5785.

Keng, Shian-Ling; Smoski, Moria J.; and Clive J. Robins. 2011. "Effects of Mindfulness on Psychological Health: A Review of Empirical Studies." *Clinical Psychology Review* 31, no. 6: 1041–1056. https://doi.org/10.1016/j.cpr.2011.04.006.

Kornfield, Jack. 2008. *The Wise Heart: A Guide to the Universal Teachings of Buddhist Psychology.* New York: Bantam Books.

Li, Jing; Long, Ling; Lin, Yu; He, Wei, He; and Min Li. 2016. "Effects of a Mindfulness-Based Intervention on Fertility Quality of Life and Pregnancy Rates Among Women Subjected to First In Vitro Fertilization Treatment." *Behaviour Research and Therapy* 77: 96–104. https://doi.org/10.1016/j.brat.2015.12.010.

Marotta, Janetti. 2013. *50 Mindful Steps to Self-Esteem: Everyday Practices for Cultivating Self-Acceptance and Self-Compassion.* Oakland, CA: New Harbinger Publications.

Marotta, Janetti. 2018. *A Fertile Path: Guiding the Journey with Mindfulness and Compassion.* North Charleston, SC: CreateSpace.

Matsubayashi, H.; Hosaka, T.; Izumi, S.; Suzuki, T. and T. Makino. 2001. Emotional distress of infertile women in Japan. *Human Reproduction* 16: 966–969.

Patel, Ansha; Sharma, P.S.V.N.; and Pratap Kumar. 2020. "Application of Mindfulness-Based Psychological Interventions in Infertility." *Journal of Human Reproductive Sciences* 13, no.1: 3–21. https://doi.org/10.4103/jhrs.JHRS_51_19.

Rooney, Kristin and Alice Domar. 2018. "The Relationship between Stress and Infertility." *Dialogues in Clinical Neuroscience* 20, no.1: 41–47. https://doi: 10.31887/DCNS.2018.20.1.

Schlaff, William D. and M. Braverman Andrea. 2015. "Introduction: Role of Mental Health Professionals in the Care of Infertile Patients." *Fertility and Sterility* 104, no. 2: 249–250. https://doi.org/10.1016/j.fertnstert.2015.06.012.

Smeenk, Jasper, M.; Verhaak, Christianne, M.; Stolwijk, Annette. M; Kremer, Jan, A.; and D.D.M. Braat. 2004. "Reasons for Dropout in an In Vitro Fertilization/Intracytoplasmic Sperm Injection Program." *Fertility and Sterility* 77: 505–510. https://doi.org/10.1016/j.fertnstert.2003.09.027.

Teasdale, John D; Segal, Zindel V.; Williams, J. Mark; Ridgeway, Valerie A.; Soulsby, Judith M.; and Mark A. Lau. 2000. "Prevention of Relapse/Recurrence in Major Depression by Mindfulness-Based Cognitive Therapy." *Journal of Consulting and Clinical Psychology* 68, no. 4: 615–623. https://doi.org/10.1037/0022-006X.68.4.615.

Verhaak, Chris M.; Smeenk, Jasper; Evers A. W. M.; Kremer, J. A. M.; Kraaimaat Floris W.; and D. D. M. Braat. 2007. "Women's Emotional Adjustment to IVF: A Systematic Review of 25 Years of Research." Human Reproduction Update 13, no 1: 27–36. https://doi.org/10.1093/humupd/dml040.

Verkuijlen, Jolijn; Verhaak, Christianne; Nelen, Willianne L. D. M.; Wilkinson, Jack; and Cindy Farquhar. 2016. "Psychological Interventions and Educational Interventions for Subfertile Men and Women." *Cochrane Database of Systematic Reviews* 3: CD011034. https://doi: 10.1002/14651858.CD011034.pub2.

7

MINDFULNESS IN CHILDBIRTH PREPARATION

Accentuating the psycho-spiritual-physiological connections

Susan Crowther and Christine Mellor

Introduction

To be thrown into the world of pregnancy either as a couple, alone, nuclear family and/or wider community can be an uncanny experience full of surprises and challenges not encountered previously. Even if this is not the first experience of journeying towards birth and the advent of new life, there is so much to consider and navigate. Antenatal, or sometimes called prenatal sessions or workshops, previously referred to as classes, can be a welcome oasis to gather with others to share the unfolding of what can feel beyond one's control. Being thrown into the new reality of pregnancy and childbirth for many can be overwhelming due to exposure to a rapidly swelling sea of myriad stories of others' experiences. These pregnancy and childbirth stories can create a background noise, a kind of idle chatter in which everyone has an opinion and claim to have the 'best' advice for what is an idiosyncratic experience across the childbirth year.

As Lesley Kay et al. (2017) found, the impact of this idle talk contributes to the ubiquitous authoritative voices of a faceless 'They' – the hum of the collective voice about what is best for everyone. For Heidegger (1927/1962), this is a phenomenological observation that is constitutive of who we are. The 'They' is a faceless voice informing who and what we do, think, say and believe. This pervasive voice of the 'They' begins steadily to penetrate into one's own private world impacting the childbirth year and entering the birthing space. The solace of antenatal sessions facilitated by a knowledgeable expert on these matters can bring great relief in the tidal wave of advice and idle talk providing opportunity to quieten the faceless voices. But is that enough? Is it simply a case of listening to the 'expert' facilitator and leaving behind the kindly often uninvited advice of the 'They' behind?

Susan's previous work has shown that the mood of the birthing experience is important because how one attunes to any experience is how one comes to

DOI: 10.4324/9781003165200-7

understand such experience (Crowther, Smythe, and Spence 2014). To put it simply, if you enter the birthing space fearfully, the world in that space will be understood as risky, dangerous and unsafe. This can lead to risk-averse behaviours and hasty choices in order to gain control or relinquish control to others if one feels paralysed by fear (O'Connell, Khashan, and Leahy-Warren 2021). This is a far cry from the empowerment and informed choice rhetoric in the milieu of westernised childbirth (McAra-Couper, Jones, and Smythe 2012). Ironically, in such risk-averse environments, intervention rates can increase in ways that women experience too much too soon in the west and in low- to middle-income countries (LMIC) too little too late (Miller et al. 2016). Perhaps unsurprisingly there is evidence that women's capacity to make informed choices in childbirth is influenced by the processes and institutional routines of birth (Bringedal and Aune 2019). So, what kind of antenatal sessions and workshops may help mitigate this – if any?

Conventional-styled antenatal educational classes have focused primarily on teaching prospective parents

- how it all works' – the anatomy and physiology of childbirth
- 'what to expect in the birthing process and initial parenting' – this may include lists of choices that inform you of the apparent pros and cons, such as where to birth, type of pain relief, types of birth, infant feeding, when to come to call the midwife or doctor and
- 'learning some coping techniques' – some breathing techniques, positions in labour and birth, and if birth partners join classes, what they can do.

These classes can be formulaic and lack the facilitative style implied when we refer to them as sessions and/or workshops (Nolan 2020). For some women and partners, childbirth can be daunting and fear inducing, and attendance at antenatal classes may lower the levels of fear associated with childbirth (Kacperczyk-Bartnik et al. 2019; Tabib et al. 2021). Yet the content and language used in sessions/classes can be a highly variable and become an overwhelming experience leading to feelings of vulnerability resulting in concerns about being in control and actually heighten anxiety about the important choices to be made (Cutajar et al. 2020). What is apparent is that one approach does not suit everyone. For example, there is also evidence that educational status has impact on participation in antenatal education sessions (Harrich and Brunschot 2022). However, the overarching desire of antenatal education is focused on lessening fear, anxiety and distress and mindfulness is showing promise in this area. Attendance at classes incorporating elements of mindfulness shows a lessening in anxiety and distress around pregnancy but does require further examination (Irving 2020).

The good or satisfactory birth experience and how that is defined is challenging because of the multilayed and contextual overlapping inter-related elements involved (Smythe et al. 2016). The importance of accentuating the psycho-spiritual-physiological connections in the childbirth year is beginning to be evidenced and the need to honour a holistic worldview is evident. For example, we know that a non-holistic approach to birth preparation can potentially lead to ongoing mood disorders affecting the postnatal period (Crowther, Stephen, and Hall 2019; Crowther et al. 2021). Likewise, a group taught structured mindfulness intervention programme[1] delivered to women suffering high levels of fear of childbirth has shown promise in lessening non-urgent obstetric interventions (Veringa-Skiba et al. 2021). It is evident that a mindfulness intervention in pregnancy may be beneficial and impact on outcomes, particularly in regard to lessening fear, stress and improve positive feelings towards childbirth (Forthcoming article 2023). Antenatal classes that incorporate mindfulness may be able to provide solace and a reprieve amongst the ceaseless background noise of the 'They'.

The inclusion of mindfulness within antenatal education may help women to relax into the childbirth experience and avoid attuning to the contagion of fear that can negate any sense of control and lead to feelings of disempowerment, vulnerability and sense of failure. There are a number of antenatal educational programmes that offer mindfulness instruction as part of the course content (e.g. Irving 2020; Pan et al. 2019; Tabib et al. 2021; Warriner et al. 2018); see box one below for more examples. Calmbirth® is one such programme that was introduced into a major tertiary hospital setting in Auckland, New Zealand and piloted. In this chapter, we explore our own journeys and present aspects of this pilot programme and the formal evaluation drawing on data highlighting mindfulness. We start by introducing ourselves and how this topic is important to us.

Our pre-understandings and situatedness

Susan and Christine live and practice/work in Aotearoa New Zealand. Christine has an Associate Director of Midwifery role at Te Toka Tumai (Auckland District Health Board). Susan is professor of midwifery at AUT University and Associate Dean of Postgraduate Studies. Both Susan and Christine have extensive experience in midwifery practice, leadership and academia.

Christine

Throughout my career, I have become increasingly conscious of how tightly interwoven the woman's mind and emotions are with her physiology, labour experience, and birth outcomes. I have also become increasingly aware of how a woman's mind and emotions during labour can influence how they perceive their birth experience in terms of how positive/safe this feels to them. In turn, this perception can have ripple effects in relation to the degree of trauma that a woman may feel post birth, and the level of fear (along with the effects of this fear) that she may carry into a subsequent birth.

I am also interested in the influence and impact that 'place' itself has in relation to labour and birth and how being within the space (for both the woman and the practitioner) can shape emotions, behaviours, practise, and ultimately the woman's labour and birth experience and outcomes. With these professional interests, married with a passion for supporting physiological birth, I conducted a hermeneutic phenomenological study exploring midwives' and obstetricians' experience of place in relation to supporting physiological birth. I will refer to this body of work in this chapter.

Prior to presenting at a conference in New Zealand, I was mistakenly introduced as being a midwife who was passionate about supporting 'psychological birth' rather than physiological. This humorous oversight undoubtedly held some truth and left me questioning that perhaps there is not enough visibility of, or focus on, the 'psychological' in view of the complex interplay that a woman's mind and emotional well-being has with her physiology during labour and birth.

Susan

I am passionate about the promotion of normal physiological birthing with a focus on exploring how we resonate with the sense of sacred in and around birth in ways that honours the celebration of natality – whatever type of birth or childbirth outcome. I am convinced that tenderness, compassion with self and others and an open awareness are qualities central to childbirth and understand that these qualities can unfold when those involved in birth value the psycho-spiritual-physiological processes that weave throughout childbirth. I consider all three of these aspects interrelated and therefore hyphenate them to show how they are in the interiority of the other, that is an inseparable whole of childbirth. Like Christine, I have become increasingly conscious of the centrality of the woman's mind and emotions for her labour and birth experience, progress, and outcomes and their strong interconnection with moods around childbirth. To deny or cover over any part is to ignore the existential and extraordinary event of birth for all involved (Crowther and Hall 2015; Wojtkowiak and Crowther 2018).

Our stories from practice

Both of us align with phenomenological inquiry and appreciate the significance of context in childbirth. We both give primacy to lived experiences and their meaningfulness. In the following section, we each narrate a story from practice to further reveal our situatedness.

Christine practice story

Rosalie was a primiparous woman who I cared for in a hospital setting. She came in and out of the birthing unit during the latent phase of her labour, checking in with us when she needed to. I thought perhaps she was anxious about her labour so needed this regular reassurance and encouragement. On her fourth visit she stayed, no longer feeling comfortable at home, and whilst her cervix was dilated to 5 cm and effaced, her contractions were not regular and there were long periods of uterine inactivity. I asked Rosalie "what do you need to help your labour"? She told me that her aunties had ceremoniously made her a birthing mat which she planned to use during her labour, but her mum had not delivered it in time. To Rosalie, this held the strength of the wāhine in her whānau[2], and the presence of her ancestors. To Rosalie this signified safety and aroha. Her partner drove across the city in the darkness to collect the mat. Shortly after it arrived Rosalie's contractions strengthened and she birthed beautifully, on the mat.

Susan practice story

I was supporting, Mary, a woman in the hospital setting having her first baby. She was labouring long and hard with her husband supporting. The lights were low, they had soft music playing and they held each other tenderly over many hours. They wanted a low intervention birth and had done childbirth classes to prepare. Mary changed position regularly as her partner supported her into positions with cushions, provided massage and continued to provide comforting affirmations. The baby's heartbeat was within normal range and the hours rolled by. On full examination, we realised the baby had rotated into a posterior position. Several hours later Mary was tired, and I repeated the assessment – no change and the head was becoming impacted. We negotiated an obstetric opinion that resulted in continuous monitoring and use of artificial oxytocin. After a few more hours there was no change with Mary exhausted. The collective decision was to have a caesarean section. The situation suddenly went from calm to hordes of people coming and going, lights turned on and a quick transfer to an operating theatre – then out of the pandemonium Mary said:

> *'is my baby okay, do I have time to do something?'* as she was being prepared for spinal analgesia. The obstetrician replied *'your baby is fine – what do you need?*

What followed can only be described as a mindful transfiguration of the physical room into a felt-space of tenderness and compassion. She asked for the phone and spoke with their church prayer group – they prayed for what seemed an eternal moment of grace. They hung up the phone and they both nodded to the surgeon to proceed. The mood of the room had palpably changed. Their baby was born into a mood of calm and peace, welcomed with such humanity touched by something unseen. Her mindful action orchestrated a psycho-spiritual-physiological connection that permeated everyone in that operating theatre – it was like witnessing a timeless holy birth. A time I have described as Kairos time at birth (Crowther et al. 2015). That was 30 years ago – it is just as real and present to me now as it was then. I reflect upon how this would play out in today's climate of risk and ongoing medicalisation? Perhaps a more mindful approach is necessary now more than ever.

Coming to understand the birth space

There is a strong body of evidence which shows that the birthplace itself influences labour and birth outcomes (e.g. Bailey 2017; Brocklehurst et al. 2011; Davis et al. 2011; Farry et al. 2019; Scarf et al. 2018) and rising rates of labour and birth intervention are causing international concern (World Health Organization [WHO] 2018). Birthplace is *experienced*; it can influence how the woman responds to her labour and impacts on her labour and birth journey.

Place and space are not neutral but are filled with discourses (Fahy, Foureur, and Hastie 2008; Hammond and Foureur 2019). Van Manen wrote about spatiality, or 'felt space', suggesting that the space that we are in is key to the way that we feel. "In general, we may say that we become the space we are in" (Van Manen 2016, 102). According to Dahlen et al. (2021), there exists a 'complex interaction' between the philosophies of the woman, the midwife, and the birthplace in relation to both maternal and midwife behaviours. Their research findings suggest that optimising physiological birth is associated with increasing distance, both physical and philosophical, from technocratic norms in relation to labour and birth. These technocratic norms may be well established within the space of some hospital settings; increasing physical distance can be challenging but distancing philosophically could be aided by a mindfulness-based programme.

Christine's hermeneutic phenomenological study (Mellor 2021) explored midwives' and obstetricians' experience of place in relation to supporting physiological birth and revealed that place influences what practitioners are attuned to, 'directed towards', and what becomes 'the path of least resistance'. Her findings show the way that practitioner's 'feel' in the space can shape how they are able to support physiological birth. It is feasible that space, and the mood within it, also influences what women attune to and how they 'feel' and this could be a key component in how they labour. The woman walks into the mood of the space and 'feels' the subtle messages about labour and birth, which may have more of an effect than we realise; creating a 'mind space' provides an element of control for the woman in relation to what she experiences.

In New Zealand, there are significant differences in the rates of spontaneous vaginal births by 'place', and also differences when benchmarking low-risk primiparae birthing in hospital maternity facilities nationally (Ministry of Health 2020). The Maternity Clinical Indicators (Ministry of Health 2020) indicate that Te Toka Tumai (Auckland District Health Board) has a relatively low rate of spontaneous vaginal birth and a correspondingly high rate of caesarean section, and this cannot be explained purely by the woman's level of 'risk'.

As part of a project to support opportunities for physiological birth at Te Toka Tumai, Christine explored the introduction of mindfulness-based childbirth preparation programmes. This decision reflected research evidence alongside anecdotal evidence of what felt to be a growing wave of fear and anxiety in relation to labour and birth. A ten-month Calmbirth® pilot programme was set up to explore and evaluate its efficacy in the hospital setting involving a cohort of over 600 women and their labour support people.

Calmbirth®

Calmbirth® is an Australian-based childbirth education programme developed in 2004. It is an antenatal educational programme specifically focused on the interrelatedness of mind and body in childbirth. Calmbirth's purpose is to improve birthing outcomes for women and their families. The programme is comprised of three major components. The first is birthing psychology and the emotional safety of women and their partners through exploration of perceptions and belief systems, and their impact on physiology. Second, the physiology of birth and how to optimally traverse labour and birth both physically and emotionally. The third aspect is what is known as the 'birth toolkit'. The toolkit comprises:

- teaching conscious breath techniques;
- visualisation and guided relaxation;
- acupressure for pregnancy and labour and birth massage;
- other comfort measures including active birth positioning;
- active the role of the birthing partner.

In our initial scoping review, no independent studies about Calmbirth® as a complete programme of antenatal education were identified (forthcoming). Most studies identified in the review only focused on single interventions and it remains unclear what, if any, the impact is when all elements of Calmbirth® are delivered together. The efficacy of such a comprehensive approach requires further research. However, evidence of specific tools in the tool kit has been previously evaluated and studied, especially mindfulness interventions. See box 1 for examples of this emergent work over the last decade.

The evaluation

An independent service evaluation was commissioned by ADHB of the pilot programme of free Calmbirth® antenatal classes delivered between September 2020 and June 2021. 438 women and 398 partners or support persons completed one of the 28 courses in this period. Due to Covid-19 restrictions attendance rates were divided between face-to-face classes (96%) online delivery (82.7%). No formal comparison between online and face-to-face was made at the time of the evaluation because the type of course delivery was dynamic due to the Covid pandemic and was not a requirement of the agreed evaluation. However, the data collection across the two deliverer styles was similar overall; in fact, some preferred the flexibility of online learning. The aim of the evaluation was to establish what standard the Calmbirth® education classes achieved over the pilot period and to inform further planning and provide recommendations for ongoing related research and

Box 7.1 Mindfulness in pregnancy studies 2011–2021[3]

Warriner, S., Crane, C., Dymond, M., Krusche, A., An evaluation of mindfulness-based childbirth and parenting courses for pregnant women and prospective fathers/partners within the UK NHS (MBCP-4-NHS). *Midwifery*, 2018. 64: p. 1–10.

Sbrilli, M.D., L.G. Duncan, and H.K. Laurent, Effects of prenatal mindfulness-based childbirth education on child-bearers' trajectories of distress: a randomized control trial. *BMC Pregnancy Childbirth*, 2020. 20(1): p. 623.

Sbrilli, M.D., L.G. Duncan, and H.K. Laurent, Effects of prenatal mindfulness-based childbirth education on child-bearers' trajectories of distress: a randomized control trial. *BMC Pregnancy Childbirth*, 2020. 20(1): p. 623.

Pan, W.L., et al., Assessing the effectiveness of mindfulness-based programs on mental health during pregnancy and early motherhood – a randomized control trial. *BMC Pregnancy Childbirth*, 2019. 19(1): p. 346.

Guardino, C.M., et al., Randomised controlled pilot trial of mindfulness training for stress reduction during pregnancy. *Psychol Health*, 2014. 29(3): p. 334–49.

Fisher, C., et al., Participant experiences of mindfulness-based childbirth education: a qualitative study. *BMC Pregnancy Childbirth*, 2012. 12(1): p. 126.

Dunn, C., et al., Mindful pregnancy and childbirth: effects of a mindfulness-based intervention on women's psychological distress and well-being in the perinatal period. *Arch Womens Ment Health*, 2012. 15(2): p. 139–43.

Duncan, L.G., et al., Benefits of preparing for childbirth with mindfulness training: a randomized controlled trial with active comparison. *BMC Pregnancy Childbirth*, 2017. 17(1): p. 140.

Byrne, J., et al., Effectiveness of a Mindfulness-Based Childbirth Education pilot study on maternal self-efficacy and fear of childbirth. *J Midwifery Womens Health*, 2014. 59(2): p. 192–7.

Beattie, J., et al., Effects of mindfulness on maternal stress, depressive symptoms and awareness of present moment experience: A pilot randomised trial. *Midwifery*, 2017. 50: p. 174–183.

Agampodi, T., et al., Feasibility of incorporating mindfulness based mental health promotion to the pregnancy care program in Sri Lanka: a pilot study. *F1000Res*, 2018. 7: p. 1850.

practice changes. The evaluation adopted a goal-free evaluation stance meaning evaluators endeavoured to perform the evaluation without rhetoric related to the programme goals. The evaluation comprised three phases:

1 a scoping review (forthcoming, currently in review),
2 online anonymous survey (qualitative and quantitative data collection)[4],
3 face-to face-individual and couple in-depth interviews (forthcoming publication).

Ethics was granted by AUTEC (AUT Ethics Committee) and ADHB Research Governance Group Meeting of Women's and Neonatal Health. In phase two 150 women completed the online Qualtrics survey. In phase three 13 interviews were conducted, 5 including partners, thus, 18 persons were interviewed. In the following sections, we focus on the mindfulness aspect of the evaluation through the qualitative data we gathered. All names are pseudonyms.

Participants voices

Participants in the evaluation interviews were asked explicitly about mindfulness. Although most did not refer to it as a tool specially it came through in how they used the technique in related tools. Here Carla talks about learning to calm down and relax more:

> I was using the breathing techniques a lot. Didn't listen to the mindfulness or meditation tracks. Started playing the sleep music a lot. I was practicing the breathing techniques a lot cause it helped me to sleep. I was having trouble sleeping. Sleeping poorly. Being in the busy lifestyle, we work, come home, do a bit of exercise, you don't think about meditating or taking some time out for yourself. I was lot more mindful and relaxed, me time, went out for massages, just relax. After doing that course I realised we needed to calm it down a bit.

Here Deborah reiterates the importance of finding time to relax and prepare and how mindfulness tools helped slow her down. With many women working until late in the third-trimester mindfulness may provide the opportunity to refocus:

> It was hard for me leading up to it, I didn't like taking day's work off, but after the first session I was like No, this is really good you know it works. ...it was great because you're like on your own coach, so you are already a little bit relaxed.

Deborah continued to use the mindfulness tools postpartum too and encouraged self-nurturing practices:

> Sometimes if [partner] has got [baby] I go to have a lie down for an hour or whatever I actually still do use those techniques, because you know if you've been running

around or you're busy it's hard to relax quickly, so I actually use some of the tricks and just the breathing just to relax and have an hour break.

For some, learning the psycho-emotional-cognitive-physiological connections inspired them. For Frances staying calm and keeping stress low to avoid complications was her inspiration to use the taught techniques:

So, one thing that really stuck with me was the fact that you know when we when you're calm in Labour like all the blood goes to your uterus and makes it a more effective. …when you start panicking your body goes into the fight or flight mode and blood will rush to your hands and your legs. You like to try and run away. … this means that your uterus isn't getting as much oxygen and blood therefore it's not going to work as efficiently as it could do. Staying calm was in my best interest to kind of make the process as quick and straightforward.

For some breathing was important, for others visualisation was a mindful practice that helped. For Mary learning to use mindful visualisation at the course was a way to enter her happy place which she found beneficial revealing the influence of integrating psycho-emotional–spiritual mindfulness practices:

I wouldn't have done it [mindfulness practices] at home myself. At first, I was a bit lost. When I think and I say 'go to visualize your happy place' – I just like, you know, go there.

For Jane, this was her first encounter with mindfulness techniques, and she found the techniques so helpful she practised them regularly after the classes finished.

Mindfulness was quite new to me … I've never really thought about like any breathing techniques and stuff like that, as part of like a pain relief or anything like that. It was more about get your stress levels down and stuff like that, but I never really thought about it, like incorporating that into like Labor. I then practised the techniques quite a lot like pretty much every other day so like three four times a week.

For Louise, there was concern about losing control and the classes gave her more confidence:

Before I've done the course and sort of thought about what kind of birth, I wanted and how I wanted to sort of take control of my birth and be in charge of it and do as much as I can to get the birth, obviously, knowing that it doesn't always go that way, but knowing I wanted to control what I could control. The classes were encouraging me to take control, but obviously talking about the way that birth can end up with intervention. I felt empowered and I felt like I was fully informed, which was what I was keen on. It felt good I felt strong – I just took control. But I think practicing them [mindfulness techniques] and having them reinforced at the course helped… and doing the breathing I found that was really helpful at calming my brain.

Additional Calmbirth® informal feedback

Gita was incredibly empowered by the birth of her first baby and so proud of what she had achieved. Gita anticipated that she would go to the hospital as soon as contractions started due to her fear of the pain, the unknown, and of being out of control. An early epidural was core to her plan, and she fully expected to mirror the traumatic, operative birth experiences of her sisters. However, when labour started Gita found herself feeling excitement instead of fear. She talked about 'relaxing into it' believing that she had the ability to cope; her body knew what to do, she just needed to nurture her mind. As she took her mind to a safe space during labour and reduced her fear Gita described being able to surrender to the process. She stayed at home for most of the day, arrived at the hospital in strong labour and went on to have a birth without intervention or pain relief. For Gita, Calmbirth® created and emanated a safe space for her mind to retreat to which allowed her to step back and let her physiology take the lead. She described taking herself to another place, being 'inside a bubble', and just 'letting it happen', holding faith in her body and feeling that she was safe.

The anecdotes gesture to some powerful outcomes from mindfulness instruction delivered as part of antenatal education. Figure 7.1 highlights the emergent six main themes in relation to the impact of mindfulness in the evaluation.

Final reflections

There is a yearning for this type of intervention and the feedback has been overwhelmingly good. Both the formal feedback through the evaluation and informal feedback clearly reveal some 'thing' we name psycho-spiritual- physiological birthing. Is this merely the soft stuff? No, we would contend it's the major stuff of birth. It is an honouring and appreciation of birth as a celebration and experience of our shared natality. The 'small things' may, in fact, represent 'big things' in relation to a woman's experience of labour, and her birth outcomes. Women are incredibly sensitive to messages that they interpret and understand; they (the women as well as their health care providers and birth partners) intuit and feel into the mood that creates the living-space around them. The impact of how a woman feels emotionally influences how labour and birth unfolds – this cannot be underestimated. The psychological, physiological and emotional-spiritual domains are inextricably interwoven. Therefore, caring for a woman's emotional well-being is also caring for her physical well-being.

Heidegger (1993), alongside 'dwelling', used the term wohnen meaning feeling at home in a place; feeling safe and at peace, which is well understood to be salient during labour and birth. Safeguarding in this context gestures to that which needs to be allowable to continue – vis-à-vis., – birthing in safe felt space

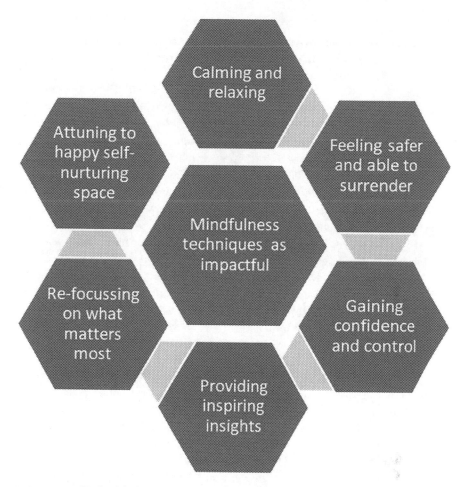

FIGURE 7.1 Six highlighted themes related to impact of mindfulness.

that feels peaceful. Heidegger also wrote that Dasein, or 'being in' the world, is always attuned towards things or situations within the world, which 'sets a tone' and can "direct oneself towards something" (1927/1962, 176). This attunement makes things 'matter' to an individual (Heidegger 1927/1962). Attuning to and 'directing towards' a focus on physiological birth and feelings of safety, peace, 'home' with the support of a mindfulness-based programme can help to create a 'space within a place' for the labouring woman. This could help quieten the ubiquitous voices of the They around childbirth (e.g. the idle talk and background risk chatty) and facilitate and nurture a peaceful homely 'mind space' — even at times when the physical birth environment is not quite as homely or /and when aspirations for a particular type of birth or birth plan is prevented due to circumstances.

We end with an example of Calmbirth® teaching incorporating mindfulness, see Box 7.2.

Box 7.2 A mindfulness activity given by Karen McClay owner and director Calmbirth Australia: reproduced with permission

This short mindfulness activity is aimed at assisting you to use your breath to hone your attention and create a calmness within your mind and body whenever you need to. Like all mindfulness activities, however, it is a practice. At first you may find yourself a little fidgety or that your mind often wanders. This is very normal so be kind to yourself and know that with time and practice this improves, and the less fidgety you will be and the less your mind will wander. It is like every skill we learn – the more we practice it, the better we get at doing it, and the bigger the benefit it has for us.

So, let us begin. You may want to record this on your phone and play it back to yourself or perhaps have someone read it to you.

When you are ready, find a comfortable position, this may-be seated, lying down or even standing. You can do this inside or outside.

Take a few moments to settle in and find your position of comfort

(Pause to allow time for this).

When you are ready allow your eyes to gently close, or if you prefer, simply soften your gaze.

And now when you are ready bring your awareness to your breath (pause).

There is no need to change it in anyway right now, just notice it, allowing each breath to flow in and out in its own natural way.

What are you noticing?

Perhaps you are aware and feeling the movement of your breath as your chest and abdomen rise and fall with each breath?

Perhaps you noticing the sensation and feeling of the breath as your breath in and breath out through your nose or gently through your mouth?

Just watch the breath breathing itself... (Pause to allow time for this)

If your mind wanders at any point, just acknowledge it without any judgement and bring your awareness back to your breath.

Now bring your awareness into your body.

Scan through and notice different feelings and sensations and start to release any tension as you go on each out-breath.

That's the way

Soften your eyes – Soften and drop your jaw and let your tongue float to your top palate...

Relax your shoulders

If you are sitting, sink into your sit bones, relaxing your spine and abdomen.

Relax your legs noticing your feet connecting with the earth.

If you are laying down, soften your whole body sinking into the bed or mat, noticing where your body most connects with the surface.

See if you can notice a comfortable heaviness developing throughout your body.

(Pause to give time to experience and be with this)

Once again if your mind wanders, acknowledge it without any judgement and bring your awareness back to your body.

Now come back to your breath

When you are ready, slow your breath down a little more now, breathing into your own natural number, perhaps to a count of 3 or 4, and breathing out to a similar count. Breathing where possible gently through your nose and into your belly.

Notes

1 The programme involved nine weekly sessions lasting three hours each delivered by experienced midwives certified in mindfulness-based childbirth interventions; sessions included mindfulness meditation practice and enquiry as well as education about psychobiological processes.

2 whānau – a te reo word meaning extended family, family group. It is a term of address to a number of people - in Māori society. wāhine – another te reo word meaning women. With the macron over the ā it becomes plural for the word wahine meaning woman.

3 Note: this is not an exhaustive list but an indication of the interest in mindfulness in this area. It is also acknowledged that some studies focused on meditation, visualisation and breathing without specifically mentioning or naming mindfulness as a key focus. Further details will be available in the forthcoming scoping review now in peer review.

4 The full report is available on request to the primary author at susan.scrowther@ aut.ac.nz . Title of full report: Service Evaluation of the Calmbirth® Antenatal Pilot Programme at Auckland District Health Board (ADHB) 2020-21. Evaluation team Crowther, S, McAra-Couper, J, Hollingshead, B., Donald, H., Hotchin, C. (Sept. 2021).

References

Bailey, David John. 2017. "Birth outcomes for women using free-standing birth centers in South Auckland, New Zealand." *Birth* 44 (3): 246–251.

Bringedal, Hilde, and Ingvild Aune. 2019. "Able to choose? Women's thoughts and experiences regarding informed choices during birth." *Midwifery* 77: 123–129.

Brocklehurst, Peter, D Puddicombe, Jennifer Hollowell, M Stewart, L Linsell, AJ Macfarlane, and C McCourt. 2011. "Perinatal and maternal outcomes by planned place of birth for healthy women with low risk pregnancies: the Birthplace in England national prospective cohort study." *British Medical Journal (BMJ)* 343: d7400.

Crowther, S. 2019. *Joy at birth: An interpretive, hermeneutic, phenomenological inquiry.* London: Routledge Taylor & Francis Group.

Crowther, S., and J. Hall. 2015. "Spirituality and spiritual care in and around childbirth." *Women and Birth* (0). http://doi.org/10.1016/j.wombi.2015.01.001.

Crowther, S., L. Smythe, and D. Spence. 2014. "Mood and birth experience." *Women and Birth: Journal of the Australian College of Midwives* 27 (1): 21–25. https://doi.org/10.1016/j.wombi.2013.02.004.

Crowther, S., L. Smythe, and D. Spence. 2015. "Kairos time at the moment of birth." *Midwifery* 31: 451–457. http://doi.org/10.1016/j.midw.2014.11.005.

Crowther, S., A. Stephen, and J. Hall. 2019. "Association of psychosocial–spiritual experiences around childbirth and subsequent perinatal mental health outcomes: an integrated review." *Journal of Reproductive and Infant Psychology* 1–26.

Crowther, Susan A., Jenny Hall, Doreen Balabanoff, Barbara Baranowska, Lesley Kay, Diane Menage, and Jane Fry. 2021. "Spirituality and childbirth: An international virtual co-operative inquiry." *Women and Birth* 34 (2):e135-e145.

Cutajar, Lisa, Michelle Miu, Julie-Anne Fleet, Allan M Cyna, and Mary Steen. 2020. "Antenatal education for childbirth: Labour and birth." *European Journal of Midwifery* 4 (11): 1–9.

Dahlen, Hannah G, Soo Downe, Melanie Jackson, Holly Priddis, Ank de Jonge, and Virginia Schmied. 2021. "An ethnographic study of the interaction between philosophy of childbirth and place of birth." *Women and Birth* 34 (6): e557–e566.

Davis, Deborah, Sally Baddock, Sally Pairman, Marion Hunter, Cheryl Benn, Don Wilson, Lesley Dixon, and Peter Herbison. 2011. "Planned place of birth in New Zealand: does it affect mode of birth and intervention rates among low-risk women?" *Birth* 38 (2): 111–119.

Fahy, Kathleen, M. Foureur, and Carolyn Hastie. 2008. *Birth territory and midwifery guardianship, Books for midwives*. London: Butterworth Heinemann Elsevier.

Farry, Annabel, J. McAra-Couper, M. Wheldon, and J.H. Clemons. 2019. "Comparing perinatal outcomes for healthy pregnant women presenting at primary and tertiary settings in South Auckland: A retrospective cohort study." *New Zealand College of Midwives Journal* 55: 5–13.

Hammond, A., and M. Foureur. 2019. "Interconnectivity in the birth room." In *Squaring the Circle: Normal birth research, theory and practice in a technological age*, edited by S. Downe and S. Byrom, 180–192. Pinter & Martin Limited.

Harrich, Friederike H. M., and Denise Özdemir-Van Brunschot. 2022. "On participation in antenatal classes depending on the academic educational status of the mother." *Indian Journal of Public Health Research & Development* 13 (1): 149–152.

Heidegger, M. 1927/1962. *Being and time*. Translated by J. Macquarrie and E Robinson. New York: Harper.

Heidegger, M. 1993. "Building, dwelling, thinking." In *Basic writings*, edited by D. Krell, 343–365. San Francisco, CA: HarperSanFrancisco.

Irving, T. A. 2020. "Mindfulness in antenatal classes: A quasi-experimental pilot study." Master of Social Sciences Thesis, University of Waikato.

Kacperczyk-Bartnik, Joanna, Paweł Bartnik, Aleksandra Symonides, Natalia Sroka-Ostrowska, Agnieszka Dobrowolska-Redo, and Ewa Romejko-Wolniewicz. 2019. "Association between antenatal classes attendance and perceived fear and pain during labour." *Taiwanese Journal of Obstetrics and Gynecology* 58 (4): 492–496.

Kay, Lesley, Soo Downe, Gill Thomson, and Kenny Finlayson. 2017. "Engaging with birth stories in pregnancy: a hermeneutic phenomenological study of women's experiences across two generations." *BMC Pregnancy and Childbirth* 17 (1): 283–283. https://doi.org./10.1186/s12884-017-1476-4.

McAra-Couper, Judith, Marion Jones, and Liz Smythe. 2012. "Caesarean-section, my body, my choice: The construction of 'informed choice' in relation to intervention in childbirth." *Feminism & Psychology* 22 (1): 81–97.

Mellor, C. 2021. Midwives' and obstetricians' experience of place in relation to supporting physiological birth: A hermeneutic phenomenological study. (Doctoral thesis, AUT University). Retrieved from https://openrepository.aut.ac.nz/bitstream/handle/10292/14780/MellorC%20%281%29.pdf?sequence=3&isAllowed=y

Miller, Suellen, Edgardo Abalos, Monica Chamillard, Agustin Ciapponi, Daniela Colaci, Daniel Comandé, Virginia Diaz, Stacie Geller, Claudia Hanson, and Ana Langer. 2016. "Beyond too little, too late and too much, too soon: a pathway towards evidence-based, respectful maternity care worldwide." *The Lancet* 388 (10056): 2176–2192.

Ministry of Health. 2020. *New Zealand maternity clinical indicators: Background document.* Wellington, New Zealand

Nolan, Mary L. 2020. *Parent education for the critical 1000 days.* London: Routledge.

O'Connell, Maeve A., Ali S. Khashan, and Patricia Leahy-Warren. 2021. "Women's experiences of interventions for fear of childbirth in the perinatal period: A meta-synthesis of qualitative research evidence." *Women and Birth* 34 (3):e309–e321. https://doi.org/10.1016/j.wombi.2020.05.008.

Pan, Wan-Lin, Meei-Ling Gau, Tzu-Ying Lee, Hei-Jen Jou, Chieh-Yu Liu, and Tzung-Kuen Wen. 2019. "Mindfulness-based programme on the psychological health of pregnant women." *Women and Birth* 32 (1):e102–e109.

Scarf, Vanessa L, Chris Rossiter, Saraswathi Vedam, Hannah G Dahlen, David Ellwood, Della Forster, Maralyn J Foureur, Helen McLachlan, Jeremy Oats, and David Sibbritt. 2018. "Maternal and perinatal outcomes by planned place of birth among women with low-risk pregnancies in high-income countries: a systematic review and meta-analysis." *Midwifery* 62: 240–255.

Smythe, Elizabeth, Marion Hunter, Jackie Gunn, Susan Crowther, Judith McAra Couper, Sally Wilson, and Deborah Payne. 2016. "Midwifing the notion of a good birth: A philosophical analysis." *Midwifery* 37: 25–31. https://doi.org/10.1016/j.midw.2016.03.012.

Tabib, Mo, Tracy Humphrey, Katrina Forbes-McKay, and Annie Lau. 2021. "Expectant parents' perspectives on the influence of a single antenatal relaxation class: A qualitative study." *Complementary Therapies in Clinical Practice* 43: 101341.

Van Manen, Max. 2016. *Researching lived experience: Human science for an action sensitive pedagogy.* London: Routledge.

Veringa-Skiba, Irena K, Esther I de Bruin, Francisca J.A. van Steensel, and Susan M. Bögels. 2021. "Fear of childbirth, nonurgent obstetric interventions, and newborn outcomes: A randomized controlled trial comparing mindfulness-based childbirth and parenting with enhanced care as usual." *Birth* 49 (1): 40–51.

Warriner, Sian, Catherine Crane, Maret Dymond, and Adele Krusche. 2018. "An evaluation of mindfulness-based childbirth and parenting courses for pregnant women and prospective fathers/partners within the UK NHS (MBCP-4-NHS)." *Midwifery* 64: 1–10.

World Health Organization. 2018. *WHO recommendations: Intrapartum care for a positive childbirth experience.* Geneva, Switzerland: Author.

Wojtkowiak, Joanna, and S. Crowther. 2018. "An existential and spiritual discussion about childbirth: Contrasting spirituality at the beginning and end of life." *Spirituality in Clinical Practice* 5 (4): 261–272. https://doi.org/10.1037/scp0000188.

8

DISRUPTING THE STATUS QUO TO CREATE THE MINDFUL BIRTH SPACE – SPACES THAT 'SING'!

Doreen Balabanoff and Maralyn Foureur

Maralyn and Doreen are academics from the disciplinary fields of midwifery and architecture, who live on opposite sides of the world in Australia and Canada. Along with many other roles, we are both mothers whose experiences of birth inspired deep curiosity and much research about the pivotal moment of childbirth in the life of a woman and her family; an experience that connects past and future in the present. We offer here our knowledge about how the design characteristics of maternity care spaces speak to women, overtly and covertly, impacting their capacities and experiences during labour and birth. We aim to consider and offer guidance on how one might create 'mindful birth spaces', and how this concept could help disrupt the status quo, the birth environment legacy of 'utility' and 'functionalism' we have inherited from the 20th century. It is time for a significant paradigm shift.

In this chapter, we take a transdisciplinary approach, which "admits and confronts complexity in science...challenges knowledge fragmentation...is the result of intersubjectivity...[and] is often action-oriented..." (Lawrence 2010). Transdisciplinarity also brings us forward to acknowledge the importance of culture and tradition, and of respecting practical and spiritual ways of knowing, along with scientific knowledge. We call upon all who design or modify maternity spaces to discover birth space design as a truly profound project – one that is *neuroarchitectural* and *phenomenological* – so that we might move beyond the paradigm of birthspace as a place that promises safety but delivers high rates of stress, interventionism, and operative birth; impacts dignity and respect negatively; and undermines women's confidence in their bodies and in giving birth. A new kind of birth space is needed that honours the physiological, emotional and spiritual needs and desires of all who participate in the personal and universal life experience of birth. Perhaps mindfulness can help us achieve it.

DOI: 10.4324/9781003165200-8

Mindfulness, as a practice of awareness – of mind–body consciousness – is centred on being fully present in the moment. As Wilson and Kabat-Zinn assert

> While we get a great deal of training in our education systems in thinking of all kinds, we have almost no exposure to the cultivation of intimacy with that other innate capacity of ours that we call *awareness*. We tend to be unaware of our awareness. We so easily take it for granted. It rarely occurs to us that it is possible to systematically explore and refine our relationship to awareness itself, or that it can be 'inhabited.' This is a profound area for both first person and third person investigation and debate
>
> *(Kabat-Zinn and Williams 2011)*

Today, neuroscientific studies are exploring how mindfulness practices impact the brain–body (Tang, Hölzel, and Posner 2015); and embodiment theories are integral to our understandings of spatial experience (Böhme 2017). The nascent fields of neuroaesthetics and neuroarchitecture and the growing evidence concerning the neurophysiology of childbirth corroborate that mind, body and environment are not disconnected (Buckley 2015; Coburn, Vartanian and Chatterjee 2017; Olza et al. 2020). Neuroscience is a rich source of knowledge about the cognitive, perceptual and phenomenological underpinnings of human spatial experience, understood as 'embodied' and 'ecological' (Palasmaa 2015).

Environment as 'felt' human experience

Our interest in 'mindful' birth spaces is thus grounded in a growing landscape of research that situates a 'new aesthetics' in architectural design – removed from aesthetics as a 'critical' or 'judgmental' arena. The new aesthetics' focus is on the environment as atmospheric, 'felt' human experience (Böhme 2021). All of the inhabitants/actors within a space are understood as part of the environment. Considering architectural settings as 'felt spaces' means we acknowledge the interrelationships between mind, body and environment.

Neuroscience and other research areas confirm that aspects of our surrounding felt environment trigger neurohormones and linked bodily systems, and these internal and interconnected activities influence and modulate our emotional landscape (Olcese, Lozier and Paradise 2013; Olcese and Beesley 2014; University of South Florida 2018; Uvnäs Moberg 2019). That is, we are engaged in a constant and intimate relationship with the built environment – and the messages it sends to us – to our minds, our bodies – are revealed in the physiological and psychological responses that we can now see and measure through MRI scans and other imaging/measuring evidence.

The current birth culture, with its focus on risk and danger, asks architects to design *from/for* 'procedural' medical perspectives or 'functionalities', rather than designing *with* awareness that mind-body-environment interwovenness could be utilized positively to support labour and birth, and to eliminate unnecessary medical interventions (Hodnett and Abel 1986; Newburn and Singh 2005; Wrønding et al. 2019). That is, the messages birth spaces convey are not yet well-attuned to optimal support for the birthing mother/child. Midwives, doulas and other supporting companions/caregivers are thus not well supported in their roles of providing continuous care during birth, which is important for positive birth experience and salutogenic outcomes. Hospital or birth centre spatial design therefore is implicated in how labour and birth progress or slow down, as the hormones of labour and birth are set in motion by spatial engagement. Within linked bodily systems, hormones kick in, and emotions are felt. Capacity for relaxation, attention and attunement are modulated by the surrounding environment.

Repeating what has gone before

Through viewing, visiting or working in birth spaces across many birth settings in Australia and New Zealand, Europe and the United Kingdom, North America and Canada and in Southeast Asia, over a timespan of four decades we have been surprised to find that built birth spaces in hospitals all look the same; no matter the culture, geography or wealth of the setting and no matter how diverse the architecture of each particular country. Images of birth rooms from early in the 20th century reveal characteristics that are echoed in images from the 21st century with only minor changes to the room's boxlike structure with its centrally placed bed and overhead operating theatre light, or cosmetic changes to the colour and decoration on the walls or furniture. What is clearly apparent is that the designers of hospital birth spaces approach the project by simply repeating what has gone before. The spaces reflect a biomedical and pathological concept of birth as dangerous and risky, best suited to constant surveillance and supervision of the woman in a room designed as a slightly modified operating theatre. It is worth reflecting on how this idea emerged (Figure 8.1).

Nearly 100 years ago, childbirth in wealthy countries moved from homes to hospitals, resulting in birth becoming firmly accommodated in the biomedical space. A focus on population-based birth outcomes rather than the personal and social experience of birth for individual women emerged as the primary goal of maternity services. Women were promised increased safety, but the cost was significant. Initially, the move resulted in a period of *increased* maternal and infant mortality due to cross-infection (Loudon 1992; de Costa 2009). It was not until life-saving antibiotics and blood transfusions became widely accessible in the late 1940s as well as a range of ecological factors (public health measures, better nutrition, and smaller families) that maternal and infant mortality began to decline (Tew 1998; Aminov 2010). However, society was seduced into assuming a causal relationship between moving to hospital and safer birth, an invalid assumption that continues to this day (Hutton et al. 2019; Reitsma et al. 2020).

Moving to the biomedical birth space resulted in important losses for women beginning with loss of privacy, intimacy, cosiness, companionship/help of other

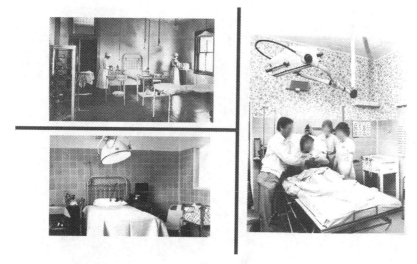

FIGURE 8.1 Historical images 20th century bio medical birth spaces.

women, ability to move according to need, a view of the external world and time passing, family presence – and loss of gentle touch, soft light, soft furnishings, familiar smells, familiar language, and sounds (Kitzinger 2011). Today, ushered into modernist biomedical/birth spaces, women find themselves swamped with anxiety-producing stimuli: an unapologetically utilitarian environment, the entire birthing suite is replete with foreign sights, smells, and noises: bright lighting to enable high visibility of occupants and the conveniently ubiquitous array of technological and discomforting objects; the lingering smells of artificial cleaning products and blood. Women are constrained through constant surveillance and limits to their freedom to move. Missing is the beauty and personal/cultural meaning that supports and enhances the emotional nature and significance of birth. But more than this, we contend that the biomedical birth environment constructed in hospitals actually alters women's instinctual birthing behaviour, leading to steadily rising rates of operative birth with both short and long-term negative consequences (Tribe et al. 2018), and rising rates of birth-related physical and psychological trauma (Beck 2018; AIHF 2021) (Figure 8.2).

The most recent decade has produced a wealth of evidence that reveals women's childbirth experiences are better when they birth at home or in freestanding birth centres (Birthplace in England Collaborative Group 2011; Hollowell et al. 2015; Homer et al. 2019). Exactly why this occurs is multifactorial and the subject of much speculation. Is it the model of birth care at home; is it the woman's ability to feel in control in her own environment; is it the lack of access to epidural anaesthetic and the much-reduced likelihood that labour will be induced, or something else? It is clear that *"aesthetic qualities of buildings have a meaningful impact on human experience"*[2]. At home the environment is already constructed or curated to be as the woman desires or, in the case of the birth centre, has

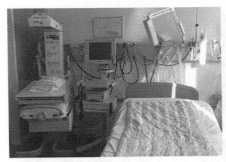

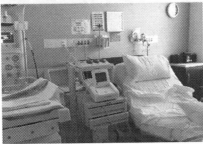

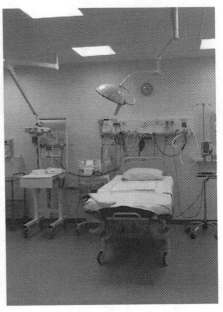

FIGURE 8.2 Focus on medical equipment and birth as a medical event.

been intentionally designed to support an understanding of the neurophysiology of birth (Odent 1992; Foureur 2008). However, even in wealthy countries few women will have the opportunity to access a birth centre (as there are few available). Fewer still will choose to birth at home as our prevailing childbirth culture wrongly believes homebirth to be fraught with danger (Scarf et al. 2018; Dahlen 2019; Hutton et al. 2019). Therefore, our focus must be on addressing the birth space in hospitals, as they so thoroughly dominate our current birth culture and health system design for maternity care.

We need to disrupt the status quo to re-imagine mindful birth spaces; spirit nourishing, spatial and sensory spaces that exemplify caring; being human in relation with and seeking harmony with all else in the universe. This will require a shift in the orientation, understanding, and enthusiasm of architects and the development of an ontological architectural awareness in birth attendants about how the birth space can and must evolve if we are to meet women's needs better (Figure 8.3).

Disrupting the status quo

New knowledge from neuroscience has enabled an increased understanding of our emotions. Neurophysiology has revealed a fundamental human need to feel safe in one's immediate surroundings – with the brain scanning the person's surrounds – moment to moment – to draw upon every sensory modality to provide input into making a judgement as to whether the environment is safe

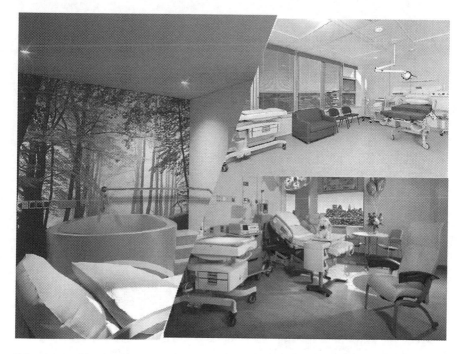

FIGURE 8.3   21st century: moving towards focus on birth experience.

or not. During childbirth, this is particularly important as the birthing woman needs to feel she is in a safe space to give birth to a vulnerable newborn. Labour will slow down or stop if the space is perceived as threatening/unsafe. We expect that women will be so reassured by the narrative of the biomedical model of childbirth and the narrative of the birth space with its ubiquitous machinery of constant surveillance – that they will feel safe. But we cannot deceive the senses for long. Unsurprisingly, the most common intervention in childbirth, once labour has begun, is to augment or speed up a slow labour that is most likely the result of a surge of adrenaline arising from the emotional perception of feeling unsafe in the biomedical birth space Buckley (2015).

There are several characteristics that architects, designers or maternity staff who are functioning mindfully can use to create birth spaces that increase womens' feelings of safety. The space must acknowledge that there is an ebb and flow to labour that needs thoughtfully designed accommodation alternatives, to which the concept of Binding can contribute. Social semiotician Maree Stenglin has identified that the way we feel in a space is influenced by how the space closes in or opens up around us, creating degrees of binding moving from bound (closes in) to unbound (opens up) (Stenglin 2004). For most of us, including women in labour, experiencing a moderately bound space appears to provide a calming and protective sense of safety. A too tightly bound space feels constrictive or claustrophobic and threatens feelings of safety. An unbound space on the other hand can also threaten safety by triggering feelings associated with exposure and insecurity. Interpretation of the degree of binding that is most comfortable can be influenced by culture or psychological makeup of the individual but also by the particular context or situation. For a woman in labour, the context changes throughout labour depending on the ebb and flow of her experience. Initially, she may feel comfortable in an unbound space as she interacts with staff, sharing the excitement of the onset of labour. As labour progresses, however, most women will want a more bound space to decrease the sense of being under constant surveillance (Stenglin and Foureur 2013) (Figure 8.4).

Most existing birth spaces embody the sense of being in highly unbound, open, brightly lit spaces that enable intense surveillance of the labouring women; there is nowhere to hide from the gaze of the healthcare professionals or her family in the room. Research has now shown us that being able to hide from the judgmental gaze of others is an important aspect of feeling safe. Immersion in water either under a shower or in a deep tub or birth pool that inevitably has high sides that surround the woman provides the opportunity to hide, which increases the sense of being in a comfortably bound, safe, and secure space (Stenglin and Foureur 2013).

Lighting is crucial to creating mood or atmosphere and contributes significantly to the concept of binding – awareness of light itself is an attunement – to locale, weather, the sky or a body of water lightening or darkening, the colour

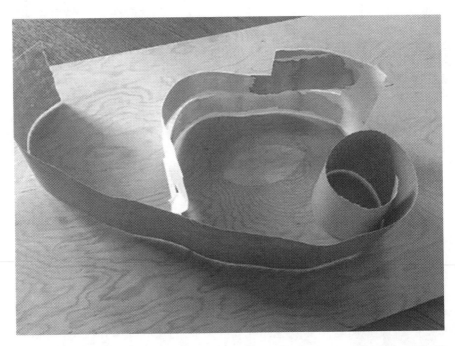

FIGURE 8.4 Conceptual Model showing spaces that are more and less bound. D. Balabanoff (2017).

of the light and vegetation shifting throughout the year, or in the course of a day. Artificial lighting for birth space has been utterly insensitive to the need for sensual lighting, minimal and flexible lighting, and privacy considerations. If nothing else is possible in an already built space, lighting can be used to create the feeling of being in an optimally bound setting through turning off overhead lighting and utilising the wide range of alternatives available today to create cosy nooks. Furthermore, startling new evidence from pineal gland research shows that the *colour* of the light in hospital entry spaces and birth environments can negatively impact the hormone melatonin, which triggers labour and works with oxytocin to sustain labour contractions (Olcese and Beesley 2014; Karpovitch et al. 2018; University of South Florida 2018).

Another characteristic that can increase feelings of being safe and secure is derived from the theoretical concept of 'Biophilia' (Wilson 1984). Biophilia explores humans' innate attraction for, indeed, need for connection to nature. 'Shinrin Yoku', or forest bathing, is one example of the important beneficial effects of connection to nature…it involves simply taking a walk and being immersed in nature, a practice that has been found to reduce heart rate, blood pressure and stress (Wen et al. 2019). If the birth environment is imagined more holistically, mindfully, biophilically, it is more than a room, it can include courtyards, forest or garden walks, views to mountains/the sea – connection to place that means home, evokes a sense of belonging, rightness, cultural significance (Figure 8.5).

In the immediate birth environment we can also experience direct, indirect, and symbolic connections to nature through providing opportunities to see and experience daylight and moonlight through openable windows that also allow for airflow; space for live plants and flowers; artwork or immersive projections; water elements; the feeling of natural materials, curved spaces and soft edges (Kellert and Wilson 2008; Vartanian et al. 2013). The cultural heritage of place, of historic and local architecture provides feelings of familiarity and security. When we are in a place that feels comfortable in these sensual and cultural ways, we can more easily settle into a private time of attunement. In a space where the surroundings have a resonant aliveness (a forest, a garden, a room with a view of the sea), we feel our own vitality in the midst of this calm, and we partake of the interconnectedness of everything (Figure 8.6).

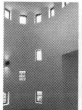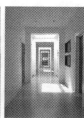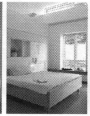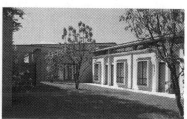

FIGURE 8.5 Brent Birth Centre, London, UK, B. Weiss Architect. photo: Gareth Gardner.

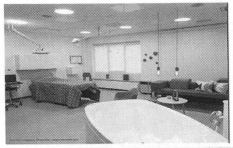
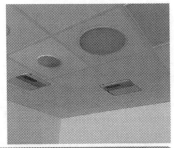
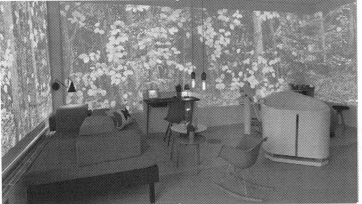

FIGURE 8.6   Immersive projection space.

Birth spaces that 'Sing'

Paul Valery asked: "Have you not noticed, about buildings: certain are mute, others speak, and others, finally – and they are the most rare - sing?" (Pallasmaa, 60). Thinking about the design of 'mindful' birth spaces we can bring together neurophysiology and poetics of space, materiality and ephemerality, science, and philosophy. 'Birth spaces that sing' would be mindful birth spaces, reminding us of breathing, of the rhythms of birth, of the resonance of our voice, our body, our attunement to being present. Birth spaces that sing would be poetic in sensibility, partaking of nature, creating delight in the sensuality of life, of birth. Birth spaces that sing might sometimes sing quietly, sometimes with vibrant energy, sometimes with melancholy. They might be serene, or full of emotion. The spatial setting is interpretable, capable of accommodating diverse ways of being… but it must not be utterly 'neutral' – a euphemism for a denial of the human spirit in all its emotional and spiritual resonance (Figure 8.7).

Each space and place of birth has not only a particular physicality composed of volumes, voids, materials, but its own ethereal resonance – made up of areas or vistas of light, colour, darkness, and of sounds and smells. Each space affords or inhibits movement; connects to or denies sunlight, vistas, and outside air. The

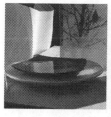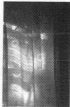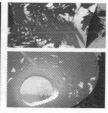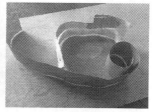

FIGURE 8.7 Sensual properties of ambient and light. D Balabanoff (2017).

space we make for birth can be open or hermetic – at best it it can offer flexible alternatives of containment or release. A mindful birth environment curates and balances the complexities of its environment to allow a focus on being in the moment, deeply aware of the power and beauty of birth.

As designers and ontological architects, we cannot avoid the time-honoured theory of Vitruvius that sets out the three fundamentals of architecture: *fitness/ structural integrity* (for site, for purpose); *functionality/commodiousness* (for use/user), and *venustas/beauty/delight* (for experiential qualities/relationships/harmonies) (Vitruvius et al. 1914)

But a new model centred on aesthetic experience is valuable for reinventing birth spaces. The 'New Aesthetics' moves beyond critical or judgemental aspects, to focus on the potency of mind–body–environment interwovenness. The experiential realm of architectural/spatial *atmosphere* brings emotional resonance, social and semiotic meanings, and opportunities for action/interaction to the discourse on aesthetic experience (Pallasmaa et al. 2015; Böhme 2017) (Figure 8.8).

In the case of birth environment design, it is precisely this concept of spatial aesthetics that is undervalued or is taken up as having to do with 'luxury' or elitist trends, or trivial desires for niceties. The notion of 'homelike' has offered a different cue, but hospitals that attempt to be 'homelike' miss the boat substantially (Bernhard et al. 2014). One needs to clarify what generates a 'homelike' spatial setting, and this is complicated (Kitzinger 2011). But as we grow in our understanding of 'felt space' as embodied experience, we can utilize what we know to make birth spaces that offer support for the emotional embodied

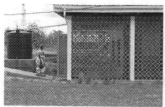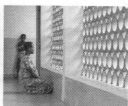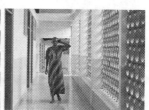

FIGURE 8.8 Kachumbala Maternity Unit, Kachumbala, Uganda HKS Architects. Photo: Peter Landers.

journey of birth. Mindfulness occurs in a space of quietude, allowing/inviting a turning/tuning to within. And we must remember the 'birth duet' that is occurring between mother and child entering the world (Leboyer 1975).

An architectural approach that considers the creation of *atmospheres* is grounded in the understanding that atmospheres exist, and we know them, feel them, can articulate them. We just don't usually think about them. Designers, working mindfully, can consider how to develop them, as Gernot Böhme has noted:

> Just as we have to learn to perceive atmospheres and to be consciously involved in them, we also need to learn the opposite, productive side of atmospheres: we have to learn to make them.
>
> *(2017: 120)*

The import of the 'new aesthetics' for mindful birth environment design is the attention to the way that spatial and material qualities provide a moodedness, a 'felt space' that matches the needs and desires of birthing women, who hope for a safe and emotionally positive personal experience.

> The experience of one's own corporeality…[is] central to bodily presence. The need to feel one's bodily presence is at once the need to feel one's own liveliness, to feel vitality.
>
> *(Böhme 2017: 95)*

Here note that 'vitality' is a remarkable atmospheric property mentioned in diverse texts as a potent aspect of our lived experience (see Balabanoff 2017: xix).

Generators of atmosphere have been described as including: (1) the geometry and configuration of the built space (e.g. layout, height, niches, expansive/contracted areas); (2) synaesthetic effects of elements of material and ambient conditions (e.g. sense of coolness created by tiling, paint colour, or air conditioning); and (3) 'social' or cultural semiotic meanings/conventions embedded in the architecture (e.g. cosiness, sacred space, medical environment, etc.) (Böhme 2017) (Figure 8.9).

Vitruvius entitled the aesthetic aspects of architecture 'Venustas', and the term literally means 'the properties of Venus" – and the goddess Venus was a personification of feminine energy and beauty – she embodied love, sexuality, and sensual aliveness. Perhaps the understanding of a mindful architecture for birth can include Venustas, in the sense of getting us away from our focus on problem-solving…of making things essentially 'structurally sound' and 'functional'. These things are necessary, but they belong to the realm of our rational busy mind. When we focus on them too intently, we can exclude Venustas, losing soulfulness, sensual aliveness, emotionality, sensory pleasure. One English translation of the Latin *Venustas* is 'delight', and Venustas includes proportional (geometric) relationships of the parts to the whole, the rhythm and form, and balancing of all the aesthetic aspects of the architecture (material, play of light, shape/form). The term Venustas evokes the beauty that architecture is capable of – the emotional resonance, the felt joy and love it can generate in

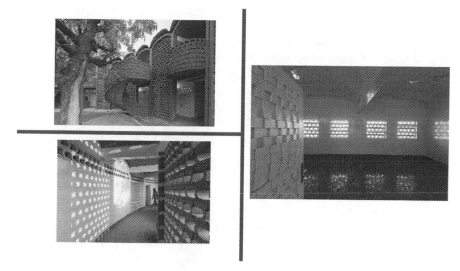

FIGURE 8.9   Tambacounda Hospital, Senegal (2021) Manuel Herz Architect w/ community consultation. Photo: Iwan Baan.

us. Such an architectural atmosphere is made by all the parts working together, and all their qualities adding to a spatial presence and meaning. But without the inhabitants/actors, and their emotional and interrelational responses/actions, a designed environment cannot actualize itself as a meaningful and delightful setting for human life (Figure 8.10).

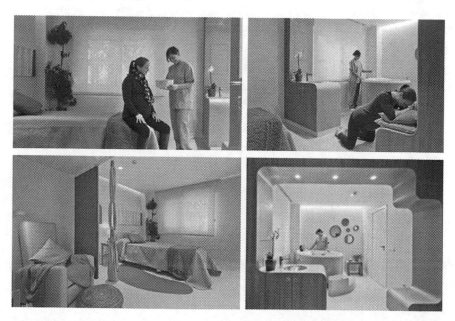

FIGURE 8.10   Natural Birth Unit Nuevo Belén Hospital, Madrid (2013) Parra-Müller Architects. Photo: David Frutos.

Conclusion

So how can existing birth rooms/units/centres, or new ones, come to be *mindful* birth spaces? We suggest that *mindfulness in the design approach* is necessary. If we take mindfulness seriously, we understand it as a way of attuning the senses to existence in the moment…seeking to being aware of and sensitive to our mind/body/environment interwovenness. But further, by contemplating birth spaces from different lenses, we learn more about how women immerse themselves in birth, and how the environment can help them achieve a deeper consciousness during birth. We begin with awareness that every sense modality counts in offering the perception and reality of emotional safety, and that the architecture/design is communicating both loud and subliminal messages directly to the brain, affecting meanings and behaviours that impact all involved.

The mindful architect, midwife, nurse, doctor, healthcare director will include *all users* of the space in creating needed change. *Cosmetic* change is not enough. We need to *all* engage deeper states of consciousness, and utilize evidence related to the mind-body-environment interrelationship in approaching and creating better birth places. It is time to make birth spaces that sing.

References

AIHF (2021). Australia's welfare 2021: In brief, summary – Australian Institute of Health and Welfare. Available: https://www.aihw.gov.au/reports/australias-welfare/australias-welfare-2021-in-brief/contents/summary.

Aminov, R.I. (2010). A brief history of the antibiotic era: Lessons learned and challenges for the future. *Frontiers in Microbiology*, 1, 134. https://doi.org/10.3389/fmicb.2010.00134.

Balabanoff, D. (2017). Light and embodied experience in the reimagined birth environment. Unpublished doctoral dissertation, University College Dublin. Available: https://www.researchgate.net/.

Beck, C. (2018). A secondary analysis of mistreatment of women during childbirth in health care facilities. *Journal of Obstetric, Gynecologic & Neonatal Nursing*, 47, 1, 94–104. https://doi.org/10.1016/j.jogn.2016.08.015.

Bernhard, C. et al. (2014). Home birth after hospital birth: Women's choices and reflections. *Journal of Midwifery & Women's Health*, 59, 2, 160–166. https://doi.org/10.1111/jmwh.12113.

Birthplace in England Collaborative Group. (2011). Perinatal and maternal outcomes by planned place of birth for healthy women with low risk pregnancies: The Birthplace in England national prospective cohort study. *BMJ*, 343, d7400. https://doi.org/10.1136/bmj.d7400.

Böhme, G. (2017). *Atmospheric architectures: The aesthetics of felt spaces*, trans./ed. Tina Engels-Schwarzpaul. London: Bloomsbury Academic.

Böhme, G. (2021). atmosphere. *Online Encyclopedia Philosophy of Nature*, 1. https://doi.org/10.11588/oepn.2021.1.80607.

Buckley, S.J. (2015). Executive summary of hormonal physiology of childbearing: Evidence and implications for women, babies, and maternity care. *The Journal of Perinatal Education*, 24, 3, 145–153. https://doi.org/10.1891/1058-1243.24.3.145.

Coburn, A., Vartanian, O. & Chatterjee, A. (2017). Buildings, beauty, and the brain: A neuroscience of architectural experience. *Journal of Cognitive Neuroscience*, 29, 9, 1521–1531.

Dahlen, H.G. (2019). Is it time to ask whether facility based birth is safe for low risk women and their babies? *EClinicalMedicine*, 14, 9–10.

De Costa, C. (2009 Autumn). Childbed fever: A major cause of maternal mortality. *Death*, 11, 1.

Foureur, M. (2008). Creating birth space to enable undisturbed birth. In Fahy, K., Foureur, M., & Hastie, C. (eds.), *Birth territory and midwifery guardianship*. Edinburgh: Elsevier.

Hodnett, E. & Abel, S.M. (1986). Person-environment interaction as a determinant of labor length variables. *Health Care for Women International*, 7, 5, 341–356, https://doi.org/10.1080/07399338609515748.

Hollowell, J. et al. (2015 August). The Birthplace in England national prospective cohort study: Further analyses to enhance policy and service delivery decision-making for planned place of birth. *Health Services and Delivery Research*, 3, 36. Southampton, UK: NIHR Journals Library. Available: https://www.ncbi.nlm.nih.gov/books/NBK311289/ https://doi.org/10.3310/hsdr03360.

Homer, C.S.E. et al. (2019). Maternal and perinatal outcomes by planned place of birth in Australia 2000 – 2012: A linked population data study. *BMJ Open*, 9, e029192. https://doi.org/10.1136/ bmjopen-2019-029192.

Hutton, E.K. et al. (2019). Perinatal or neonatal mortality among women who intend at the onset of labour to give birth at home compared to women of low obstetrical risk who intend to give birth in hospital: A systematic review and meta-analyses. *EClinicalMedicine*, 14, 59–70.

Kabat-Zinn, J. & Williams, M. G. (2011). Mindfulness: Diverse perspectives on its meaning, origins, and multiple applications at the intersection of science and dharma. *Contemporary Buddhism*, 12, 1, 1–18. https://doi.org/10.1080/14639947.2011.564811.

Karpovitch, A. E., Inna, E. & Moiseevich, K.I. (2018). In melatonin: Pregnancy and childbirth. *MOJ Current Research & Reviews*, 1, 5, 206–210.

Kellert, S.R. & Wilson, E.O. (2008). Biophilia. *Human Ecology*, 2008, 462–466.

Kitzinger, S. (2011). *Rediscovering birth, 2nd edition*. London: Pinter & Martin Ltd.

Lawrence, R. J. (2010). Deciphering interdisciplinary and transdisciplinary contributions. *Transdisciplinary Journal of Engineering & Science*, 1, 1, 125–130.

Leboyer, F. (1975). *Birth without violence*. New York: Knopf/Random House.

Loudon, I. (1992). *Death in childbirth. An international study of maternal care and maternal mortality 1800–1950*. Oxford: Clarendon Press.

Newburn, M. & Singh, D. (2005). Are women getting the birth environment they need. *Report of a national survey of women's experiences*. London: National Childbirth Trust.

Odent, M. (1992). *The nature of birth and breast-feeding*. Westport, CT: Bergin & Garvey.

Olcese, J. & Beesley, S. (2014). Clinical significance of melatonin receptors in the human myometrium. *Fertility and Sterility*, 102, 2, 329–335.

Olcese, J., Lozier, S., & Paradise, C. (2013). Melatonin and the circadian timing of human parturition. *Reproductive Sciences*, 20, 2, 168–174.

Olza, I. et al. (2020). Birth as a neuro-psycho-social event: An integrative model of maternal experiences and their relation to neurohormonal events during childbirth. *PLoS One*, 15, 7, e0230992. https://doi.org/10.1371/journal.pone.0230992.

Palasmaa, J. (2015). *Body, mind and imagination: The mental essence of architecture. In Mind in architecture: Neuroscience, embodiment and the future of design*, ed. Robinson, S. & Pallasmaa, J. Cambridge, MA: MIT Press, 51–74.

Pallasmaa, J., Mallgrave, H.F., Robinson, S. & Gallese, V. (2015). *Architecture and empathy*. Finland: Tapio Wirkkala Rut Bryk Foundation.

Reitsma, A. et al. (2020). Maternal outcomes and birth interventions among women who begin labour intending to give birth at home compared to women of low obstetrical risk who intend to give birth in hospital: A systematic review and meta-analyses. *EClinicalMedicine*, 21 (April), 100319. https://doi.org/10.1016/j.eclinm.2020.100319.

Scarf, V.L. et al. (2018). Maternal and perinatal outcomes by planned place of birth among women with low-risk pregnancies in high-income countries: A systematic review and meta-analysis. *Midwifery*, 62, 240–255.

Stenglin, M.K. (2004). Packaging curiosities: Towards a grammar of three-dimensional space. Unpublished doctoral dissertation. Department of Linguistics, Faculty of Arts, University of Sydney. Available: https://ses.library.usyd.edu.au/bitstream/2123/635/1/adt-NU20050909.16134302whole.pdf.

Stenglin, M.K. & Foureur, M. (2013). Designing out the fear cascade to increase the likelihood of normal birth. Midwifery, 29, 8, 819–825.

Tang, Y., Hölzel, B.KL., & Posner, M.I. (2015). The neuroscience of mindfulness meditation. *Nature*, 16, 21225. https://doi.org/10.1038/nrn3916.

Tew, M. (1998). *Safer childbirth? A critical history of maternity care*. London: Free Association Books ISBN 10: 1853434264; ISBN 13: 9781853434266.

Tribe, R.M. et al. (2018 December). Parturition and the perinatal period: Can mode of delivery impact on the future health of the neonate? *The Journal of Physiology*, 596, 23, 5709–5722. https://doi.org/10.1113/JP275429. Epub 2018 Apr 15. PMID: 29533463; PMCID: PMC6265543.

University of South Florida. (2018). Nightly suppression of contractions in at-risk pregnancies by the infusion of defused blue light. Clinical trial registration NCT03691740. clinicaltrials.gov.

Uvnäs Moberg, Kerstin. (2019). *Why oxytocin matters*. London: Pinter & Martin Ltd.

Vartanian, O. et al. (2013). Impact of contour on aesthetic judgement and approach-avoidance decisions in architecture. *Proceedings of the National Academy of Science, USA*, 110, 2, 10446–10453.

Vitruvius Pollio et al. (1914). Vitruvius: The ten books on architecture. Translated by Morris Hicky Morgan. [Edited and translation completed by Albert A. Howard]. Cambridge, MA: Harvard University Press.

Wen, Y. et al. (2019). Medical empirical research on forest bathing (Shinrin-yoku): A systematic review. *Environmental Health and Preventive Medicine*, 24, 70.

Wilson, E.O. (1984). *Biophilia*. Cambridge, MA: Harvard University Press.

Wrønding, T. et al. (2019). The aesthetic nature of the birthing room environment may alter the need for obstetrical interventions – an observational retrospective cohort study. *Scientific Reports*, 9 (January), 303.

Bibliography

Betran, A.P. et al. (2021). Trends and projections of caesarean section rates: Global and regional estimates. *BMJ Global Health*, 66, e005671. https://doi.org/10.1136/bmjgh-2021-005671. PMID: 34130991; PMCID: PMC8208001.

Bowden, C., Sheehan, A. & Foureur, M. (2016). Birth room images: What they tell us about childbirth. A discourse analysis of the birth environment in developed countries. *Midwifery*, 35, 71–77.

Chien, P. (2021). Global rising rates of caesarean sections. *BJOG*, 128, 5, 781–782.

Euro-Peristat. (2018). Euro-Peristat project. European perinatal health report. Core indicators of the health and care of pregnant women and babies in Europe in 2015. https://www.europeristat.com.

Hammond, A., Foureur, M. & Homer, C.S.E. (2014). The hardware and software implications of hospital birth room design: A midwifery perspective. *Midwifery*, 30, 7, 825–830.

Hammond, A., Homer, C.S.E. & Foureur, M. (2017). Friendliness, functionality and freedom: Design characteristics that support midwifery practice in the hospital setting. *Midwifery*, 50, 133–138.

Lepori, R.B. (1992). *La nascita e i suoi luoghi*. Como: Red Edizioni.

Lorentzen, I.P. et al. (2021). Does giving birth in a 'birth environment room' versus a standard birth room lower augmentation of labor? – Results from a randomized controlled trial. *European Journal of Obstetrics & Gynecology and Reproductive Biology*, X, 10 (April), 100125.

Mondy, T. et al. (2016). How domesticity dictates behaviour in the birth space: Lessons for designing birth environments in institutions wanting to promote a positive experience of birth *Midwifery*, 43, 37–47.

Setola, N. et al. (2019). The impact of the physical environment on intrapartum maternity care: Identification of eight crucial building spaces. *Health Environments Research & Design Journal*, 12, 4, 67–98.

Singh, D. & Newburn, M. (2006). Feathering the nest: What women want from the birth environment. *RCM Midwives: The Official Journal of the Royal College of Midwives*, 9, 7, 266–269.

9
BRINGING PRESENCE TO THE INTRAPARTUM EXPERIENCE

Mo Tabib and Tracy Humphrey

We have worked together as midwifery practitioners, educators and researchers for nearly 15 years. Our interest in 'relaxation' and its use in childbirth stemmed from our growing focus on women's experiences and a recognition of the increased incidence of anxiety and fearfulness of the birthing process. Having sought training in meditation and hypnosis, we incorporated many of the principles into our own practice. The results were astounding, with most women embracing this approach and many using no pharmaceutical or regional anaesthesia during childbirth. We also observed that their labour was often quicker than the average for their parity. We went on to work with a colleague to establish a dedicated service for women who had a fear of childbirth and were seeking to avoid a vaginal birth to overcome this. The content of the service focused on the principles of relaxation to make it more accessible and useful for childbirth. Women and clinicians were so positive about this service that it demanded an expansion of the provision and also warranted the training of more midwives. This service has now been accessible to any woman in this particular Health Board in Scotland for the last eight years. During this time thousands of women and many partners have attended and most completed an evaluation. This has provided us with rich insights into their experiences of the Service and how this has impacted their birth experience. We are now exploring this further in primary research and disseminating this widely. As midwifery educators and researchers, we recognised that we also needed to prepare midwives to support women using these techniques and have incorporated this into undergraduate, pre-registration curricula for student midwives. This has also been rolled out into continuous professional development for midwives building capacity and acceptability in the workforce. This chapter will examine the influence that meditation and relaxation, may have on childbirth experiences. We will draw on the existing literature and reflect on our experience of embedding the

DOI: 10.4324/9781003165200-9

knowledge and skills of meditation and relaxation within the context of antenatal education and midwifery practice in NHS maternity services in the UK. By describing the processes of development, service delivery and sharing research and evaluation, we will bring new insights to this important area of childbirth practice.

Introduction

Contemporary childbirth practices and culture across the globe with an over reliance on technology, stem from a medical model of health rooted in Cartesian medicine. Descartes the French philosopher (1596–1650) exerted a profound influence on modern Western thought and medicine with the birth of philosophical systems known as Cartesianism. Understanding the mind and the body as two distinct entities was the prominent conclusion of Descartes's work which has profoundly permeated the current health care systems including childbirth practices (Davis-Floyd 1994; Mehta 2011). In Cartesian philosophy, the birthing experience is understood as dysfunction, the pain as pathology, and the birthing body as an object requiring medical treatment and management at the discretion of the technology and childbirth experts (Goldberg 2002). It disregards the close connectedness between the woman's spirit, psyche and biological functions of her birthing body. Both health care system provision and cultural perceptions are entrenched in this paradigm. As a result, women themselves may perceive their bodies as merely a collection of mechanical systems composed of cells, tissues and biochemistry (Benner 2000). Hence, they may feel alienated and disconnected from their own bodies (Young 1998), perceiving 'here I am and there is my body' at the mercy of the health care system, medical procedures and medications.

This perceived separation from one's own body diminishes women's confidence in their birthing capability (Reed, Barnes and Rowe 2016), hence generating fear and anxiety around childbirth (Neerland 2018). There is a growing body of evidence suggesting an association between maternal feelings of fear and anxiety with a diverse range of adverse physical and psychological health outcomes for women and their offspring (Kenny et al. 2014). These include rising rates of obstetric interventions, well beyond WHO recommendations (Miller et al. 2016) with escalating and unsustainable costs for health systems (Shaw et al. 2016).

As opposed to a Cartesian paradigm, a holistic paradigm transcends the mind-body dichotomy, recognising childbirth as a biopsychosocial event shaped by the interplay of biological, psychological and cultural processes (Saxbe 2017). As such, incorporating approaches that enhance maternal emotional wellbeing in and around childbirth may play an influential role on the holistic health of the mother and child. Integrating the ancient practices of meditation and relaxation within childbirth practices and culture may offer a new possibility of shifting the current paradigm underpinning maternity care to a holistic and health-enhancing one.

Defining key terms

As the result of our exposure to the feedback collected from thousands of women and hundreds of birth attendants, our understanding of the phenomena of **'relaxation'** and **'relaxation techniques'** has evolved over years. In this chapter, we present our current understanding of such phenomena and recognise that this is still evolving. Throughout this chapter, the term 'relaxation' refers to a 'particular state of consciousness' in which the mind is still and the body is relaxed. The 'relaxation techniques', on the other hand, are considered as the gateways or tools for entering this state. The techniques we have mainly used in our teaching, research and practice include conscious breathing, body scanning, meditation, visualisation, use of silence and hypnosis. However, we also appreciate other approaches such as yoga, aromatherapy and many more as alternative gateways to the same state. To us, the tools and techniques are secondary to the primary aim of stepping into 'relaxation'.

Ella's story

Please try to engage with the following script, allow the words to become carriers of the presence and allow the silence between the words to create stillness inside you.

> '... Breathe in slowly and easily... and breathe out gently and patiently... and listen to the sound of your breathing... allow your outbreath to softly flow over your whole body... inviting the body to relax, to let go. now, feel the sensations of settling in your body... your forehead... eyelids... your jaw... allowing a gentle relaxing wave to softly flow to your neck... shoulders.... arms... your back muscles... thighs... calves... feet..., and... toe tips, relaxing your toe tips one by one... and now allow the visualisation to begin... just turn your gaze to the image of the vast calm ocean in front of you... the clear blue sky above... sense the soft powdery sand beneath and the cool breeze on your skin... remember you don't need to do anything or go anywhere right now... but 'to just be'... to be present and to be at ease with yourself and the universe around you... and to gently breathe with the slow motion of the ocean waves...".

This script is a brief reflection from a midwife caring for 17-year-old Ella[1], when she arrived at the midwife-led unit in the middle of night in a state of utter fear and distress. Ella was in the very early stage of labour and the priority was to calm her down. The midwife describes what she did:

> As I used the calm slow voice, just using the tone, the pace, I could see her going quiet, her eyes closing, her breathing slowing down, completely sinking into the bed. Then I knew she'd got it and I could go quiet.
>
> *(Louise, the midwife)*

Ella narrates her experience:

> At the beginning, I was terrified, imagining all the things that could go wrong and the pain, aye, even thought I could die… I was surprised when Louise asked me if I'd seen a cat in labour, what a strange thing to say, I thought. But it made total sense when she explained for the cat's labour to go smoothly, she hides in a dark and quiet place, you know then something clicked, I wanted to be like the cat… then I went with that meditation thing… it was a strange feeling… my body became a bit lighter and I was like 100% focused on breathing and going into myself… every pain was then a wave bringing my baby a bit closer to me, nothing to be feared… at some point it was just me and him (baby) and nothing else, it felt like everything else had faded away…
>
> *(Ella)*

Louise continues:

> with each contraction, she was just going down into herself, really shutting out the world…just disappearing into this little bubble…
>
> *(Louise, the midwife)*

Ella remained in the midwife-led unit. Her labour progressed quickly, and she gave birth to a healthy baby boy. Louise adds:

> When I handed her the baby, she looked into my eyes and said, 'that was amazing', and I felt this lump in my throat… it reminded me why I became a midwife…
>
> *(Louise, the midwife)*

Ella's journey and experience describes a childbirth experience with a seamless flow of physiological processes with a positive psychological transformation to motherhood. This points to a particular state of consciousness, when Ella was highly focused and intensely present in her own body. This has been recognised as an 'Altered State of Consciousness' (ASC) in childbirth literature (Reed, Barnes and Rowe 2016; Olza et al. 2020; Dahan 2021), a state significantly different from our habitual, day-to-day state of consciousness.

An altered state of consciousness (ASC) in physiological childbirth

ASC remains an underexplored phenomenon in childbirth research. This state is often experienced spontaneously, during physiological, unmedicated and undisturbed childbirth. The heightened senses and change in the perceptions of time and space are often the characteristics of this state (Olza et al. 2018). It is suggested that this state may well be the hallmark of childbirth as a physiological, psychological and spiritual event in humans (Olza et al. 2020). Dramatic changes in neurohormonal mechanisms including peaks in endogenous oxytocin mark ASC. The rise in endogenous oxytocin during labour is perceived to be the major factor activating the neurohormonal mechanisms involved in ASC (Uvnäs Moberg et al. 2019). Oxytocin rise activates the parasympathetic system (Davis 2017), induces pain relief, and decreases fear and stress levels (Uvnäs Moberg 2014). The neurobiological processes orchestrated by endogenous oxytocin release are considered to be responsible for transformative psychological experiences of labour and a positive transition to motherhood (Davis 2017; Hoekzema et al. 2017).

Hyperactivity of the neocortex (the part of the brain responsible for higher cognitive functions) coupled with elevated stress hormones could interrupt oxytocin release during labour, hence disrupting a positive psychological experience of childbirth for the birthing woman (Odent 2001). A risk averse and fear-driven culture in contemporary maternity services with increasing maternal surveillance during labour tends to inadvertently stimulate neocortical activity (Odent 2017). The use of bright lights, the foreign environment of the hospital, the presence of unfamiliar birth attendants, restriction to bed and medical interventions are also recognised as the stimulants of a stress response (Harris and Ayres 2012; Downe et al. 2018). All can potentially impede the health-enhancing effects of oxytocin on maternal physical and psychological wellbeing.

Downe et al. (2020) view a shift of paradigm from the current prevailing technocratic childbirth to a salutogenic one as essential for reversing the trend of escalating interventions and negative psychological outcomes of childbirth. A salutogenic perspective aims to enhance wellbeing first by understanding the origins of health and the assets for it (contrary to the origins of disease and risk factors) (Mittelmark et al. 2017). If ASC is understood as a health generating, health-enhancing state in childbirth, the salutogenic enquiry should be at the forefront of childbirth care provision. So, the question is '*how could childbirth education and practices prepare women for experiencing an ASC and foster this state during childbirth even when birth interventions are used?*'

Physiology of meditation and relaxation

Through the millennia of human evolution, the remarkable development of the neocortex has resulted in high cognitive functioning of the human brain. Whilst such high cognitive functioning or sophisticated levels of thinking have brought us cultural and technological advances, involuntary and compulsive thinking experienced in everyday life has had limiting impacts (Tolle 2001). Continuous neocortical hyperactivity in involuntary thinking is often followed by emotional arousal (Krans, Bree and Moulds 2015) that could impede the optimum physiological functions within the body. Some commentators suggest this hyperactivity could be at least partially responsible for the reduced birthing capacity of our species compared with other mammals (Odent 2019). During childbirth, neocortical activity is naturally reduced in the absence of external and internal stimuli, allowing the primitive parts of the brain to drive the process. Pre-existing fear and anxiety around childbirth are considered as examples of internal stimuli, whilst feeling of being observed and monitored, birth attendants' inappropriate comments, lack of privacy, and need for birth interventions may constitute external stimuli (Odent 1991).

Ancient practices of meditation and relaxation are known for their enabling potential in reducing mental noise, the hyperactivity of the neocortex and inducing an altered and focused state of consciousness similar to the spontaneous ASC experienced during physiological childbirth. Meditation is professed to be accompanied by the release of oxytocin in the brain which in turn contributes to an emotional sense of safety and trust (Ito et al. 2019). During meditation[2], one's attention is deliberately guided towards the breath and the body, thus shifted away from the thoughts. The awareness of a sense of presence in the body is usually experienced.

In spiritual terms, this state of presence is interpreted as connection with self and the universe, sensing self as a part of the totality of existence (Tolle 2006). Often, a subtle sense of stillness and calmness is experienced. In physiological terms, meditation is predominantly associated with reduced sympathetic activity and dominance of the parasympathetic nervous system (Manocha 2000). This effect is known as 'Relaxation Response'.

The term 'Relaxation Response' was first coined by Herbert Benson (1975; Benson and Proctor 2011). He explained that when the mind is focused or silenced through meditation, the body reacts with a dramatic response in heart rate, breathing rate, blood pressure and metabolic rate, the exact opposite effects of the fight-or-flight response. Evoking the relaxation response seems to facilitate the flow of physiological functions in the body of which childbirth is one. Figure 9.1 intends to demonstrate the proposed relationship between practice of meditation and an ASC during childbirth.

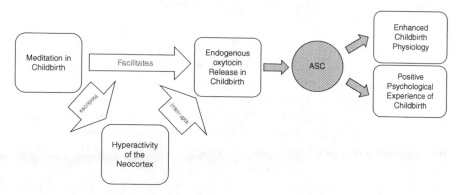

FIGURE 9.1 The proposed relationship between meditation and an ASC during childbirth.

Antenatal education: a window of opportunity

All education provided during pregnancy is recognised as a window of opportunity to make a positive impact on women's health behaviour and prepare expectant parents for childbirth (see also Chapter 7). However, a more holistic approach that is mindful of the interconnectedness between body, mind and spirit may have the potential to enhance both birth experiences and outcomes. Current Education for Pregnancy, Birth and Parenting in the context of NHS maternity services in the UK is primarily focused on providing information regarding childbirth processes and parenthood. Education on childbirth physiology and self-help methods such as meditation or hypnosis are not generally included in the mainstream antenatal education (NCT 2021). In 2011, a single-session Antenatal Relaxation Class (ARC), was introduced in our local NHS tertiary maternity hospital. The class was first established in response to the increasing number of women seeking medical interventions in the absence of clinical indicators, due to a fear of childbirth. Over time, the class has evolved into a three-hour session which is underpinned and continually improved based on theoretical and empirical literature and evidence from evaluations. The class is now available to all women and their birth partners during the third trimester of pregnancy with a maximum of 16 participants per session. It is delivered by midwives trained in relaxation techniques. ARC does not overlap with routine antenatal classes and is supplementary to them. The class starts with a comprehensive explanation of the physiological responses of the body to emotions particularly during childbirth. This is underpinned by theories of Fear-Tension-Pain (Dick-Read 2013) and physiological/hormonal processes in childbirth (Buckley 2015). The theory is then followed by several relaxation exercises including breathing and visualisation meditation, hypnosis and meditation in labour. In addition, two one-minute on-the-go techniques are introduced to allow practice during the busy daily life too, particularly when encountering anxiety-provoking situations.

Related research and service evaluation of ARC

Our ongoing primary research suggests the theory on childbirth physiology presented in ARC is seen by participants as new, liberating and challenging the traditional societal and health professionals' views (Tabib et al. 2021). This theory is filled with the notion of 'lived body' (Merleau-Ponty 1965/2013) underpinned by a holistic paradigm, evidencing how intertwined the emotions and physiological functions of the body in childbirth are. Women report that understanding the self as a lived body that is capable of influencing the physical body at a physiological level shifted their thinking about childbirth and led to feelings of confidence and empowerment whilst alleviating fear and anxiety. Lara describes:

> '...realising that the womb is a muscle, and you can work with it' as 'liberating'.

Sara comments,

> I felt really nervous and truthfully scared of labour, but after the class I felt much more confident, labour became something I looked forward to experiencing and was no longer fearful of it.

Whilst the theory provided an intellectual understanding, practice of the exercises in the class led to an appreciation and experience of their ability to step into an ASC. They describe this ASC as '*a heavy feeling, a deep sense of calmness*' (Charlotte), or a sense of '*physical presence and awareness of my body*' (Lara). Some depict it as the cessation of compulsive mind activity resulting in a sense of relaxation in the body,

> To start off, my mind goes like 20 million places but then I get to the point that I stop having such an active mind, I then feel my whole body relaxes with it.

> *(Rosie)*

This state was considered a 'respite' that they could enter whenever they experienced fear or anxiety. The 'Fear–Confidence Seesaw' (Figure 9.2) may well describe the relationship between the two phenomena of fear and confidence that are indeed two sides of the same coin. The gained confidence from the combination of theory and practice in the class seems to be alleviating fear. Furthermore, as fear is a product of mind activity, a mental project of something that 'might' happen, deliberate diversion of the attention from the thoughts to the breath and body during the meditative practices creates pauses in the thoughts stream, thus easing fear.

During pregnancy, the techniques were used for a wide range of purposes of which management of anxiety, panic attacks, insomnia, minor ailments of pregnancy and preparation for childbirth were a few examples. The practice of meditation was also associated with a rise in positive feelings, a sense of wellness, "*you could just switch off and feel good about being pregnant, so it's just a lovely experience.*" *(Angela)*

Women reported approaching childbirth feeling equipped, empowered and excited about the upcoming birth.

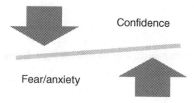

Confidence

Fear/anxiety

FIGURE 9.2 Fear–confidence seesaw.

> Having attended the class, I felt reassured, positive, and equipped to give birth. I was given that confidence, kind of, I was almost given a toolkit of how to mentally prepare myself for the birth, whatever scenario.
>
> *(Liz)*

Although discussion on birthplace is not included in ARC, some women related their eventual choice of homebirth to their understanding of childbirth physiology discussed in the class.

> Something clicked, and it was just like, you know…this is not an illness, like you go into hospital when you're ill…this is natural, this is what I was born to do.
>
> *(Louise)*

Those whose labour started spontaneously at home felt confident to apply relaxation techniques for some time at home before seeking hospitalisation. Auditing electronic notes of 93 ARC participants having their first baby showed 74% of them with spontaneous onset of labour were admitted to hospital with cervical dilatations of 5 cm or more, with some being in advanced stage of labour (Stevenson and Tabib 2020). These women expressed feelings of pride and satisfaction with their own performance.

Women used the terms '*the zone*' or '*the mood*' spontaneously and repeatedly to refer to an ASC which seemed to be the ultimate aim of using the techniques. Amy describes this state as,

> For me, labour was like a tornado, the force of it was really powerful … getting myself into the zone was like moving to the centre, to the eye of tornado and find that sacred space that nothing could touch me.
>
> *(Amy)*

Taking oneself to '*the zone*' was to allow and trust the body to do whatever it needed to do, gaining control by relinquishing control, a conscious transfer of control from the mind to the body. Conscious meditative breathing was repeatedly identified as a simple yet powerful technique influencing the experience of labour pain. Angela explains,

> …the whole experience was so positive…pain was there, but not nearly as bad as when I first gave birth. Throughout the breathing, I couldn't believe how much it did help with the pain. The first pregnancy the pain at the time seemed extreme 10 out of 10. This time, five.
>
> *(Angela)*

Likewise, women who underwent medical interventions, such as induction of labour, reported feeling confident in excerpting their learnt skills to alleviate labour pain. Charlotte, a primiparous woman whose labour was induced and had an instrumental birth comments,

> I really felt I got myself into the zone, went into a total, really focused, a calm kind of state. I took gas and air but, that was it, I didn't have anything else. I never ever felt the need to ask for anything stronger. I think I could've coped with more. I do put it down to the breathing techniques.
>
> *(Charlotte)*

What was noticeable in our research findings was that all women who were contacted after birth, irrespective of their mode of birth and the clinical picture of their childbirth experience, had creatively applied the relaxation techniques for a range of purposes including coping with stressful medical procedures and emergency situations. Liz who underwent a planned Caesarean Section, explains how the breathing techniques she used helped her to cope with the epidural insertion,

> Another thing that I practiced and used when I was getting the epidural, was the breathing exercises. I didn't feel anything, and I am not good with needles. I can hardly get bloods and I do think a lot of that was just being in the right mental space, just letting go, letting go of the idea of pain, just allowing things to happen, almost like turning it off, I suppose it (breathing exercise) just helped me do that.
>
> *(Liz)*

Another finding was that all participants described their overall experience of childbirth as positive, despite some experiencing a range of childbirth complications. Neave who underwent an emergency c-section and a major haemorrhage in the theatre comments,

> …we went through a lot, but I feel quite pragmatic about it. It was something that happened, people helped me, and I helped myself with using different techniques …I think because I had so much that I could use and rely on, I feel like I've had a really positive experience from the start.
>
> *(Neave)*

The literature suggests women experiencing childbirth complications are at greater risk of developing negative psychological outcomes such as posttraumatic stress (PTSD) or increased fear and anxiety following birth (Olde et al. 2006). Our service evaluation (Tabib and Crowther 2018) and primary research (Tabib et al. 2021) to date indicate that the practice of meditation and relaxation techniques in and around childbirth may have a buffering influence against the adverse effect of childbirth complications on maternal psychological wellbeing.

Ito et al. (2019) suggest psychological effects of oxytocin (released during meditation) as upregulating wellbeing and downregulating stress and anxiety. This makes one wonder whether it is plausible that inducing an ASC (through meditative practices) in complicated births imitates the same health-enhancing effects of a spontaneously occurring ASC during undisturbed childbirth. Is it a plausible conjecture that the endogenous oxytocin released through practice of meditation could compensate for the neurohormonal interruption occurring during complicated births? Such questions seem to be highly relevant in the context of contemporary maternity services particularly in light of increasing medical interventions and their subsequent influence on maternal psychological wellbeing.

Although the data suggested that women were capable of inducing an ASC for short episodes of time for a range of purposes during childbirth, maintaining this state through the whole labour process was highly dependent on the birth space. The birth space is defined as, '*the physical environment, people who are with the woman and what happens and is done to her*' (Joyce 2021). Physical surroundings such as lighting, privacy, or an environment that allowed freedom of movement were frequently highlighted as influential factors on women's ability to sustain that state. The space was also influenced by the clinical picture of the experience including procedures such as induction of labour. Nonetheless, midwives' impact on the space was perceived as the most influential factor, a '*game changer*' (Sandra) (see also Chapter 3).

Midwife, the game changer

In the UK and many other countries, midwives are the primary care providers for all women during labour and birth. The significant impact of the midwife on childbirth experience and environment has been well demonstrated throughout the childbirth literature. The word 'midwife' means 'to be with woman', to be attentive to her needs including the subtle psychological needs. In the context of dominant biomedical childbirth care, however, the role of the midwife is more focused on 'the doing' and what she is expected to do from institutional and medicolegal perspectives. Midwives often find the two roles of 'being with the woman' and 'the doing' in conflict, particularly when providing care in obstetric-led units, most likely to reduce their ability to 'be fully there'. Meeting the institutional expectations and performing the exhaustive list of to do tasks, naturally demands the midwife to be in a sympathetic-dominant state with the rise in stress hormones. Now, s/he is occupied, stuck in a utilitarian mood, in a conditioned pattern of behaviour to meet the obvious job demands, compromising her full attentiveness to the subtle emotional needs of the woman in her care.

In addition, emotions are contagious (Hatfield, Rapson, and Narine 2009); the midwife's sympathetic-dominant state is likely to be transmitted to the woman within the birth space and impede the physiological processes in her body (Fahy et al. 2011). Creating a birth space that radiates calmness and emotional safety, particularly in the context of obstetric-led units, requires an extraordinary level of emotional intelligence in the midwife. Emotional intelligence comprises the ability of being aware of one's own emotions and managing them effectively, recognising the emotions in others and developing nourishing relationships with others (modified from Goleman 1996). A high level of moment-to-moment awareness of own emotions and having the skills to manage these emotions, enables the midwife to be mentally and emotionally present, open, available and attuned to the woman, recognising her emotions and responding to them consciously (see also Chapter 3). This creates reciprocity and nourishing relationships that foster a health-enhancing birth space (Crowther et al. 2019). Emotional intelligence can be learned and developed (Serrat 2017) and practice of meditation is suggested to increase emotional intelligence and reduce perceived stress in workplace (Valosek et al. 2018). Meditation creates mental space for conscious responses instead of conditioned reactions.

Despite the ethos of midwifery discipline being deeply grounded in a holistic model of care, in line with the dominant technocratic birth culture, the focus of both undergraduate midwifery programs and midwives' mandatory continuous professional development (CPD) programs seem to be more on 'the doing'. This culture does not seem to recognise that 'doing' is never enough if 'being' is neglected (Tolle 2006). We started implementing education on the concepts of emotional intelligence, meditation and involved psychological and physiological processes in both undergraduate Midwifery programme and CPD programmes for midwives in 2014. It includes educating the practitioners on how 'to be' in the world and how 'to be' with others, a state of 'being' out of which a different quality of 'the doing' can flow. A practical example of such an approach is dealing with and managing an obstetric emergency whilst remaining attuned to the psychological needs of the woman in the moment. Such an approach to care may reduce women's fears and anxieties. The positive influence of this approach for many women including those at risk of birth trauma became evident in the data collected from hundreds of women, midwives and student midwives.

To date approximately 100 midwives and over 400 student midwives have undertaken the education. The feedback collected suggests that, similar to ARC participants, they had applied their learning to their personal lives for a wide range of purposes such as dealing with anxiety, conflicting relationships at work or home and even insomnia. In their practice, they had creatively tailored the skills to different clinical scenarios. Helping women with needle phobia, providing psychological support prior to or during the medical procedures, facilitating physiological childbirth and use of the techniques as a pain relief method were a few examples. Midwives' ability to contribute to women's positive experiences seemed to have contributed to a high level of satisfaction with their own performance.

I started to use my relaxation skills with her, in this situation we ended up being transferred to theatre but even in there, we did the gentle breathing techniques, and it was the nicest c-section I had been in, as it felt like we were in our own little bubble…

(Megan, the student midwife) (see Chapter 15 for further discussion on mindfulness in education)

Implications for practice

The contemporary role of the midwife is identified as emotionally demanding with many midwives across the UK experiencing high levels of stress, burnout, anxiety and depression (Hunter et al. 2019), and a great number considering leaving the profession (Harvie et al. 2019). This is of critical concern to the profession and has serious implications for the delivery of high-quality, safe maternity care. One of the major factors compromising the midwives' emotional wellbeing and contributing to their intention to leave the profession is the conflict between midwives' aspiration of truly 'being with the woman' and the medicalised and mind-dominated institutional expectations of the role which is mainly focused on 'the doing' aspects of the job. The current medicalised culture has led to rising rate of unnecessary childbirth interventions coupled with adverse health outcomes, unsustainable costs and an emotionally exhausted workforce. A substantial shift in this risk-focused, fear-generating culture to a holistic, health-focused and health-enhancing one is deemed to be long overdue.

The philosophical essence of meditation is to recognise an ASC, a state altered from our habitual and mind-dominated state. Stepping into an ASC is to be here in the now, is to step back from conditioned thoughts, judgements and interpretations, and all those mind-made stories. It is to consciously see the self and the world as they really are, with fresh eyes. This new and pristine way of seeing then opens us up to new possibilities, we become more aware of the conditioned patterns of the mind and 'the doing', not only at an individual level but at organisational scales too.

Embedding the philosophy of meditation and relaxation in maternity services at an organisational level has the potential to permeate the 'being' of the system and that of the humans operating in it. Such an overarching approach could create and protect 'the space' where the health and wellbeing of the workforce, childbearing women, their families and the next generation can flourish in. After all, we are all connected!

Implications for future research

To date, the research in the field has mainly concentrated on the effect of antenatal relaxation (or meditation) education on short-term childbirth outcomes. There is little known about the potential influence of such education on long-term health outcomes for the mother and child. In addition, there is a paucity of evidence around the influence of all-encompassing and complex interventions comprising antenatal education, education for the birth practitioners and revisiting institutional ethos. Such overarching interventions are more likely to meaningfully impact the outcomes at statistically significant levels. They would also allow investigating the impact on workforce's emotional wellbeing, emotional intelligence and their job satisfaction levels. Nonetheless, simultaneous implementation of and researching such complex and overarching interventions demands a strong will and support from the policy makers and funding bodies.

Conclusion

In this chapter, we have introduced the concept and theories behind maternity care provision leading to the medicalisation of childbirth and subsequently a lack of confidence in women's ability to birth without it being distressing or requiring unnecessary or iatrogenic childbirth interventions. This means that some women approach childbirth with emotions of fear and anxiety. Relaxation and meditation could improve women's confidence and experiences of childbirth. As demonstrated by our own initiative, even a single session on bringing meditation and relaxation into childbirth can bring women back into the presence of their own birthing experience without apprehension. If such education is to be effectively translated into practice, then midwives must be adequately prepared to facilitate a birthing space that is conducive to the sense of presence. Incorporating education on the ancient practices of meditation along with the contemporary understanding of their physiological, psychological and spiritual impact into pre-registration midwifery curricula and post-registration professional development will build and sustain midwifery capability and capacity in this area. Of course, more research is needed; particularly into the longer-term or unintended benefits to women, families as well as health professionals providing maternity care.

Notes

1 All names in this chapter, other than the authors and cited sources have been given pseudonyms to ensure anonymity.
2 Meditation in this sense refers to mindfulness practice.

References

Benner, Patricia. "The roles of embodiment, emotion and lifeworld for rationality and agency in nursing practice." *Nursing Philosophy* 1, no. 1 (2000): 5–19.

Benson, H. "with Klipper MZ. *The relaxation response.* New York: William Morrow and Co." (1975).

Benson, Herbert, and William Proctor. *Relaxation revolution: The science and genetics of mind body healing.* New York: Simon and Schuster, 2011.

Buckley, Sarah J. "Executive summary of hormonal physiology of childbearing: Evidence and implications for women, babies, and maternity care." *The Journal of Perinatal Education* 24, no. 3 (2015): 145–153.

Crowther, Susan, Cary L. Cooper, Fiona Meecham, and Neal M. Ashkanasy. "The role of emotion, empathy, and compassion in organisations." In *Squaring the circle: Normal birth research, theory and practice in a technological age*, edited by S. Byrom and S. Downe, pp. 111–119. London: Pinter and Martin, 2019.

Dahan, Orli. "Birthing consciousness: A lacuna in evolutionary psychological science." *New Ideas in Psychology* 60 (2021): 100822.

Davies, Lorna. "Biobehavioural aspects of parenting." In *Physiology in Childbearing*, 4th ed., edited by Jean Rankin, pp. 597–603. Edinburgh: Elsevier, 2017.

Davis-Floyd, Robbie. "Culture and birth: The technocratic imperative." *International Journal of Childbirth Education* 9, no. 2 (1994): 6–7.

Dick-Read, Grantly. *Childbirth without fear: The principles and practice of natural childbirth.* London: Pinter & Martin Publishers, 2013.

Downe, Soo, Jean Calleja Agius, Marie-Clare Balaam, and Lucy Frith. "Understanding childbirth as a complex salutogenic phenomenon: The EU COST BIRTH Action Special Collection." *PLoS One* 15, no. 8 (2020): e0236722.

Downe, Soo, Kenneth Finlayson, Olufemi Oladapo, Mercedes Bonet, and A. Metin Gülmezoglu. "What matters to women during childbirth: A systematic qualitative review." *PLoS One* 13, no. 4 (2018): e0194906.

Fahy, Kathleen, Jenny Parratt, Maralyn Foureur, and Carolyn Hastie. "Birth territory: A theory for midwifery practice." In *Theory for Midwifery Practice*, 2nd ed., edited by R. Bryar and M. Sinclair, pp. 215–240. Basingstoke: Palgrave, 2011.

Goldberg, Lisa. "Rethinking the birthing body: Cartesian dualism and perinatal nursing." *Journal of Advanced Nursing* 37, no. 5 (2002): 446–451.

Goleman, Daniel. *Emotional Intelligence: Why it can matter more than IQ.* London: Bloomsbury, 1996.

Harris, Rachel, and Susan Ayers. "What makes labour and birth traumatic? A survey of intrapartum 'hotspots'." *Psychology & Health* 27, no. 10 (2012): 1166–1177.

Harvie, Karina, Mary Sidebotham, and Jennifer Fenwick. "Australian midwives' intentions to leave the profession and the reasons why." *Women and Birth* 32, no. 6 (2019): e584-e593.

Hatfield, Elaine, Richard L. Rapson, and Victoria Narine. "Emotional contagion and empathy." In *The social neuroscience of empathy*, edited by Jean Decety and Ickes William, pp. 19–30. Boston, MA: MIT Press, 2009.

Hoekzema, Elseline, Erika Barba-Müller, Cristina Pozzobon, Marisol Picado, Florencio Lucco, David García-García, Juan Carlos Soliva et al. "Pregnancy leads to long-lasting changes in human brain structure." *Nature neuroscience* 20, no. 2 (2017): 287–296.

Hunter, Billie, Jennifer Fenwick, Mary Sidebotham, and Josie Henley. "Midwives in the United Kingdom: Levels of burnout, depression, anxiety and stress and associated predictors." *Midwifery* 79 (2019): 102526.

Ito, Etsuro, Rei Shima, and Tohru Yoshioka. "A novel role of oxytocin: Oxytocin-induced well-being in humans." *Biophysics and Physicobiology* 16 (2019): 132–139.

Joyce, Sarah. "Re-naming the 'birth environment' an architect's view." *The Practising Midwife* 24, no. 1 (2021): 23–28.

Kenny, Louise C., Claire Everard, and Ali S. Khashan. "Maternal stress and in utero programming." In *Hormones, intrauterine health and programming*, edited by J. Seckl and Y. Christen, pp. 41–55. Cham: Springer, 2014.

Krans, Julie, June de Bree, and Michelle L. Moulds. "Involuntary cognitions in everyday life: Exploration of type, quality, content, and function." *Frontiers in Psychiatry* 6 (2015): 7.

Manocha, Ramesh. "Why meditation?." *Australian Family Physician* 29, no. 12 (2000): 1135–1138.

Mehl-Madrona, Lewis E. "Hypnosis to facilitate uncomplicated birth." *American Journal of Clinical Hypnosis* 46, no. 4 (2004): 299–312.

Mehta, Neeta. "Mind-body dualism: A critique from a health perspective." *Mens Sana Monographs* 9, no. 1 (2011): 202.

Merleau-Ponty, Maurice. *Phenomenology of perception*. London: Routledge, 2022.

Miller, Suellen, Edgardo Abalos, Monica Chamillard, Agustin Ciapponi, Daniela Colaci, Daniel Comandé, Virginia Diaz et al. "Beyond too little, too late and too much, too soon: A pathway towards evidence-based, respectful maternity care worldwide." *The Lancet* 388, no. 10056 (2016): 2176–2192.

Mittelmark, Maurice B., Shifra Sagy, Monica Eriksson, Georg F. Bauer, Jürgen M. Pelikan, Bengt Lindström, and Geir Arild Espnes. *The handbook of salutogenesis*. Cham (CH): Springer, 2017.

NCT. 2021. "Hypnobirthing: Where to start." 1st 1,000 Days, Natural Childbirth Trust, last revised March 2021. https://www.nct.org.uk/labour-birth/getting-ready-for-birth/hypnobirthing-where-start

Neerland, Carrie E. "Maternal confidence for physiologic childbirth: A concept analysis." *Journal of Midwifery & Women's Health* 63, no. 4 (2018): 425–435.

Odent, Michel. "New reasons and new ways to study birth physiology." *International Journal of Gynecology & Obstetrics* 75 (2001): S39–S45.

Odent, Michel. *The Birth of Homo, the Marine Chimpanzee*. London: Pinter & Martin, 2017

Odent, Michel. *The Future of Homo*. London: Pinter & Martin, 2019

Odent, Michel R. "Fear of death during labour." *Journal of Reproductive and Infant Psychology* 9, no. 1 (1991): 43–47.

Olde, Eelco, Onno van der Hart, Rolf Kleber, and Maarten van Son. "Posttraumatic stress following childbirth: A review." *Clinical Psychology Review* 26, no. 1 (2006): 1–16.

Olza, Ibone, Patricia Leahy-Warren, Yael Benyamini, Maria Kazmierczak, Sigfridur Inga Karlsdottir, Andria Spyridou, Esther Crespo-Mirasol et al. "Women's psychological experiences of physiological childbirth: A meta-synthesis." *BMJ Open* 8, no. 10 (2018): e020347.

Olza, Ibone, Kerstin Uvnas-Moberg, Anette Ekström-Bergström, Patricia Leahy-Warren, Sigfridur Inga Karlsdottir, Marianne Nieuwenhuijze, Stella Villarmea et al. "Birth as a neuro-psycho-social event: An integrative model of maternal experiences and their relation to neurohormonal events during childbirth." *PLoS One* 15, no. 7 (2020): e0230992.

Reed, Rachel, Margaret Barnes, and Jennifer Rowe. "Women's experience of birth: Childbirth as a rite of passage." *International Journal of Childbirth* 6, no. 1 (2016): 46–56.

Saxbe, Darby E. "Birth of a new perspective? A call for biopsychosocial research on childbirth." *Current Directions in Psychological Science* 26, no. 1 (2017): 81–86.

Serrat, Olivier. "Understanding and developing emotional intelligence." In *Knowledge solutions*, pp. 329–339. Singapore: Springer, 2017.

Shaw, Dorothy, Jeanne-Marie Guise, Neel Shah, Kristina Gemzell-Danielsson, K. S. Joseph, Barbara Levy, Fontayne Wong, Susannah Woodd, and Elliott K. Main. "Drivers of maternity care in high-income countries: Can health systems support woman-centred care?." *The Lancet* 388, no. 10057 (2016): 2282–2295.

Stevenson, Geraldine, and Tabib Mo. An audit of electronic maternity records for the participants of Antenatal Relaxation Classes (2019 data). Unpublished raw data. 2020

Tabib, Mo, and Susan Crowther. "Service evaluation of relaxation workshops for pregnant women." *The Journal of Perinatal Education* 27, no. 1 (2018): 10–19.

Tabib, Mo, Tracy Humphrey, Katrina Forbes-McKay, and Annie Lau. "Expectant parents' perspectives on the influence of a single antenatal relaxation class: A qualitative study." *Complementary Therapies in Clinical Practice* 43 (2021): 101341.

Tolle, Eckhart. *The power of now: A guide to spiritual enlightenment.* London: New World Library, 2001.

Tolle, Eckhart. *A new earth: Awakening to your life's purpose.* New York: Penguin Group, 2006.

Uvnäs-Moberg. *Oxytocin: The biological guide to motherhood.* Amarillo, TX: Praeclarus Press, LLC, 2014.

Uvnäs-Moberg, Kerstin, Anette Ekström-Bergström, Marie Berg, Sarah Buckley, Zada Pajalic, Eleni Hadjigeorgiou, Alicja Kotłowska et al. "Maternal plasma levels of oxytocin during physiological childbirth–a systematic review with implications for uterine contractions and central actions of oxytocin." *BMC Pregnancy and Childbirth* 19, no. 1 (2019): 1–17.

Valosek, Laurent, Janice Link, Paul Mills, Arthur Konrad, Maxwell Rainforth, and Sanford Nidich. "Effect of meditation on emotional intelligence and perceived stress in the workplace: A randomized controlled study." *The Permanente Journal* 22 (2018): 17–172.

Young, Iris Marion. "Pregnant embodiment." In *Body and flesh: A philosophical reader*, edited by Donn Welton, pp. 247–285. Oxford: Blackwell, 1998.

10

PARADIGM OF PAIN IN THE BIRTH SPHERE

Liz Newnham, Laura Whitburn and Lester Jones

Introduction

It is challenging to understand someone else's pain and predict its effect on them. With increasing questions about the relationship between pain and tissue damage, pain is now understood to be complex, individual, contextual and subjective experience that defies objective evaluation (Whitburn 2013). It is the result of complex central processing, largely attributed to the brain. Pain emerges when this complex processing identifies the need for a person to address a threat to safety, and is shaped by sensory, emotional, cognitive and social inputs. Pain triggers us to take notice of our body and our environment and motivates us to do something to either protect ourselves or escape, or alert others of our plight (Whitburn 2013).

The experience of pain as part of the normal physiology of labour is somewhat unique. Typically, pain is associated with states of ill-health, such as injuries, pathologies and diseases, and in these contexts, pain alerts us that something is wrong. However, uncomplicated labour is not a state of ill-health – labour is part of the normal and essential function of childbirth that promotes the survival of our species. What, then, is the function of pain in the labour and birth context?

As authors, our interest in this topic has arisen as birthing women (LW and EN), supporters of birthing women (LJ), midwives (EN) and birth and pain researchers (LW, EN and LJ). Our collective experiences have led us to believe that there is an association between the relevance of pain and the concept of a state of mindfulness. We feel that mindfulness can be viewed as a state where a person lets their body find its normal or even primal state, unaffected by expectations, fears or external influences and influencers. This accepting and non-reactive state is not passive but allows normal physiological processes such as labour to calibrate to basic instincts and drives. Pain is a first-person experience that cannot be directly known, observed or measured by another. Pain only exists in the conscious

DOI: 10.4324/9781003165200-10

mind of the person experiencing it, therefore, consideration of the concept of the human mind is pivotal to understanding the human experience of pain. Our previous research has demonstrated that women in labour have the innate capacity to adopt a state of mind that we describe as mindful, and this influences their experience of labour pain (Whitburn et al. 2014). During our own labours, we have experienced the power of birthing hormones, and their effect on our consciousness, awareness of space and time, thoughts and feelings, and our perception of pain. A better understanding of these processes provides important clues to how to better support women to work with their birthing hormones, and tap into this primal state of mindfulness; to change their experience of pain and enhance their capacity to cope.

To understand the human experience of pain, and the role of pain in the context of labour and birth, we will explore a number of topics in this chapter. We will review the current definitions of pain and consider how labour pain fits into accepted theoretical frameworks of pain. We will examine how birthing hormones may alter the consciousness of a labouring woman and consider how the experience of pain in childbirth might be moderated if she achieves a state of mindfulness. Finally, we will consider how this knowledge is relevant practically, informing including the critical role that supports people can play in shaping a woman's experience of labour pain.

Pain definitions – What does labour pain fit in?

A view of labour pain as anything other than a sign of suffering challenges many preconceptions held regarding what pain is, how it comes about, and its role in our lives. According to the International Association for the Study of Pain (IASP), pain is: "An unpleasant sensory and emotional experience associated with, or resembling that associated with, actual or potential tissue damage" (Raja et al. 2020) (see Box 1 for accompanying notes).

Box 10.1 Six key notes accompanying the IASP definition (Raja et al. 2020)

- Pain is always a personal experience that is influenced to varying degrees by biological, psychological and social factors.
- Pain and nociception are different phenomena. Pain cannot be inferred solely from activity in sensory neurons.
- Through their life experiences, individuals learn the concept of pain.
- A person's report of an experience as pain should be respected.
- Although pain usually serves an adaptive role, it may have adverse effects on function and social and psychological well-being.
- Verbal description is only one of several behaviours to express pain; inability to communicate does not negate the possibility that a human or a nonhuman animal experiences pain.

Despite this definition being broadly accepted in clinical and academic contexts, it presents challenges when applied to the context of labour. The challenges relate to the focus on, and reliance of, tissue *damage* – actual or perceived – in the definition, and its implication that the function of pain is to indicate damage to the body. We agree that there is a tissue component to pain experienced in labour as various body structures are stretched and compressed beyond normal, causing nociception. However, this is not necessarily tissue *damage* and particularly not in the sense of a pathological change to the tissues (Whitburn et al. 2017). Labour is a healthy physiological process, and so the pain that occurs in an uncomplicated labour is uniquely different from the pain that is associated with pathology. Also missing from the definition is acknowledgement of the significant role of cognitions and the social environment in shaping a person's pain experience – variables that are particularly important in the context of childbirth (Whitburn et al. 2017).

We suggest that labour pain is different from other kinds of pain. Tissue changes that occur during an uncomplicated labour are not pathological. In this sense, pain in labour is unique in that it is associated with a healthy physiological process and a positive outcome – the birth of a baby. The growing intensity of pain during normal labour generally indicates that this process is functioning well. Importantly, pain in labour helps drive the neurohormonal events required to make labour efficient and effective (Buckley 2015). As we will examine in the next section, this hormonal cascade helps the woman manage the growing intensity of pain and contributes to her and her baby's well-being.

Pain and the neurohormonal cascade

To fully understand the pain associated with labour, we believe it is critical to understand the hormonal sequence that drives normal physiological childbirth because pain forms part of the complex hormonal feedback loop, both affecting and being alleviated by labour hormones. The sensations of labour, including those characterised as pain, help to drive this process which ultimately facilitates an efficient and effective birth (Buckley 2015). To understand how these processes affect the way women perceive their childbirth experience, we will first explore the basic neurophysiology of brain evolution and function.

In a simplistic model of the brain, we can divide it into three areas that have developed sequentially through evolution – the brainstem, limbic system and cortex. The brainstem is described as controlling basic survival or primal functions including the sympathetic 'fight, flight or freeze' stress response. Importantly, actions driving the birthing process will be controlled by the brainstem. The limbic system mediates human emotion – such as fear (via the amygdala) and joy. It also generates motivational states and appraises incoming information, giving it meaning and determining if it is worth paying attention to (Legrain et al. 2009, Shackman et al. 2011). This part of the brain also includes our social engagement system – the part that motivates us as social beings to connect with others and form attachments to caregivers (Amodio and Frith 2006, Porges

2005). Finally, there is the neocortex, which consists of the top layer of the cerebral hemispheres and is involved in higher-order functions including thinking and judgement, language and self-awareness.

During normal physiological childbirth, three hormonal systems play critical roles in driving labour and, in doing so, affect these brain regions: oxytocin, beta-endorphins and stress hormones (adrenaline, noradrenaline, cortisol). We have summarised the effects of these hormones in Table 10.1. **Oxytocin** is released by the maternal brain and has systemic (bodily) and central (brain) effects. Systemically, oxytocin is released (by the pituitary gland) into the bloodstream in pulses, causing the rhythmic uterine contractions of labour. Centrally, oxytocin is released into the limbic system. Here, it attenuates activity in the amygdala and sympathetic nervous system (SNS), to reduce fear and stress (Riem et al. 2011). Oxytocin also activates the parasympathetic nervous system (PNS), social neural pathways and dopamine-associated brain reward pathways to trigger pleasure, promote calmness and social connection (Uvnäs Moberg 2003). These psychological and emotional effects support the labouring woman to manage the growing intensity of her labour and prepares her to bond with her new-born.

Through a positive feedback mechanism, oxytocin levels build throughout labour. This mechanism depends on feedback from nerve endings in the uterus, which are stimulated by pressure and stretch of tissues during contractions and signal to the hypothalamus to trigger further oxytocin. As labour progresses into the second stage, the foetal head stimulates receptors in the vagina and cervix that trigger a flood of oxytocin release. Known as the Ferguson reflex (Ferguson 1941), this triggers stronger contractions that facilitate a swift and effective birth, while at the same time giving the birthing woman a flood of oxytocin in the brain.

As oxytocin works to increase the intensity of uterine contractions, the powerful stretch and compression of abdominal and pelvic tissues will activate nociceptors. Nociceptors are 'danger' receptors located in our bodily tissues that respond to noxious (potentially dangerous) tissue changes. Nociception is one of the many inputs the brain uses to shape a pain experience. Nociceptive input into the central nervous system, as well as stress and oxytocin, triggers the release of **beta-endorphins**. These endogenous opioids have an analgesic effect by attenuating nociceptive transmission and enhancing descending inhibition (Basbaum and Fields 1984). Beta-endorphins also subdue the neocortex and activate brain rewards centres, inducing a euphoric and altered state of mind (Sauriyal, Jaggi, and Singh 2011). Inhibition of acoustic and visual information by beta-endorphins may further contribute to this altered state of consciousness, facilitating the woman to become inwardly focussed (Hartwig 1991). This dynamic link between beta-endorphins and oxytocin helps the woman manage the mounting intensity of uterine contractions and associated psycho-emotional stresses. Often, in early labour, women report fearing that they will not be able to cope with any further rises in intensity. By considering the neurohormonal cascade here, it is apparent that in those moments, these women may not yet be benefiting from the beta-endorphin release that is soon to come.

Women whose labour is driven by their birthing hormones will experience associated shifts through three brainwave states: beta waves, associated with the 'thinking' neocortex (e.g. language, self-awareness and active problem solving); alpha waves, associated with inward focus and relaxation; and theta waves, the deepest we can experience when awake and associated with an unfocussed state where time can feel elastic and experience is driven by the emotional limbic system (Davis and Pascali–Bonaro 2010).

Finally, it is important to consider the role of the **stress hormones**, particularly adrenalin and noradrenalin (referred to from here on as adrenalin), in labour progress and labour pain. Adrenalin is released in response to stress, perceived threats or fear. It activates the fight–flight–freeze response of the SNS and shuts down the calming and connecting PNS. We can consider childbirth to be a 'healthy' eustress, where adrenalin levels start low, then gradually rise as labour becomes more intense. Rising adrenalin levels may help to mobilise metabolic fuels for the physical effort of labour, as well as keep a woman's senses on high alert, helping her remain vigilant to possible dangers. As a result, despite the dream–like and drowsy effects of beta-endorphins, she will remain sensitive to sounds around her – including comments from those caring for her. Adrenalin levels then peak towards the end of the first stage, stimulating the neocortex and priming the woman for the physical effort required in the second stage. This can often be observed by those caring for birthing women as the women suddenly become highly alert (due to adrenalin countering the drowsy effects of beta-endorphins) and capable of the huge physical effort of the second stage (Buckley 2015), despite their seemingly exhausted state just moments before (Dixon, Skinner, and Foureur 2013).

Adrenalin levels that are elevated prematurely by stress or fear can interfere with labour progress by inhibiting oxytocin, decreasing uterine blood flow and slowing contractions (Newton, Foshee, and Newton 1966). This phenomenon may be seen as a woman moves from home to the birthing hospital – an unfamiliar space with unfamiliar caregivers and usually associated with a reduction in privacy. In the context of a mammal in the wild who is faced with a perceived threat, slowing and/or stopping labour to facilitate escape is appropriate. However, in the modern-day context of a woman moving to a hospital for care, this response is unhelpful and may lead to intervention to help stimulate her stalled labour. High adrenalin levels also increase alertness (Tsigos and Chrousos 2002), making a woman more aware of her surroundings and stimulating her 'thinking' neocortex – *Is my baby okay? Can I cope? When will this end?* These future-oriented thoughts become perceived threats that may further trigger the stress response. Ultimately, adrenalin will interrupt the dynamic interplay of oxytocin and beta-endorphins that are calming the mother and helping her to manage pain.

Many other common interventions, such as inductions, augmentations, opioid analgesic drugs and epidurals, as well as the type of care provided and the labour environment, have been shown to further interrupt these hormonal mechanisms and affect a woman's experience and birth, and postnatal outcomes, including attachment between mother and baby (Buckley 2015).

TABLE 10.1 Effects of Birthing Hormonal Systems on Cognitions, Emotions and Pain Perception

Hormonal System	Effect
Oxytocin	• Reduces stress, fear and anxiety • Promotes calmness and social connection • Activates dopamine-associated brain reward pathways, triggering pleasure and driving attachment • Analgesia – decreases pain
Beta-endorphins	• Inhibits thinking brain (neocortex) – induces altered state of consciousness • Inhibits acoustic and visual information processing – attention inwardly focussed • Stimulate reward and pleasure centres • Analgesia – decreases pain
Stress hormones (in excess)	• Increases alertness – attention outwardly focussed • Triggers fear regions (amygdala) in brain • Redirects blood flow away from uterus • Inhibits oxytocin – slows labour • Inhibits analgesic effects of oxytocin and beta-endorphins – increases pain perception • Increases attention to pain experience – can trigger pain catastrophising

Pain vulnerability

In the context of labour, the woman's prior exposure to painful experiences and adverse life events, including previous traumatic labour, may prime her system to be more pain reactive. The relatively recent idea of *pain vulnerability* is worth mentioning here. Pain vulnerability was proposed as an explanation of why some people might be more susceptible to developing a painful condition. Three components are used to explain this susceptibility: inherited *genetic profile, environmental influences*, and *gene and environment interactions* (Denk, McMahon, and Tracey 2014). This neurobiological explanation describes processes that prime the nociceptive system to be more reactive. Influences on the expression of pain include previous painful experiences and stressful events. It has been demonstrated that the number of adverse life events experienced is associated with the development of ongoing painful conditions (Generaal et al. 2016). This is important knowledge for those responsible for supporting women in labour as it provides an explanation for the variability in the intensity of pain that is not associated with tissue changes.

Current discourses of childbirth pain

Given the powerful effects of labour hormones in supporting women through labour and promoting hers and her baby's wellbeing, why are physiological birth rates declining? Although there are women opting for physiological birth uninterrupted by pharmacological or medical intervention, it is increasingly common for women to request pharmacological analgesia such as nitrous oxide gas, opioids and epidural, and even surgical births without a medical indication, to avoid pain (McAra-Couper, Jones, and Smythe 2012). While desire or request for analgesia during birth may be understandable, particularly if labour is not straightforward, it is also occurring because practices and environments that support physiological birth are not always prioritised (Newnham, McKellar, and Pincombe 2018). In addition, there are competing social discourses about labour pain, which are based on a variety of assumptions and knowledge claims (Newnham, McKellar, and Pincombe 2016).

Current discourses of childbirth and pain include such ideas as:

- Women are unable to tolerate labour pain
- It is of utmost importance (to women, and above all else) to relieve women of labour pain
- Medicine rescues women from labour pain
- Pain relief is a human right
- Pain relief is associated with progress and modernity (experiencing pain is therefore 'archaic')
- Pain relief is safe (Newnham, McKellar, and Pincombe 2016).

These ideas, which float through the ether of late modernity, signal to women that labour analgesia, specifically epidural analgesia, is a panacea that can relieve the 'barbaric' torture of birth pain and replace it with a risk-free, pleasant experience. Opioids have long been used as labour analgesia, but have moderate analgesic effect and bring more well-known side effects such as sedation, nausea and vomiting, and risks of respiratory depression (Smith, Burns, and Cuthbert 2018). This has led to a preference towards epidural analgesia, where it is available, as the more effective analgesia (Madden et al. 2013). However, what women are often not aware of is that epidural analgesia actually does come with significant possible adverse effects (Smith, Burns, and Cuthbert 2018). Some of these are negligible, but risks include: maternal fever (pyrexia) which can lead to maternal and infant separation at birth and the use of antibiotics; instrumental birth, which in turn increases the risk of a severe perineal tear, and the possibility for severe pathological pain, for months, even years after the birth of the baby; and decreased success in breastfeeding, leading to maternal distress and disturbance to the microbiome and future wellbeing of the infant (Anim-Somuah et al. 2018, Newnham, McKellar, and Pincombe 2016, Newnham et al. 2020). Epidural analgesia also halts or greatly diminishes maternal oxytocin production, which interrupts the feedback loop of labour hormones (Buckley 2015). Effects of this can mean stalled labour and the use of synthetic oxytocin, which does not cross the blood-brain barrier and therefore does not stimulate beta-endorphins in the same way. In addition, despite epidural analgesia being very effective at relieving pain, women who use this form of pain relief are not necessarily more satisfied with their birth experience and some studies have reported decreased satisfaction and a more distinct memory of the pain of labour (Hodnett 2002, Uvnäs Moberg 2016). These findings are likely due to this interference with birth hormones, although there is a lack of research in this area. However, it is enough to cast doubt on the widespread availability of epidural analgesia as a routine labour analgesia.

In addition, these factors are not usually acknowledged within the medical literature, which is broadly dismissive of the pain caused by iatrogenic harm or intervention, and often does not address long-term outcomes or the effect of outcomes on a woman's life and wellbeing. The emphasis rests exclusively on relieving labour pain (at any cost)—and is underpinned by a science that has as its basis a historic mistrust of women's bodies, a belief that (physiological) birth is dangerous, that pain is detrimental and that women cannot cope with it, and that medicine provides rescue (Newnham, McKellar, and Pincombe 2018).

It is clear, however, that despite its intensity, women can experience labour pain without distress or suffering (Whitburn et al. 2019), and this can be more easily understood when considering the positive effects of oxytocin and beta-endorphins on activating pleasure and reward centres in the brain during labour and birth to promote psychological wellbeing.

What matters: Women's experiences

It has only been within recent history that researchers have started asking women themselves how they feel about pain in labour, and this has formed an alternative discourse. In our recent review of the literature, labour pain was consistently described by women as intense, unique, and meaningful (Whitburn et al. 2019). Women often describe labour pain as different from other experiences of pain because of the unique and positive outcome – the birth of a child. Many women see the pain of childbirth as transformative, joyful and a necessary part of this significant rite of passage. Moreover, women appear to expect to feel some kind of pain in labour (Karlsdottir, Halldorsdottir, and Lundgren 2014, Newnham, McKellar, and Pincombe 2018, Van der Gucht, and Lewis 2014). Labour pain is not necessarily talked about as their greatest concern, with women reporting that fears surrounding birth include fear of intervention, of loss of control and of the unknown (Newnham, McKellar, and Pincombe 2018).

In a large randomised controlled trial in Australia (the COSMOS trial), women who were cared for by a primary midwife during the antenatal, intra-partum and postpartum periods (continuity of care model) were more likely to have a positive experience of pain (McLachlan et al. 2016) while also requesting epidural analgesia less often (McLachlan et al. 2012). A systematic review of factors influencing women's birth experiences demonstrated that the attitudes and behaviours of caregivers are more powerful than pain intensity, pain relief or medical interventions (Hodnett 2002). Bohren et al. (2017) also found that women who have continuous support in labour were less likely to use analgesia or report a negative experience of childbirth. Another Australian study looking at the pain relief preferences of women, midwives and obstetricians found that the highest preference for all groups (>90%) was the inclusion of a support person in labour (Madden et al 2013). If women are provided with information and relational support during the antenatal period, then it can decrease pharmacological analgesia use (Leap et al. 2010, Levett et al. 2016).

This research promoting continuity of care and emphasising the quality of relationships with supportive caregivers, provides support for what many midwives have known about, practiced, and passed on. The midwifery literature about labour pain talks about it being salutogenic, meaning that it has the capacity to increase wellbeing (Downe and McCourt 2019, Karlsdottir et al. 2019). This epitomises the concerns we raised earlier about the IASP definition with its focus on tissue damage. People who have given birth, or who work with birth, make the link between pain and power (Dempsey 2020). This link is significant because the power of birth-giving – both individually and collectively – and the knowledge (and power) that this afforded midwives is a likely part of the reason why childbirth became of such great interest to men from the middle of the 18th century, as social, economic, industrial structures shifted in the wake of the Renaissance (Newnham, McKellar, and Pincombe 2018). This history influenced the way in which knowledge about women's bodies, birth and pain was produced (Newnham, McKellar, and Pincombe 2016).

Mindfulness and pain catastrophising in labour

In our research (Whitburn et al. 2014), we identified an 'optimal' state of mind with similarities to the concept of a state of *mindfulness*. Mindfulness has been described by Jon Kabat-Zinn (2003) as

> the awareness that emerges through paying attention on purpose, in the present moment, and nonjudgmentally to the unfolding of experience moment by moment.

In other pain contexts, mindfulness training has been shown to decrease pain ratings and sensitivity by reducing anxiety and increasing focus on the present moment (Zeidan et al. 2010). From the narratives that the women shared, it was apparent that their state of mind shaped their experiences of pain during labour and the role of birthing hormones. The hormonal systems engaged in labour trigger a state of mind that has much in common with mindfulness. We also identified key distractors that could draw a woman out of a mindful state, including environmental stressors, that ultimately affected her capacity to persist with labour (Whitburn et al. 2014).

In labour, oxytocin induces a similar calm and non-reactive state to mindfulness by downregulating the SNS and upregulating the PNS. Beta-endorphins attenuate the activity of the labouring woman's neocortex to suppress thoughts, including judgemental and future-oriented thoughts. These hormones work together to enable the woman to become inwardly focussed and create the circumstances for a 'mindful' state. There are, however, notable differences between mindfulness and the mindful state of a woman working with her birthing hormones. While mindfulness engages metacognition to actively notice thoughts, feelings and sensations, the mind of a labouring woman may be better characterised by a loss of metacognition. Under the influence of beta-endorphins, the swamped neocortex has less capacity to actively observe thoughts and emotions, or to reflect on the self. This subduing of the rational neocortex is particularly useful when the woman is working with the growing intensity of contractions – instead of 'thinking' about pain, the woman just experiences it.

Our research on the state of mind of women in labour labelled this state as 'mindful acceptance.' Women described this as a state of intense focus, during which their mind remained in the present moment. They attended to bodily sensations, including pain, without reaction or self-judgement. Importantly, pain was accepted as part of the labour process and there was no attempt to ignore or dismiss it. Critically, women reported a greater capacity to work with the growing intensity of labour when in a 'mindful acceptance' state.

There was, however, great effort to engage and maintain this state – women described the mental work of 'staying focussed' during their labour. As one woman explained, '*I was putting a lot of attention to my breath… If I wasn't so focussed, I think I would have just felt a blanket of pain*' Participant 12 (Whitburn et al. 2014). If this focus was interrupted, a labouring woman could be drawn towards what we labelled a 'distracted and distraught' state (Whitburn et al. 2014). Distractors included an unfamiliar birthing space, unfamiliar people that made her feel uncomfortable and/or observed and being asked questions or attempting to make sense of information. When in this state, women reported thought processes that suggested a stimulated neocortex, including self-judgement ('*I'm so weak, I can't do this!*'), self-consciousness ('*Am I making too much noise?*') and pain catastrophising ('*Will this get worse!?*').

Pain catastrophising is described as "a tendency to focus on and exaggerate the threat value of pain and negatively evaluate one's ability to deal with it" (Whitburn et al. 2014). The communal coping model suggests that catastrophising helps an individual to elicit support and assistance from others (Sullivan 2012), and in this sense can be seen to be useful to help women communicate their needs when in the vulnerable state of giving birth. Pain catastrophising is a neocortical process where unhelpful thoughts amplify the pain experience and make it feel more threatening. Our research suggests that, in labour, pain catastrophising may be an indicator that a woman's neocortex is overstimulated leading her to negatively evaluate her capacity to cope (Whitburn et al. 2014).

Reconceptualising birth: pleasure and pain

Reframing the concept of 'labour pain' can help set it apart from the pain of injury, disease, or pathology. Childbirth educator Rhea Dempsey uses the terms 'functional' or 'physiological' pain to describe the pain of childbirth as that associated with 'a healthy body working at high intensity' (Dempsey 2013, 56). Sanders (2015) proposes the term 'functional discomfort' to shift the focus from pain and its association with pathology, and encourages midwives to *ease* rather than *relieve* labour pain in the way they facilitate birth and support birthing women. Another description we have offered for labour pain is 'productive and purposeful.' Describing labour pain as productive suggests that this pain is not associated with a passive need to rest or avoid (as may be appropriate with tissue injury or disease) but an active need to engage and produce (to birth a child). The pain is purposeful in that there is a known reason for the intense feelings and the reason is anticipated: it is signalling the onset and progress of this normal physiological process to the woman and her caregivers, a healthy process that is working to birth her baby.

Working with pain and supporting birth hormones

Nicky Leap has conceptualised the way in which midwives work with women in labour as either presenting a pain relief menu, or as having a 'working with pain' approach (Leap 1997). Midwives who work with this latter approach see the positive aspects of labour pain and support women to work with their bodies, with minimal disturbance, in order not to interrupt the hormonal cascade. The 'pain relief menu' approach, Leap says, is where midwives list a series of coping mechanisms beginning with physiological (movement, warmth, water) then progressing through pharmacological options, ending with epidural analgesia as the most effective, yet most complex intervention with the most side effects. This approach may unwittingly imply to women that they will be unable to cope with labour pain—and will need to resort to *something,* unsure if that something is going to be a warm bath or an epidural.

Leap and Hunter (2016) suggest that rather than teaching women specific strategies, reassuring them they will find their own ways of coping, and supporting them in this, is more effective, and we agree. What is needed is not necessarily a specific knowledge or tool – although these may be helpful to some women (2016) – but supporting the woman to get into that mindful space, whatever that feels like for her. Therefore, we suggest that a different way of discussing non-pharmacological coping strategies is to describe them as mechanisms that increase a woman's receptiveness to a state of mindfulness, associated with her birthing hormones, rather than as mechanisms of coping with pain. In this way, these mechanisms can be discussed without reference to the 'pain relief menu,' and supports ideas of working with pain (Leap and Hunter 2016), and the power and physiology of birth. In light of this, rather than listing a series of practical exercises that women can do, or that caregivers can suggest, we present four practices that are probably as ancient as childbirth itself, which promote these hormonal responses and therefore help women to access the state of 'mindful acceptance.'

Breath and vocalisations

Breathing techniques have been included in techniques of 'natural' childbirth since the mid-20th century. Antenatal yoga classes often teach women how to be in touch with their breath, and how to focus on deep breathing while the body is in exertion. Paying attention to the breath is a central feature of mindfulness meditation, as a strategy to keep the focus on the natural movements of the body and in the present moment (Baer 2003). In labour, attending to the breath may help keep the woman's mind in the present moment, to minimise worrying or catastrophising thoughts that may lead to feelings of helplessness and distress (Whitburn et al. 2014). There is a connection between breath and vocalisation, and those who attend women in labour will be familiar with the different sounds women make, from the almost melodic singsong of early labour contractions to the much lower moans that often come with the transition to the second stage. High-pitched noises or shallow breath can signal to caregivers that the woman may be experiencing fear or panic and needs help to re-establish a more relaxed state. This can sometimes be achieved by gently reminding them to take their breath right down into the abdomen, or by encouraging deep vocalisation. Some women have described vocalisations useful as a way to manage the intensity of contractions – the sound of their voice and the effort to produce the sound become the focus point, and avoids their mind wandering to less helpful thoughts or fears (Whitburn et al. 2014). This does, however, depend upon a woman feeling uninhibited to do so, which will be influenced, in part, by not feeling observed or judged by those around her.

Movement

Women who are given the space and encouragement to move in labour will do so instinctively in varied and individual ways. This might include position changes, rocking the pelvis, swaying, walking, or pacing, squatting (moving the hips downwards with a contraction), and other movements. In one study, 90% of women in spontaneous labour used rhythmic movements and 50% used gripping actions (Cheyne and Duff 2019). Conversely, women whose movement is limited, for example by monitors, report greater difficulty in managing their pain (Whitburn et al. 2014). Free and uninhibited movement in labour encourages upright positions, which increases labour effectiveness by working in line with gravity, facilitating optimal foetal positioning and widening the pelvic outlet (Perez-Botella et al. 2019). Movement may also help women stay inwardly focussed and attuned to their bodies – the rhythm of swaying or walking (Simkin 2007) can become the focus point. This is akin to mindful movement, where the woman uses rhythmic movements matched to her breath to work through the rise and fall of each contraction. Caregivers can help women by giving them space and reassurance to move in whichever way feels best to them.

Water/touch

The use of warm water promotes a relaxed state and has the added benefit of offering women privacy. As well as stimulating oxytocin release (Uvnäs Moberg 2003), the sound of the shower or water may help quiet a woman's neocortex, by muffling other sounds that may otherwise interrupt her focus. Showers in labour have been shown to decrease pain and anxiety and increase relaxation, also delaying the use of pharmacological analgesia and helping to maintain upright labour positioning (Stark and Remynse 2016). Women often report having more control over their immediate environment when in the shower or bath because of the fluid barrier surrounding their body (Feeley, Cooper, and Burns 2021, Maude and Foureur 2007). Immersion in water can reduce uptake of epidural (Cluett, Burns, and Cuthbert 2018) and is associated with high levels of pain relief satisfaction and positive birth experience, with higher rates of an intact perineum (Nutter et al. 2014), and no increase in adverse outcomes (Cluett, Burns, and Cuthbert 2018, Nutter et al. 2014). Supportive and welcomed touch in labour is another common midwifery practice and offers opportunity for connection as well as being therapeutic, reducing pain and anxiety (Walsh 2012). Welcomed touch is a strong trigger for oxytocin release and brings associated reduction in stress and higher tolerance for pain (Uvnäs Moberg 2003). Both water and touch may further act as sensory cues to help a woman stay mindful and inwardly focussed during her labour.

Support

As Michel Odent says, 'a labouring woman first needs to feel secure. This feeling of security is a prerequisite for the changing level of consciousness which characterises the birth process' (Odent 1999, p. 30). This makes sense in light of the neurophysiology of childbirth, and is perhaps why, in a systematic review of over 15,000 women, continuous support during labour (from any source, including midwives, friends, partners or doulas) resulted in a greater number of women having a spontaneous vaginal birth, a reduction in analgesia requirements and decreased caesarean section rates. Labour length was shorter and women were more satisfied with their birth experience (Bohren et al. 2017). Having a known midwife has also been shown to decrease epidural rates, increase rates of spontaneous vaginal birth (fewer instrumental births), and reduce the chance of having a pre-term or stillborn baby (Sandall et al. 2016). One likely contributing factor is the influence of supportive interpersonal relationships on oxytocin production with its beneficial effects (Uvnäs Moberg 2003). Support people provide emotional comfort and act as motivators and companions. They can play a pivotal role in 'protecting' a woman's birthing space, advocating for her, and helping her, control variables that may otherwise distract her, or stimulate her neocortex, disrupting the optimum level of consciousness.

Final thoughts

Pain is an individual and subjective experience. With the knowledge that pain in labour is healthy, the confidence that women are capable, and the trusting presence of human care, labour pain can be experienced as a positive component to a transformative life event. In our current medicalised setting for birth, continuous, deep, human support is often not prioritised. The possibilities for stress-triggering distractions in combination with fragmented care leave women feeling emotionally unsupported and interrupt the flow of birthing hormones. In these contexts, in particular, the need for approaches that can preserve a mindful state of consciousness through labour is even greater. Modalities that quiet the neocortex and focus attention on the present moment, facilitated by an emotionally connected caregiver who acts to protect the birthing woman's 'space,' may assist in preserving a mindful state, making a woman feel secure and providing the foundation for effective coping with the intensity of the birthing experience.

References

Amodio, David M., and Chris D. Frith. 2006. "Meeting of minds: the medial frontal cortex and social cognition." *Nature Reviews Neuroscience* 7 (4):268–277.

Anim-Somuah, Millicent, Rebecca M.D. Smyth, Allan M. Cyna, and Anna Cuthbert. 2018. "Epidural versus non-epidural or no analgesia for pain management in labour." *Cochrane Database of Systematic Reviews* (5): 1–149. doi: 10.1002/14651858.CD000331.pub4.

Baer, Ruth A. 2003. "Mindfulness training as a clinical intervention: a conceptual and empirical review." *Clinical Psychology: Science and Practice* 10 (2):125–143.

Basbaum, Allan I., and Howard L. Fields. 1984. "Endogenous pain control systems: brainstem spinal pathways and endorphin circuitry." *Annual Review of Neuroscience* 7 (1):309–338.

Bohren, Meghan A., G. Justus Hofmeyr, Carol Sakala, Rieko K. Fukuzawa, and Anna Cuthbert. 2017. "Continuous support for women during childbirth." *Cochrane Database of Systematic Reviews* (7). doi: 10.1002/14651858.CD003766.pub6.

Buckley, Sarah. 2015. *Hormonal physiology of childbearing: evidence an implications for women, babies, and maternity care.* Washington, DC: Childbirth Connection Programs, National Partnership for Women & Families.

Cheyne, Helen, and Margie Duff. 2019. "Anatomy and physiology of labour and associated behavioural cues." In *Squaring the Circle: researching normal childbirth in a technological world,* edited by S. Downe and S. Byrom. London: Pinter and Martin.

Cluett, Elizabeth R., Ethel Burns, and Anna Cuthbert. 2018. "Immersion in water during labour and birth." *Cochrane Database of Systematic Reviews* (5). doi: 10.1002/14651858.CD000111.pub4.

Davis, Elizabeth, and Debra Pascali-Bonaro. 2010. *Orgasmic birth: your guide to a safe, satisfying, and pleasurable birth experience*. New York: Rodale.

Dempsey, Rhea. 2013. *Birth with confidence: savvy choices for normal birth*. Fairfield: Boathouse Press.

Dempsey, Rhea. 2020. *Beyond the birth plan: getting real about pain and power*. Fairfield: Boathouse Press.

Denk, Franziska, Stephen B McMahon, and Irene Tracey. 2014. "Pain vulnerability: a neurobiological perspective." *Nature Neuroscience* 17 (2):192.

Dixon, Lesley, Joan Skinner, and Maralyn Foureur. 2013. "The emotional and hormonal pathways of labour and birth: integrating mind, body and behaviour." *Journal-New Zealand College of Midwives*.

Downe, Soo, and Christine McCourt. 2019. "From being to becoming: reconstructing childbirth knowledge." In *Squaring the circle: normal birth research, theory, and practice in a technological age*, edited by S. Downe and S. Byrom, 69–99. London: Pinter & Martin.

Feeley, Claire, Megan Cooper, and Ethel Burns. 2021. "A systematic meta-thematic synthesis to examine the views and experiences of women following water immersion during labour and waterbirth." *Journal of Advanced Nursing* 77:2942–2956.

Ferguson, James K.W. 1941. "A study of the motility of the intact uterus at term." *Surgery, Gynecology and Obstetrics* 73:359–366.

Generaal, Ellen, Nicole Vogelzangs, Gary J. Macfarlane, Rinie Geenen, Johannes H. Smit, Eco J.C.N. De Geus, Brenda W.J.H. Penninx, and Joost Dekker. 2016. "Biological stress systems, adverse life events and the onset of chronic multisite musculoskeletal pain: a 6-year cohort study." *Annals of the Rheumatic Diseases* 75 (5):847–854.

Hartwig, A.C. 1991. "Peripheral beta-endorphin and pain modulation." *Anesthesia Progress* 38 (3):75.

Hodnett, Ellen D. 2002. "Pain and women's satisfaction with the experience of childbirth: a systematic review." *American Journal of Obstetrics and Gynecology* 186 (5):160–172.

Kabat-Zinn, Jon. 2003. "Mindfulness-based interventions in context: past, present, and future." *Clinical Psychology: Science and Practice* 10 (2):144–156.

Karlsdottir, Sigfríður Inga, Sigridur Halldorsdottir, and Ingela Lundgren. 2014. "The third paradigm in labour pain preparation and management: the childbearing woman's paradigm." *Scandinavian Journal of Caring Sciences* 28 (2):315–27. doi: 10.1111/scs.12061.

Karlsdottir, Sigfríður Inga, Elizabeth Newnham, Hildur Kristjansdottir, and Ruth Sanders. 2019. "Decision-making around pain and its management during labour and birth." In *Empowering decision-making in midwifery: a global perspective*, edited by E. Jefford and J. Jomeen, 141–152. Abingdon: Routledge.

Leap, Nicky, and Billie Hunter. 2016. *Supporting women for labour and birth: a thoughtful guide*. Abingdon, Oxon: Routledge.

Leap, Nicky, Elizabeth Newnham, and Sigfríður Inga Karlsdottir. 2019. "Approaches to pain in labour: implications for midwifery practice." In *Squaring the Circle: researching normal childbirth in a technological world*, edited by S. Downe and S. Byrom, 193–203. London: Pinter & Martin.

Leap, Nicky, Jane Sandall, Sara Buckland, and Ulli Huber. 2010. "Journey to confidence: women's experiences of pain in labour and relational continuity of care." *Journal of Midwifery & Women's Health* 55 (3):234–42. doi: 10.1016/j.jmwh.2010.02.001.

Leap, Nicky. 1997. "Being with women in pain—do midwives need to rethink their role?" *British Journal of Midwifery* 5 (5):263.

Legrain, Valéry, Stefaan Van Damme, Christopher Eccleston, Karen D. Davis, David A. Seminowicz, and Geert Crombez. 2009. "A neurocognitive model of attention to pain: behavioral and neuroimaging evidence." *Pain* 144 (3):230–232.

Levett, Kate M., C.A. Smith, Alan Bensoussan, and Hannah G. Dahlen. 2016. "Complementary therapies for labour and birth study: a randomised controlled trial of antenatal integrative medicine for pain management in labour." *BMJ Open* 6 (7):e010691.

Madden, Kelly L., Deborah Turnbull, Allan M. Cyna, Pamela Adelson, and Chris Wilkinson. 2013. "Pain relief for childbirth: the preferences of pregnant women, midwives and obstetricians." *Women and Birth* 26 (1):33–40.

Maude, Robyn, and Maralyn Foureur. 2007. "It's beyond water: stories of women's experience of using water for labour and birth." *Women and Birth* 20 (1):17–24.

McAra-Couper, Judith, Marion Jones, and Liz Smythe. 2012. "Caesarean-section, my body, my choice: the construction of 'informed choice' in relation to intervention in childbirth." *Feminism & Psychology* 22 (1):81–97.

McLachlan, Helen L., Della A. Forster, Mary-Ann Davey, Tanya Farrell, Margaret Flood, Touran Shafiei, and Ulla Waldenström. 2016. "The effect of primary midwife-led care on women's experience of childbirth: results from the COSMOS randomised controlled trial." *BJOG: An International Journal of Obstetrics & Gynaecology* 123 (3):465–474.

McLachlan, Helen L., Della A. Forster, Mary-Ann Davey, Tanya Farrell, Lisa Gold, Mary Anne Biro, Leah Albers, Maggie Flood, Jeremy Oats, and Ulla Waldenström. 2012. "Effects of continuity of care by a primary midwife (caseload midwifery) on caesarean section rates in women of low obstetric risk: the COSMOS randomised controlled trial." *BJOG: An International Journal of Obstetrics & Gynaecology* 119 (12):1483–1492.

Newnham, Elizabeth C., Lois V. McKellar, and Jan I. Pincombe. 2016. "A critical literature review of epidural analgesia." *Evidence Based Midwifery* 14 (1):22–28.

Newnham, Elizabeth C., Lois V. McKellar, and Jan I. Pincombe. 2018. *Towards the humanisation of birth: a study of epidural analgesia and hospital birth culture.* Cham: Palgrave Macmillan.

Newnham, Elizabeth C., Patrick S. Moran, Cecily M. Begley, Margaret Carroll, and Deirdre Daly. 2020. "Comparison of labour and birth outcomes between nulliparous women who used epidural analgesia in labour and those who did not: a prospective cohort study." *Women and Birth* In press. doi: 10.1016/j.wombi.2020.09.001.

Newton, Niles, Donald Foshee, and Michael Newton. 1966. "Experimental inhibition of labor through environmental disturbance." *Obstetrics & Gynecology* 27 (3):371–377.

Nutter, Elizabeth, Shaunette Meyer, Jenna Shaw-Battista, and Amy Marowitz. 2014. "Waterbirth: an integrative analysis of peer-reviewed literature." *Journal of Midwifery & women's Health* 59 (3):286–319.

Odent, Michel. 1999. *The scientification of love.* London: Free Association Books

Perez-Botella, M., L. van Lessen, S. Morano, and A. de Jonge. 2019. "What works to promote physiological labour and birth for healthy women and babies?" In *Squaring the circle: normal birth research, theory, and practice in a technological age*, edited by S. Downe and S. Byrom, 54–66. London: Pinter & Martin.

Porges, Stephen W. 2005. "The role of social engagement in attachment and bonding." *Attachment & Bonding* 3:33–54.

Raja, Srinivasa N., Daniel B. Carr, Milton Cohen, Nanna B. Finnerup, Herta Flor, Stephen Gibson, Francis J. Keefe, Jeffrey S. Mogil, Matthias Ringkamp, Kathleen A. Sluka, Xue-Jun Song, Bonnie Stevens, Mark D. Sullivan, Perri R. Tutelman, Takahiro Ushida, and Kyle Vader. 2020. "The revised International Association for the Study of Pain definition of pain: concepts, challenges, and compromises." *PAIN* 161 (9):1976–1982. doi: 10.1097/j.pain.0000000000001939.

Riem, Madelon M.E., Marian J. Bakermans-Kranenburg, Suzanne Pieper, Mattie Tops, Maarten A.S. Boksem, Robert R.J.M. Vermeiren, Marinus H. van IJzendoorn, and Serge A.R.B. Rombouts. 2011. "Oxytocin modulates amygdala, insula, and inferior frontal gyrus responses to infant crying: a randomized controlled trial." *Biological psychiatry* 70 (3):291–297.

Sandall, Jane, Hora Soltani, Simon Gates, Andrew Shennan, and Declan Devane. 2016. "Midwife-led continuity models versus other models of care for childbearing women." *Cochrane Database of Systematic Reviews* (4): 1–122.

Sanders, Ruth. 2015. "Functional discomfort and a shift in midwifery paradigm." *Women Birth* 28 (3):e87–e91.

Sauriyal, Dharmraj Singh, Amteshwar Singh Jaggi, and Nirmal Singh. 2011. "Extending pharmacological spectrum of opioids beyond analgesia: multifunctional aspects in different pathophysiological states." *Neuropeptides* 45 (3):175–188.

Shackman, A.J., Tim V. Salomons, Heleen A. Slagter, Andrew S. Fox, Jameel J. Winter, and Richa J. Davidson. 2011. "The integration of negative affect, pain and cognitive control in the cingulate cortex." *Nature Reviews Neuroscience* 12 (3):154–167.

Simkin, Penny. 2007. Comfort in labour: how you can help yourself to a normal satisfying childbirth. https://www.nationalpartnership.org/our-work/resources/health-care/maternity/comfort-in-labor-simkin.pdf

Smith, Lesley A., Ethel Burns, and Anna Cuthbert. 2018. "Parenteral opioids for maternal pain management in labour." *Cochrane Database of Systematic Reviews* (6). doi: 10.1002/14651858.CD007396.pub3.

Stark, Mary Ann, and Marshe Remynse. 2016. "Comparison between therapeutic showering and usual care during labor." *Journal of Obstetric, Gynecologic & Neonatal Nursing* 45 (3):S43.

Sullivan, Michael J.L. 2012. "The communal coping model of pain catastrophising: clinical and research implications." *Canadian Psychology* 53 (1):32–41.

Tsigos, Constantine, and George P. Chrousos. 2002. "Hypothalamic–pituitary–adrenal axis, neuroendocrine factors and stress." *Journal of Psychosomatic Research* 53 (4):865–871.

Uvnäs Moberg, Kerstin. 2003. *The oxytocin factor: tapping the hormone of calm, love, and healing.* Cambridge, MA: Da Capo Press.

Uvnäs Moberg, Kerstin. 2016. "The oxytocin factor [Keynote presentation]." Normal Labour and Birth Conference, Sydney, Australia.

Van der Gucht, R.M. Natalie, and Kiara Lewis. 2014. "Women's experiences of coping with pain during childbirth: a critical review of qualitative research." *Midwifery* 31 (3):349–358.

Walsh, Denis. 2012. *Evidence and skills for normal labour and birth: a guide for midwives.* 2nd ed. London: Routledge.

Whitburn, Laura Y. 2013. "Labour pain: from the physical brain to the conscious mind." *Journal of Psychosomatic Obstetrics & Gynaecology* 34 (3):139–143. doi: 10.3109/0167482X.2013.829033.

Whitburn, Laura Y., Lester E. Jones, Mary-Ann Davey, and Rhonda Small. 2014. "Women's experiences of labour pain and the role of the mind: an exploratory study." *Midwifery* 30 (9):1029–1035.

Whitburn, Laura Y., Lester E. Jones, Mary-Ann Davey, and Susan McDonald. 2019. "The nature of labour pain: an updated review of the literature." *Women and Birth* 32 (1):28–38.

Whitburn, Laura Y., Lester E. Jones, Mary-Ann Davey, and Rhonda Small. 2017. "Supporting the updated definition of pain. But what about labour pain?" *Pain* 158 (5):990–991.

Zeidan, Fadel, Nakia S. Gordon, Junaid Merchant, and Paula Goolkasian. 2010. "The effects of brief mindfulness meditation training on experimentally induced pain." *The Journal of Pain* 11 (3):199–209.

11

BREASTFEEDING

The ultimate mindful practice?

Ira Kantrowitz-Gordon and Anna Byrom

Introduction

In this chapter, the question 'can breast/chest-feeding be considered the ultimate mindful practice?' is considered. This includes an exploration of the benefits of breastfeeding alongside some of the bio-psycho-social barriers. There is a review of key evidence associated with mindfulness and breastfeeding alongside a proposed conceptual framework for supporting mindful mother/parent-infant feeding. There are critical considerations made throughout, with regards to concepts of motherhood, parenting and the impact of research, practice and care on outcomes and experiences.

Personal perspectives

Anna's reflection

Preparing to write this chapter I was called to reflect on my own experiences of breastfeeding, as a mother, health professional, educator and researcher. I brought to mind memories of supporting new parents and infants navigating early breastfeeding experiences, leading and researching infant feeding services. These were recalled alongside moments of being with my own children as we journeyed our way to and through the ups and downs and in-betweens of our Earth-side relationships. As someone who might be referred to as 'fast and furious', breastfeeding called me to a more 'calm and curious' state with all the force of physiology; an evolutionary instruction passed on to ensure our survival and success (Buckley, 2015). As the pace of life surges on, I feel an ever-growing desire to slow down and simply 'be' in the present, just as I experienced nourishing my own and other's breastfeeding moments.

DOI: 10.4324/9781003165200-11

Ira's reflection

My experiences with breastfeeding have necessarily been vicarious through my support of my wife in breastfeeding our four children, as well as listening to the joys and struggles of my patients during many years as a perinatal nurse and nurse-midwife. Whereas the feeding journeys of our first three children proceeded with expected challenges, our fourth presented new challenges after her unexpected birth at 28-week gestation. The prolonged hospitalization in neonatal intensive care, nearly six months of pumping milk and the struggle to achieve feeding at the breast forced us to slow down, refocus priorities and work together in new ways to support a vulnerable child in partnership. This was the beginning for me in a professional journey to focus my efforts on understanding how mindfulness can be developed further as a strategy to help mothers with their symptoms during pregnancy and postpartum.

Shared insights

Collectively, through our professional and personal experiences, we have both come to see the joy and anguish, the pain and pride parents can experience across their infant feeding journeys. As with any human-life experience, breast/–chest-feeding is nuanced, contextual and uniquely interpreted. Whilst research can capture normative values, impacts and consequences of breast/chest-feeding, how it is 'lived' out, across the fabric of our personal life course is subjective and will always vary.

As captured, throughout this book, the growing interest in mindfulness training during pregnancy began as an adaptation of mindfulness-based stress reduction (MBSR) for childbirth preparation (Kabat-Zinn, 2003; Lönnberg et al., 2020). The perinatal period is an ideal time for future parents to develop new skills because pregnancy is a strong motivator for personal growth and behaviour change. Mindfulness-Based Childbirth and Parenting (MBCP) is an example of an in-person, group intervention to help couples prepare for childbirth and the transition to parenting using mindfulness as a skill to foster calm, acceptance and wisdom with benefits extending into parenthood (Bardacke, 2012; Duncan and Bardacke, 2010). During the postpartum period, mindfulness-based interventions have not included infant feeding or breastfeeding; instead, they have focused on parenting skills, emotional regulation and interpersonal relationships (Fernandes et al., 2022). The postpartum period is also an appropriate time to incorporate mindfulness skills because of the embodied physical changes. Postpartum experiences, including breastfeeding and infant feeding are activities that could be enhanced by mindfulness approaches because it is an opportunity for the parent to engage the infant with attention and awareness (Babbar et al., 2021). The potential for enhancing the breastfeeding and infant feeding experience for early parenthood has not yet been realized as the research in this area is in its infancy.

Breastfeeding continues to be levied as a global public health priority, with established evidence highlighting broad population-level benefits for infants, mothers, families and society (Renfrew et al., 2006; World Health Organisation [WHO], 2020). Despite significant investment in interventions to support breast-feeding, rates continue to decline, with wide variations in initiation and continuation rates around the world (Victora et al., 2016). In general, breastfeeding rates appear to be lower in high-income countries when compared to low- and middle-income countries (UNICEF, 2018). There are multiple, complex and nuanced bio-psycho-social barriers to enabling optimal infant feeding outcomes and experiences (Brown, 2018). Some key, evidence-informed barriers to successful breastfeeding rates and experiences are captured in Table 11.1, synthesised from a range of evidence sources (Brown, 2018; Rollins et al., 2016; Victora et al., 2016).

With appropriate support, many of the physical challenges cited in Table 11.1, can be overcome and successful breastfeeding can be experienced for the parent-infant dyad and wider family. Beyond the physical, the psycho-social and cultural barriers are more pervasive and challenging to overcome. Many interventions have been developed to promote, protect and support breastfeeding for example the UNICEF UK BFI, peer support programmes, breastfeeding education programmes and specialist health professional support (Sinha et al., 2015; Trickey et al., 2018).

Increased mindfulness has the potential to address common challenges to early breastfeeding success to improve breastfeeding rates and satisfaction with breastfeeding (Kantrowitz-Gordon, Abbott and Hoehn, 2018). Breast and nipple pain are among the most common reasons why women stop breastfeeding early (Morrison, Gentry and Anderson, 2019). Pain during breastfeeding can elicit disappointment because of the difficulty in handling an expected maternal function or guilt from negative feelings towards the baby. Mindfulness-based interventions have the potential to improve coping and appraisal of pain across a variety of contexts, including chronic pain (Hilton et al., 2017), acute pain (McClintock et al., 2019) and labour pain (Duncan et al., 2017). If the pain leads to early cessation of breastfeeding, women may judge themselves for failing to meet societal expectations for being a good mother by providing the best infant nutrition (Jackson, Mantler and O'Keefe-McCarthy, 2019). The mindfulness focus on non-judgement and self-compassion may be especially helpful in letting go of these negative appraisals of breastfeeding pain.

Morrison, Gentry and Anderson (2019) found that perceived insufficient milk supply is another common reason for early breastfeeding cessation that could potentially be addressed with mindfulness. The perception of insufficient milk supply is related to a combination of psychological and physiological factors (Kent et al., 2021) and may be unrelated to actual milk supply (Galipeau, Dumas and Lepage, 2017). Breastfeeding self-efficacy is an important correlate of maternal perception of producing sufficient milk (Menekse et al., 2021) and interventions to increase breastfeeding self-efficacy have been shown to increase

TABLE 11.1 Reported Barriers to Successful Breastfeeding Rates and Experiences

Physical Barriers	Psychological Barriers	Social Barriers	Cultural Barriers
Neonatal • Structural anomalies, e.g. cleft palate • Pre-existing health conditions, e.g. genetic syndrome • Prematurity • Growth restriction • Neonatal medications, e.g. sedation • Neonatal conditions, e.g. jaundice, hypoglycaemia *Maternal* • Nipple pain, engorgement, mastitis, thrush, abscess • Pre-existing medical or obstetric conditions, e.g. breast cancer, diabetes, massive haemorrhage • Actual insufficient milk supply • Structural anomalies, e.g. inverted nipples *Birth Interventions* • Anaesthetics, analgesics, e.g. opiods/narcotics • Instrumental/operative birth • Separation of mother and baby at birth • Restricted skin contact	• Poor attachment • Maternal mental health illness, e.g. Posttraumatic Stress Disorder, anxiety, depression • Perceived insufficient milk supply • Guilt and shame • Lack of emotional support	• Returning to work • Limited social support • Restrictive or unsupportive/ limited health and social policy and legislation • Lack of healthcare support • Negative social media influences • Access to education and educational attainment • Health inequities • Structural racism • Unconscious and conscious bias	• Sexualisation of breasts • Bottlefeeding cultures • Artificial milk advertising • Personal, family and society values

breastfeeding rates at one and two months postpartum (Brockway, Benzies and Hayden, 2017). Mindfulness-based interventions are an untested approach to improving breastfeeding self-efficacy, although limited studies suggest that mindfulness-based interventions can increase childbirth self-efficacy (Duncan et al., 2017) and maternal self-efficacy in breastfeeding mothers (Perez-Blasco et al., 2013) – (see Chapters 7 and 8 for examples of mindfulness and childbirth self-efficacy). Mindfulness has the potential to help breastfeeding mothers increase their attention and awareness towards newborn cues that indicate a satisfactory milk supply, such as satiety at the end of a feeding (Shloim et al., 2017).

There is some evidence that relaxation (changing the state of one's mind) may have an effect on milk ejection and milk supply and infant growth (Mohd Shukri et al., 2019). In a small randomized clinical trial, infants of mothers randomized to relaxation therapy had decreased milk cortisol and increased growth compared to control mothers (Mohd Shukri et al., 2019).

Stress and mood symptoms are another set of negative postpartum experiences that have been associated with reduced breastfeeding success and could be improved with a mindfulness approach. The correlation between depression and breastfeeding has been established in multiple studies (Dias and Figueiredo, 2015; Slomian, 2019). Lower oxytocin levels may have a mediating effect on this relationship (Lara, 2017). Similarly, there is an association between breastfeeding duration, pain and depression symptoms (Brown, 2018) (see Chapter 13). Stressful life events such as divorce or separation, financial difficulties and moving during pregnancy were associated with increased odds of early cessation of breastfeeding in a longitudinal cohort study in Australia (Li et al., 2008). Mindfulness, due to its efficacy in helping with perinatal depression, stress reduction and pain has the potential to ameliorate these symptoms factors that can be considered barriers to successful breastfeeding (Dozier, Nelson and Brownell, 2012).

Mindfulness also has the potential for facilitating positive relationships between the mother and the infant. For example, mindfulness prenatally was associated with increased postpartum responsiveness to infant needs for both secure and insecure infant attachment styles (Pickard et al., 2017). Similarly, mothers with increased mindfulness scores were more responsive to infant distress when teaching them a developmentally appropriate new task at six months old (Pickard et al., 2018). The contribution of mindfulness to responsiveness to infant cues and distress has the potential to be extended to the interaction during breastfeeding, both as a way to enhance the positive aspects of the interaction in response to infant cues (positive and negative), as well as helping the mother navigate challenges. These studies suggesting the relationship between mindfulness and mother-infant attunement as well as with maternal psychological symptoms are descriptive in nature. It remains to be seen whether interventions to increase mindfulness can be successful at increasing the mother's ability to navigate the challenges of breastfeeding and improve breastfeeding outcomes and experiences.

Reviewing the literature on breastfeeding and mindfulness

There are limited studies that have examined, directly, the link between mindfulness and mindful practice and the physiology of lactation. However, it is useful to consider the theoretical knowledge of lactation physiology, specifically the ecologically responsive hormonal physiology of lactation that helps us to understand how breastfeeding success can be sensitive to psycho-social, cultural and environmental contextual influences. In her report on the 'Hormonal Physiology of Childbearing' Sarah Buckley reviews the available evidence, describing the physiologic roles of four essential hormone systems and how they influence maternal–newborn adaptations around the time of birth (Buckley, 2015). Buckley (2015, p. viii) argues that 'despite research gaps, a consistent and coherent mosaic is coming into view, of a finely tuned hormonal physiology of childbearing, active from pregnancy to lactation and beyond which supports health, connection and well-being for mother and baby, in the short term and even lifelong'; see Figure 11.1 for more details.

From a hormonal perspective, considering the interconnectedness of breastfeeding and maternal–neonatal adaptations along the childbearing, birth and transition to life continuum, breastfeeding could be considered a mindful practice. It certainly offers some of the physiological benefits that mindful meditation practice aims to achieve, namely, stress and anxiety reduction, awareness and alertness. In relation to parenting and breastfeeding, mindfulness could help to stimulate and sustain physiology; specifically, the hormones needed for attachment, alertness, connectedness and well-being.

Yet, the perinatal period is highly sensitive for the parent-infant, in relation to hormonal and other biologic processes. A series of bio-psycho-social and cultural factors have been identified that can create barriers to effective breastfeeding. Therefore, it is essential that practices that support and protect physiological processes and are developed and sustained.

Little research has been done to understand the role of mindfulness in the experience of breastfeeding, contributions to breastfeeding outcomes (duration, exclusivity, others). The nonreacting facet of mindfulness was independently associated with the intention to breastfeed in 790 pregnant women in the Netherlands (OR, 1.09; 95% CI, 1.03–1.15) (Hulsbosch et al., 2021). A new mindful

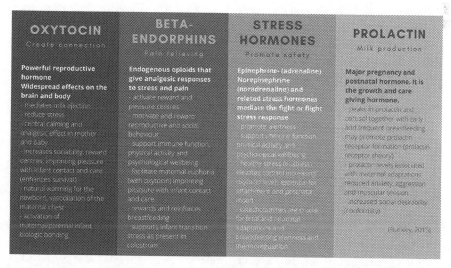

FIGURE 11.1 Hormonal physiology of childbearing, lactation and attachment (content adapted from Buckley, 2015).

breastfeeding scale showed a positive correlation with breastfeeding self-efficacy in newly postpartum women in Turkey (Korukcu et al., 2021). Mindfulness-based interventions (MBIs) during the perinatal (pregnancy, postpartum and early parenting) have primarily focused on stress reduction, alleviation of symptoms of depression and anxiety and preparation for labour and birth. Some interventions have included limited content on breastfeeding. For example, MBCP covers in the eighth class session how mindfulness skills can be used to support breastfeeding and the development of a maternal-infant relationship after birth (Duncan and Bardacke, 2010). However, breastfeeding outcomes have not been measured in randomized clinical trials of MBCP and similar MBIs in pregnancy.

The experiences of women postpartum using mindfulness skills have been described in qualitative research studies. Qualitative data from follow-up of mindfulness-based interventions provide support for the benefits of mindfulness skills during the postpartum period and for breastfeeding. Often participants used formal and informal mindfulness practices to increase their attention to the present moment. The benefits included staying present during breastfeeding sessions and letting go of intrusive negative thoughts and self-judgements about breastfeeding difficulties. Using mindfulness during breastfeeding enabled increased relaxation and an antidote to the draw of smartphones and other distractions (Kantrowitz-Gordon, Abbott and Hoehn, 2018; Lönnberg, Nissen and Niemi, 2018; Roy Malis, Meyer and Gross, 2017).

A 3-week breastfeeding educational program developed in Taiwan using self-efficacy theory and mindfulness was tested during pregnancy to improve breastfeeding rates (Tseng et al., 2020). The antenatal classes included didactic content, simulation and mindfulness training. In a randomized controlled trial, women ($n = 50$) who completed the training had higher breastfeeding self-efficacy compared to women who received routine care ($n = 43$). Breastfeeding rates were significantly higher through six months of follow-up. Because the intervention included only one class on mindfulness among other content and trait mindfulness was not measured before or after the intervention, it is not clear that the improved breastfeeding outcomes can be attributed to increased mindfulness skills. Nevertheless, the results show promise for a mindfulness approach toward improving breastfeeding outcomes.

Based on the limited research on mindfulness and breastfeeding, there are significant gaps in the literature. First, there is a need for observational studies to examine the relationship between mindfulness and breastfeeding, looking at the process and infant outcomes, such as growth and duration of breastfeeding. It is likely that these relationships are complex as they relate to interpersonal factors such as maternal-infant attachment, as well as external environmental factors. Second, mindfulness-based intervention trials need to robustly test feasible and accessible interventions that can prepare women for breastfeeding either during pregnancy or early in the postpartum period. This can be approached as a targeted intervention specific to breastfeeding or as part of a larger intervention to prepare for childbirth and parenting. An advantage of mindfulness as an intervention is the adaptability of the practice to multiple contexts. Recorded mindfulness meditations can be used to focus attention during breastfeeding episodes. However, a formal meditation may not be necessary for a woman with general mindfulness training, as they can informally use each feeding session as an opportunity to focus their attention on their infant.

There are some philosophical challenges towards advancing the science of mindful lactation. First, mindfulness is based on a core value of acceptance without judgement. This leads to one of the paradoxes of mindfulness: acceptance versus change (Shapiro, Siegel and Neff, 2018). Whereas the two concepts seem contradictory, acceptance of the way things are is often the first step towards initiating change. When a woman faces extreme challenges with breastfeeding, such as unresolved pain, intractable difficulties in achieving a latch, or prolonged mastitis, acceptance may lead to a mindful choice out of self-compassion to discontinue breastfeeding. In such a situation, the benefit of mindfulness is not from continuing to breastfeed, but through gaining acceptance and peace in the rational choice to stop breastfeeding. Mindful acceptance of a discontinued lactation journey, rather than self-judgement, can therefore be framed as a positive outcome. This may require an expanded notion of how success is defined when testing interventions. Second, measuring breastfeeding outcomes such as duration, or overcoming negative symptoms such as pain, does not encompass the more positive aspects of breastfeeding. There is a need to measure the improvement in the parent-child relationship from breastfeeding, including bonding/attachment, enjoyment and being present to engage with the child and feeding. Third, the mindfulness approach to improving breastfeeding focuses on the individual and interpersonal aspects of breastfeeding. This puts additional pressure on the performance of motherhood while ignoring the lack of structural support for breastfeeding across society, health-systems, in the workplace and home (Byrom, 2013; Thomson et al., 2015). Individually focused pressures can contribute to negative emotional responses such as guilt, shame, anxiety and depression (Byrom, 2013; Jackson et al., 2021; Thomson et al., 2015). It is recommended that approaches to supporting optimal infant feeding outcomes and experiences, including mindful breastfeeding approaches, consider the wider picture, including environmental, family, societal and policy influences (Brown and Shenker, 2019).

The environment is an important determinant of lactation duration, with a large drop-off of lactation upon the return to work (Hamner et al., 2021). Mindfulness-based lactation interventions can be more supportive of women across the lactation and infant feeding journey if they are presented as applicable for all feeding experiences including after weaning and this time frame should be included in intervention assessment.

Despite some of the challenges and cautions discussed here, mindfulness practice has been shown to improve satisfaction through the postnatal transition to parenthood which offers promise for all parents, regardless of feeding choices and experiences (Kantrowitz-Gordon, Abbott and Hoehn, 2018). There is an ongoing need to improve social support for breastfeeding, parenting and changing institutional environments and policies and shift modern, western cultural attitudes and expectations. Mindful breastfeeding approaches could be considered within this broader context and factored into frameworks for breastfeeding and wider infant-feeding support. In the next section of this chapter, a conceptual model for mindful breastfeeding is presented, to move towards practical implications for everyday practice.

A conceptual model for mindful breastfeeding

Breastfeeding is a culturally mediated bio-psycho-social activity. It is more than a merely physiological act focused on provided infant nutrition. Breastfeeding is relational with Jackson, Mantler and O'Keefe-McCarthy (2019, p. 67) argue that 'breastfeeding is a complex, learned behaviour that is imbedded in a gendered, social and cultural context' and challenge the notion that breastfeeding is 'easy', especially in societies or cultures where breastfeeding is not the 'norm'. As highlighted, in the sections above, mindfulness practice may offer a way to promote, protect and support breastfeeding and optimal infant feeding practices and experiences. In this section, a conceptual model for mindful breastfeeding, offering practice considerations and implications, is presented.

Mindful breastfeeding can be defined as *feeding the infant at the breast/chest with deliberate attention and awareness of the physical, emotional and relational experience without judgement.* During the feeding, the mother/parent strives to not be distracted by phones, worries, or work and household responsibilities. Mindful feeding can be a moment of solace and respite from the daily worries and experiences. This allows the mother/parent to remain focused in the moment of feeding, in a reciprocal relationship with the infant's focus. Through the mental well-being benefits of breastfeeding, negative mood symptoms are reduced and oxytocin is increased with benefits to lactation and sense of well-being and connection. As a practice, mindfulness does not require perfection – if the mother/parent notices their attention wandering, then they gently and without judgement return their attention back to being with their baby. See Figure 11.2 for a graphical representation of this model of mindful breastfeeding. The diagram captures how mindful awareness shields the mother/parent-infant/child from wider judgements, worries and distractions which helps to support and sustain reciprocity and the physiology associated with breastfeeding, e.g. oxytocin release.

Pickard et al. (2017) describe mindfulness as a vehicle for maternal responsiveness that promotes attuned mother-infant interaction (e.g., through maternal response to distress and positive effects on developmental outcomes). *Trait mindfulness* can be described as a specific person characteristic, that has been associated with breastfeeding intention and practice, defined as 'someone's predisposition to be mindful' (Hulsbosch et al., 2021, p. 2). As already presented above and in earlier chapters of the book, mindfulness can be defined as an awareness that arises from our intentional presence, in the moment, paying attention non-judgementally to our ever-revealing experiences. Pickard et al. (2017)

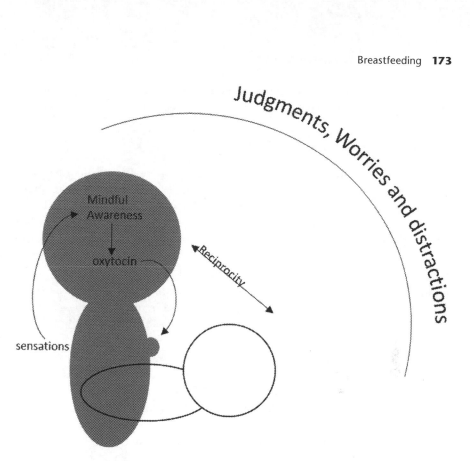

FIGURE 11.2 Graphical representation of a novel conceptual model of mindful breastfeeding.

propose that mindful awareness enables people to process current experiences affording choice over behavioural responses reflective of the context rather than preconceived beliefs. This could support enhanced meaning and behaviours with breastfeeding and wider infant feeding experiences.

Bandura's (2012) self-efficacy account, grounded in social cognitive theory has been developed by Dennis and Faux (1999) and further reviewed by Brockway et al. (2017) who found that increased breastfeeding self-efficacy [BSE] was positively associated with increased breastfeeding rates. Mindful practice has been shown to improve BSE, making it a useful approach to consider, when supporting breastfeeding women, parents and families. Interestingly, *trait mindfulness* defined above as our predisposition to being mindful, whilst thought to be stable, can be strengthened over time through *state mindfulness*. State mindfulness is described as a situationally variable psychological process that can be practiced, for example during mindful meditation (Kiken et al., 2015). This has been shown to reduce preoccupation, especially the preoccupation brought on by acute and chronic pressures which can result in stress, anxiety and/or depression (Hughes et al., 2009). Mindful awareness can help parents to reduce the preoccupations and enable greater levels of response to child–infant behaviour strengthening secure attachment and breastfeeding initiation and continuation, as previously demonstrated in Figure 11.2.

Practical implications

Although typical mindfulness-based interventions can feel time-intensive with weekly classes, daily practice and all-day silent retreats, it is possible to offer more accessible mindfulness resources and practices. Meaningful increases in mindfulness have been demonstrated in brief interventions and mobile approaches (Cavanagh et al., 2018; Mikolasek et al., 2018). While unproven in supporting lactation, health professionals can provide a script or audio recording of mindful breastfeeding or infant feeding practice, prenatally or postnatally as support. A sample meditation is provided here, which applies to breast or bottle feeding. This can be used by any parent or caregiver involved in infant feeding.

BOX 11.1 EXCERPT FROM LOVING KINDNESS WHILE FEEDING BABY BY BECCA CALHOUN (HTTPS:// CCFWB.UW.EDU/RESOURCE/LOVING-KINDNESS-WHILE-FEEDING-BABY/)

Taking a moment now to bring your attention into the body,
Noticing the weight of your body on the surface beneath you,
feeling all of those points of contact.
Maybe releasing or letting go a little bit more into the surface beneath you.
Observing the weight of your baby,
Cradled in your arms or across your lap against your chest.
Noticing all the points of contact with baby.
Inviting a sense of settling into this time together.
Maybe aware of sounds of baby eating in this moment.
Aware of the two of you, together.
Now, intentionally connecting with baby.
Maybe choosing to open your eyes if they've been closed.
Taking a moment to soak in baby visually.
Aware of sensations of holding baby.
Aware of how baby looks.
Intentionally inviting a sense of tenderness for your baby.
A sense of care and love.
Beginning to extend the phrases of loving kindness to your baby.
May you be safe and protected.
May you be healthy in body and mind.
May you be happy.
May you live in peace.

The intention behind developing mindfulness practice centred on breastfeeding is to remain present during each feeding, increase connection with the infant and to accept and let go of any associated discomfort. Because infants are only cognitively able to focus on the present moment, they offer meaningful reminders to parents and caregivers on the importance of presence and reciprocity.

Breast/chest-feeding creates a space to 'be': to be with our newborns, our children and ourselves. Yet, the stillness breastfeeding instils can be challenging in this post-modern world full of interruptions driven by capitalist call for pace, competition and insufficient material and social support for breastfeeding and parenting. Mindful mother/parent-hood does not aim to transform personalities or foster perfect parents but offers an approach that facilitates presence, awareness of unique experiences and perspectives and connection to their infant and others (Vieten, Laraia and Kristeller, 2018).

This chapter has explored how mindfulness can support those experiencing pain during breastfeeding offering a way to mediate the pain. However, it is important to remember that those experiencing breastfeeding pain frequently use words such as 'dreadful', 'being in hell' or 'indescribable' to describe their discomfort (Kronborg, Harder and Hall, 2015). Yet discontinuing breastfeeding results in feelings of guilt and shame leaving parents feeling pressured and trapped (Byrom, 2013; Thomson, Ebisch-Burton and Flacking). Mindfulness may have benefit for those who are unable to continue with breastfeeding to adapt and manage negative thoughts, feelings and emotions. Caregivers can offer compassion as well as foster self-compassion in mothers who have made this transition. Mindfulness should be further extended to any mode of infant feeding, as this is one of the most important interactions between parents and infants. More research is needed to examine and explore the impact, influences and experiences of parents using mindfulness practices on both their state and trait mindfulness and how this can support, protect and promote optimal feeding practice and experiences for all.

References

Babbar, S., Oyarzabal, A. J., & Oyarzabal, E. A. (2021). Meditation and mindfulness in pregnancy and postpartum: A review of the evidence. *Clinical Obstetrics and Gynecology*, 64(3): 661–682 https://doi.org/10.1097/GRF.0000000000000640

Bandura, A. (2012). On the functional properties of perceived self-efficacy revisited. *Journal of Management*, 38(1): 9–44.

Bardacke, N. (2012). *Mindful birthing: Training the mind, body and heart for childbirth and beyond*. New York: HarperOne.

Brockway, M., Benzies, K., & Hayden, K. A. (2017). Interventions to improve breastfeeding self-efficacy and resultant breastfeeding rates: A systematic review and meta-analysis. *Journal of Human Lactation*, 33(3): 486–499. https://doi.org/10.1177/0890334417707957

Brown, A. (2018). *The positive breastfeeding book*. London: Pinter and Martin.

Brown, A., & Shenker, N. (2019). Midwifery basics 8: What can we do to better support breastfeeding mothers? *The Practising Midwife*, 22(4). https://www.all4maternity.com/-midwifery-basics-8-what-can-we-do-to-better-support-breastfeeding-mothers/

Buckley, S. J. (2015). *Hormonal physiology of childbearing: Evidence and implications for women, babies, and maternity care.* Washington, D.C.: Childbirth Connection Programs, National Partnership for Women & Families.

Byrom, A. (2013). Feeding guilt. *The Practising Midwife*, 16(3): 18–23.

Cavanagh, K., Churchard, A., O'Hanlon, P., Mundy, T., Votolato, P., Jones, F., & Strauss, C. (2018). A randomised controlled trial of a brief online mindfulness-based intervention in a non-clinical population: Replication and extension. *Mindfulness (N Y)*, 9(4): 1191–1205. https://doi.org/10.1007/s12671-017-0856-1

Dennis, C. L., & Faux, S. (1999). Development and psychometric testing of the breast-feeding self-efficacy scale. *Research in Nursing Health*, 22(5): 399–409. https://doi.org/10.1002/(sici)1098-240x(199910)22:5<399::aid-nur6>3.0.co;2-4. PMID: 10520192.

Dias, C. C., & Figueiredo, B. (2015). Breastfeeding and depression: A systematic review of the literature. *Journal of Affective Disorders*, 171: 142–154. https://doi.org/10.1016/j.jad.2014.09.022

Dozier, A. M., Nelson, A., & Brownell, E. (2012). The relationship between life stress and breastfeeding outcomes among low-income mothers. *Advances in Preventive Medicine*, 902487. https://doi.org/10.1155/2012/902487

Duncan, L. G., & Bardacke, N. (2010). Mindfulness-based childbirth and parenting education: Promoting family mindfulness during the perinatal period. *Journal of Child and Family Studies,* 19(2): 190–202. https://doi.org/10.1007/s10826-009-9313-7. http://www.ncbi.nlm.nih.gov/pubmed/20339571

Duncan, L. G., Cohn, M. A., Chao, M. T., Cook, J. G., Riccobono, J., & Bardacke, N. (2017). Benefits of preparing for childbirth with mindfulness training: A randomized controlled trial with active comparison. *BMC Pregnancy Childbirth*, 17(1): 140. https://doi.org/10.1186/s12884-017-1319-3. https://www.ncbi.nlm.nih.gov/pubmed/28499376

Fernandes, D. V., Martins, A. R., Canavarro, M. C., & Moreira, H. (2022). Mindfulness- and compassion-based parenting interventions applied to the postpartum period: A systematic review. *Journal of Child & Family Studies*, 31(2): 563–587. https://doi.org/10.1007/s10826-021-02175-z

Galipeau, R., Dumas, L., & Lepage, M. (2017). Perception of not having enough milk and actual milk production of first-time breastfeeding mothers: Is there a difference? *Breastfeeding Medicine*, 12: 210–217. https://doi.org/10.1089/bfm.2016.0183. https://www.ncbi.nlm.nih.gov/pubmed/28326807

Hamner, H. C., Chiang, K. V., & Li, R. (2021). Returning to work and breastfeeding duration at 12 months, WIC infant and toddler feeding practices study-2. *Breastfeeding Medicine*, 16(12): 956–964. https://doi.org/10.1089/bfm.2021.0081

Hilton, L., Hempel, S., Ewing, B. A., Apaydin, E., Xenakis, L., Newberry, S., … Maglione, M. A. (2017). Mindfulness meditation for chronic pain: Systematic review and meta-analysis. *Annals of Behavioral Medicine*, 51(2): 199–213. https://doi.org/10.1007/s12160-016-9844-2

Hughes, A., Williams, M., Bardacke, N., Duncan, L. G., Dimidjian, S., & Goodman, S. H. (2009). Mindfulness approaches to childbirth and parenting. *British Journal of Midwifery*, 17(10): 630–635

Hulsbosch, L. P., Potharst, E. S., Boekhorst, M. G., Nyklíček, I., & Pop, V. J. (2021). Breastfeeding intention and trait mindfulness during pregnancy. *Midwifery*, 101: 103064. https://doi.org/10.1016/j.midw.2021.103064. https://www.ncbi.nlm.nih.gov/pubmed/34161916

Jackson, K. T., Mantler, T., & O'Keefe-McCarthy, S. (2019). Women's experiences of breastfeeding-related pain. *MCN: The American Journal of Maternal/Child Nursing*,

44(2): 66–72. https://doi.org/10.1097/NMC.0000000000000508. https://www.ncbi.nlm.nih.gov/pubmed/30688667.

Jackson, L., De Pascalis, L., Harrold, J., & Fallon, V. (2021). Guilt, shame, and postpartum infant feeding outcomes: A systematic review. *Maternal & Child Nutrition*, 17(3): e13141. https://doi.org/10.1111/mcn.13141

Kabat-Zinn, J. (2003). Mindfulness-based interventions in context: Past, present, and future. *Clinical Psychology: Science and Practice*, 10: 144–56. https://doi.org/10.1093/clipsy.bpg016

Kantrowitz-Gordon, I., Abbott, S., & Hoehn, R. (2018). Experiences of postpartum women after mindfulness childbirth classes: A qualitative study. *Journal of Midwifery & Women's Health*. In press.

Kent, J. C., Ashton, E., Hardwick, C. M., Rea, A., Murray, K., & Geddes, D. T. (2021). Causes of perception of insufficient milk supply in Western Australian mothers. *Maternal & Child Nutrition*, 17(1): e13080. https://doi.org/10.1111/mcn.13080. https://www.ncbi.nlm.nih.gov/pubmed/32954674

Kiken, L. G., Garland, E. L., Bluth, K., Palsson, O. S., & Gaylord, S. A. (2015). From a state to a trait: Trajectories of state mindfulness in meditation during intervention predict changes in trait mindfulness. *Personality and Individual Differences*, 1(81): 41–46. https://doi.org/10.1016/j.paid.2014.12.044. PMID: 25914434; PMCID: PMC4404745.

Korukcu, O., Kabukcuoğlu, K., Aune, I., & Haugan, G. (2021). Development and psychometric testing of the 'mindful breastfeeding scale' (mindf-bfs) among postpartum women in turkey. *Current Psychology: A Journal for Diverse Perspectives on Diverse Psychological Issues*. https://doi.org/10.1007/s12144-021-01858-6. http://offcampus.lib.washington.edu/login?url=https://search.ebscohost.com/login.aspx?direct=true&db=psyh&AN=2021-49463-001&site=ehost-live.oznurkorukcu@akdeniz.edu.tr

Kronborg, H., Harder, I., & Hall, E. O. C. (2015). First time mothers' experiences of breastfeeding their newborn. *Sexual & Reproductive Healthcare*, 6(2): 82–87.

Lara-Cinisomo S, McKenney K, Di Florio A, Meltzer-Brody S. (2017). Associations Between Postpartum Depression, Breastfeeding, and Oxytocin Levels in Latina Mothers. *Breastfeed Med.*, 12(7): 436–442. doi: 10.1089/bfm.2016.0213. Epub 2017 Jul 27. Erratum in: *Breastfeed Med.* (2020); 15(1): 65–66. PMID: 28749705; PMCID: PMC5646739.

Li, J., Kendall, G. E., Henderson, S., Downie, J., Landsborough, L., & Oddy, W. H. (2008). Maternal psychosocial well-being in pregnancy and breastfeeding duration. *Acta Paediatrica*, 97(2): 221–225. https://doi.org/10.1111/j.1651-2227.2007.00602.x. https://www.ncbi.nlm.nih.gov/pubmed/18254911

Lönnberg, G., Jonas, W., Unternaehrer, E., Bränström, R., Nissen, E., & Niemi, M. (2020). Effects of a mindfulness based childbirth and parenting program on pregnant women's perceived stress and risk of perinatal depression-results from a randomized controlled trial. *Journal of Affective Disorders*, 262: 133–142. https://doi.org/10.1016/j.jad.2019.10.048

Lönnberg, G., Nissen, E., & Niemi, M. (2018). What is learned from mindfulness based childbirth and parenting education? Participants' experiences. *BMC Pregnancy Childbirth*, 18(1): 466. https://doi.org/10.1186/s12884-018-2098-1. https://www.ncbi.nlm.nih.gov/pubmed/30509218

McClintock, A. S., McCarrick, S. M., Garland, E. L., Zeidan, F., & Zgierska, A. E. (2019). Brief mindfulness-based interventions for acute and chronic pain: A systematic review. *Journal of Alternative and Complementary Medicine*, 25(3): 265–278. https://doi.org/10.1089/acm.2018.0351

Menekse, D., Tiryaki, Ö., Karakaya Suzan, Ö., & Cinar, N. (2021). An investigation of the relationship between mother's personality traits, breastfeeding self-efficacy, and perception of insufficient milk supply. *Health Care for Women International*, 42(4–6): 925–941. https://doi.org/10.1080/07399332.2021.1892114

Mikolasek, M., Berg, J., Witt, C. M., & Barth, J. (2018). Effectiveness of mindfulness- and relaxation-based ehealth interventions for patients with medical conditions: A systematic review and synthesis. *International Journal of Behavioral Medicine*, 25(1): 1–16. https://doi.org/10.1007/s12529-017-9679-7

Mohd Shukri, N. H., Wells, J., Eaton, S., Mukhtar, F., Petelin, A., Jenko-Pražnikar, Z., & Fewtrell, M. (2019). Randomized controlled trial investigating the effects of a breastfeeding relaxation intervention on maternal psychological state, breast milk outcomes, and infant behavior and growth. *American Journal of Clinical Nutrition*, 110 (1): 121–130. https://doi.org/10.1093/ajcn/nqz033. https://www.ncbi.nlm.nih.gov/pubmed/31161202

Morrison, A. H., Gentry, R., & Anderson, J. (2019). Mothers' reasons for early breastfeeding cessation. *MCN: The American Journal of Maternal/Child Nursing*, 44 (6): 325–330. https://doi.org/10.1097/NMC.0000000000000566

Perez-Blasco, J., Viguer, P., & Rodrigo, M. (2013). Effects of a mindfulness-based intervention on psychological distress, well-being, and maternal self-efficacy in breastfeeding mothers: Results of a pilot study. *Archives of Women's Mental Health*, 16(3): 227–236 210p. https://doi.org/10.1007/s00737-013-0337-z

Pickard, J. A., Townsend, M., Caputi, P., & Grenyer, B. F. S. (2017). Observing the influence of mindfulness and attachment styles through mother and infant interaction: A longitudinal study. *Infant Mental Health Journal*, 38(3): 343–350. https://doi.org/10.1002/imhj.21645

Pickard, J. A., Townsend, M. L., Caputi, P., & Grenyer, B. F. S. (2018). Top-down and bottom-up: The role of social information processing and mindfulness as predictors in maternal–infant interaction. *Infant Mental Health Journal*, 39(1): 44–54. https://doi.org/10.1002/imhj.21687

Renfrew, M. J., McFadden, A., Dykes, F., Wallace, L., Abbott, S., Burt, S. & Kosmala-Anderson, J. (2006). Addressing the learning deficit in breastfeeding: Strategies for change. *Maternal and Child Nutrition*, 2: 239–244.

Rollins, N., Bhandari, N., Hajeebhoy, N., Horton, S., Lutter, C., Martines, J. C., Piwoz, E. G., Richter, L. M., & Victora, C. G. (2016). Why invest, and what it will take to improve breastfeeding practices? *The Lancet*, 387(10017): 491–504.

Roy Malis, F., Meyer, T., & Gross, M. M. (2017). Effects of an antenatal mindfulness-based childbirth and parenting programme on the postpartum experiences of mothers: A qualitative interview study. *BMC Pregnancy Childbirth*, 17 (1): 57. https://doi.org/10.1186/s12884-017-1240-9. https://www.ncbi.nlm.nih.gov/pubmed/28173769

Shapiro, S., Siegel, R., & Neff, K. D. (2018). Paradoxes of mindfulness. *Mindfulness*, 9(6): 1693–1701. https://doi.org/10.1007/s12671-018-0957-5. http://offcampus.lib.washington.edu/login?url=https://search.ebscohost.com/login.aspx?direct=true&db=psyh&AN=2018-26744-001&site=ehost-live. slshapiro@scu.edu

Shloim, N., Vereijken, C. M. J. L., Blundell, P., & Hetherington, M. M. (2017). Looking for cues - infant communication of hunger and satiation during milk feeding. *Appetite*, 108: 74–82. https://doi.org/10.1016/j.appet.2016.09.020

Sinha, B., Chowdhury, R., Sankar, M. J., Martines, J., Taneja, S., Mazumder, S., Rollins, N., Bahl, R., & Bhandari, N. (2015). Interventions to improve breastfeeding outcomes: A systematic review and meta-analysis. *Acta Paediatrica*, 104(467): 114–134.

Slomian, J., Honvo, G., Emonts, P., Reginster, J.Y., & Bruyère O. (2019). Consequences of maternal postpartum depression: A systematic review of maternal and infant outcomes. *Women's Health*, 15. https://doi.org/10.1177/1745506519844044

Thomson, G., Ebisch-Burton, K., & Flacking, R. (2015). Shame if you do—Shame if you don't: Women's experiences of infant feeding. *Maternal & Child Nutrition*, 11: 33–46. https://doi.org/10.1111/mcn.12148

Trickey, H. et al. (2018). A realist review of one-to-one breastfeeding peer support experiments conducted in developed country settings. *Maternal and Child Nutrition*, 14(-1): e12559.

Tseng, J. F., Chen, S. R., Au, H. K., Chipojola, R., Lee, G. T., Lee, P. H., Shyu, M. L., & Kuo, S. Y. (2020). Effectiveness of an integrated breastfeeding education program to improve self-efficacy and exclusive breastfeeding rate: A single-blind, randomised controlled study. *International Journal of Nursing Studies*, 111: 103770. https://doi.org/10.1016/j.ijnurstu.2020.103770. https://www.ncbi.nlm.nih.gov/pubmed/32961461

United Nations Children's Fund (UNICEF) (2018). *A mother's gift for every child*. New York: UNICEF's Nutrition Section, Programme Division. https://www.unicef.org/media/48046/file/UNICEF_Breastfeeding_A_Mothers_Gift_for_Every_Child.pdf

Victora, C. G., Bahl, R., Barros, A. J. D., França, G. V. A., Horton, S., Krasevec, J., Murch, S., Sankar, M. J., Walker, N., & Rollins, N. C. (2016). Breastfeeding in the 21st century: Epidemiology, mechanisms, and lifelong effect. *The Lancet*, 387(10017): 475–490.

Vieten, C., Laraia, B. A., Kristeller, J. et al. (2018). The mindful moms training: Development of a mindfulness-based intervention to reduce stress and overeating during pregnancy. *BMC Pregnancy Childbirth*, 18: 201. https://doi.org/10.1186/s12884-018-1757-6

WHO (2020). *Infant and young child feeding*. https://www.who.int/en/news-room/factsheets/detail/infant-and-young-child-feeding (Accessed 20th January 2022).

12

THE VALUE OF MINDFULNESS IN THE NICU

Dan MacKay and Maggie Meeks

Introduction

This chapter provides insights into mindfulness within the context of Neonatal Intensive Care (NICU). It also explores how mindfulness can support the provision of positive experiences within pregnancy, parenting and early childhood to lay the foundation for optimal health outcomes for parents and their baby. As authors of this chapter, we do not claim to be highly experienced mindfulness practitioners and our context of learning has been predominantly biomedical. However, we are both highly reflective individuals who have an interest in the psychology of human experiences and behaviour. These traits together with our own life experiences have fostered an interest in a mindful approach that we remain keen to continue to develop. We believe that our ideas align both with previous chapters and with the influential text 'The Art and Science of Mindfulness' (Shapiro and Carlson 2009). In this book, mindfulness is described as both a process and an outcome; the concept of a mindfulness *process* is a practice that involves being clear about one's intentions and cultivating sustained and concentrated attention with a compassionate attitude.

The concept of mindfulness as an *outcome* may be considered as a *way of being* with the development of increased awareness of both internal and external contexts. One of us is an educator within healthcare and believes that mindfulness as an outcome can be considered as having a relationship with reflection as described by Schon (1983). Schon originally described reflection as both 'reflection in action' and 'reflection on action'. 'Reflection in action' describes the ability to consciously reflect on an action whilst performing that action whereas 'reflection on action' refers to the more commonly applied reflection for learning which occurs after the event. The relationship with mindfulness is primarily with 'reflection in action' to encourage both an

DOI: 10.4324/9781003165200-12

awareness of internal context on the outside world as well as that of the outside world in the internal context.

Our ideas presented in this chapter have been informed by recognition of the emotional and moral exhaustion that occurs in healthcare practitioners as well as by our own clinical practice, reading, social interactions and discussions. We hope that our perspectives are complementary, with one of us (MM) nearing the end of her clinical career while the other (DM) is just about to transition into his first consultant role. As Neonatologists, our primary intention within this chapter is to consider the integration of mindfulness practice into newborn care, particularly newborn intensive care, as this is critically important to the long-term health of this potentially vulnerable population. There should be a collaboration between the medical or scientific approaches and the psychological and socio-cultural approaches needed to support each baby and family interacting with the NICU. Our own philosophical understanding of health is that it is a complex interaction between physical health, community and family health, mental and emotional health, and spiritual health which fits with the Maori Te Whare Tapa Whā model of healthcare referred to in New Zealand (see Chapter 4 for further information and diagram). The importance of 'fetal programming' and relevance of maternal mental and physical wellbeing on infant mental health, childhood development and long-term adult mental and physical health have also been increasingly recognised (Barker 1995, 2000; Pereira et al. 2012; DeSocio 2018; Porter et al. 2019). Of interest, there is also increasing concern about the concepts of intergenerational trauma which has long been acknowledged by many indigenous societies (Please see Chapter 4).

The definition of trauma is one of a deeply disturbing or distressing experience (see Chapter 14) and the admission of a newborn to the NICU can be considered a potential psychological trauma for the baby, family (Fowler et al. 2019; Dickinson, Vangaveti, and Browne 2022) and to a lesser extent the staff. In this chapter, we will begin with a brief description of the medical reality of NICU before considering the perspectives of the babies, families and staff themselves. We will then reflect on what is done well and what could be done better before proposing how a combination of organisational and individual mindfulness-based practice can continue to improve the NICU experience for both families and staff. We will also consider how mindfulness awareness may also have a role, particularly in preventing staff suffering emotional and moral exhaustion.

The medical reality of NICU

Neonatology established itself as a separate Paediatric Speciality in the middle to the latter part of the 20th century with the first NICU having been established in the United Kingdom in 1946 and the United States in 1960 (Alberman et al. 2001). Some of the foundational concepts included temperature regulation, infection prevention, providing breathing support and ensuring optimal nutrition, which included the importance of breastmilk in this context. These concepts remain equally as valid today. The current NICU environment can also be considered as full of contrasts; there are the babies born only shortly before their due date that have no significant medical concerns but require physiological support regarding temperature and nutrition as well as psychosocial support, and there are those with complicated medical diagnoses at a very real risk of dying. The percentage of births that may result in an admission to NICU has been quoted as up to 14% and it is often not recognised that term babies (37–42 weeks) make up the largest group of these neonatal admissions (Tracy, Tracy, and Sullivan 2007; Braun et al. 2020). Of these, some will only be admitted for a few days with problems of initial adaptation to extra uterine life while others will have more complicated medical diagnoses. The remaining admissions are likely to have been born preterm and their gestation may range from 23 weeks (or even younger) to 36 weeks + 6 days.

The practice of neonatal medicine, like other areas, epitomises the science versus art conundrum of medicine. The understanding of the science of physiology and pathophysiology have contributed to the evidence for effective treatments such as surfactant (lung detergent that helps maintain lung inflation in preterm babies) and cooling for babies that have suffered an ischemic (lack of blood flow) or hypoxic (lack of oxygen) injury around the time of birth. Science has also contributed to the development of increasingly complex technical support such as non-invasive and invasive ventilator breathing support. In contrast, the art of medicine remains a critical component of care which aligns with the humanistic psychological theories, into which mindfulness can be incorporated (Shapiro 2009). However, it would seem that some practitioners have temporarily lost sight of the fact that the development of a neuroscientific approach in psychology has also provided the scientific evidence for the benefits of 'human' touch on long-term optimal neurodevelopmental survival (Bergman 2014; Bergman et al. 2019).

The experiences of NICU

Baby's Experience and potential consequences

An admission to NICU may lead to long-term physical and mental wellbeing effects, both because of the reasons for admission and the experiences or consequences of the admission itself. NICU staff need to become more reflective practitioners, mindful of both the physical and psychological impacts of a neonatal admission on the baby for whom they are providing aspects of care and this is an important area of learning. The long-term physical or medical sequelae of experiences prior to birth are well known; Barkers original 'fetal origins' hypothesis proposed in 1995 suggested that poor nutrition prior to birth, shown by low birthweight, predisposed to the metabolic syndrome of obesity, diabetes, hypertension and hyperlipidaemia in adulthood (Barker 1995). It is now known that fetal and early life experiences of natural events such as earthquakes and human-constructed trauma, also have long-term emotional and mental health sequelae (Pesonen et al. 2006; Lombardo et al. 2012; Liberty et al. 2016; Tarren-Sweeney 2018). This is now also referred to as fetal programming. Additionally, it is increasingly understood that the newborn is not a 'blank slate'; the expression of their unique genetic code is likely to have been influenced by the experiences of past generations and will influence the way in which each baby constructs its own unique understanding of the world in response to its present experiences (see Chapter 4).

The NICU nurseries can be full of potentially distressing sensory experiences for the newborn baby and many of these experiences may occur without the presence of a parent or guardian. These include unfamiliar sensations such as bright light, noise, smell and touch that may be occurring at unexpected times (e.g. during rest or sleep) as well as more invasive procedures such as blood tests. There has been significant work by several neurodevelopmental advocates regarding the importance of minimising exposure to excessive light and noise but the area of touch has been more complex. The professional touch of the nursing and medical staff, while intended to be as supportive as possible, can contribute to the stress of the infant's experience (Weber and Harrison 2019). This includes even gentle and appropriate handling in response to the baby's cues. The importance of parental touch such as skin-to-skin or kangaroo care from the mother and family members is well documented but is not always implemented as much as intended (Campbell-Yeo et al. 2019; Coutts et al. 2021). The parents may receive conflicting messages and may be unsure of when and how they should touch their fragile baby and may be unaware of the enormous value of providing comforting familiar sensations such as their voice, smell and their very presence in providing the foundation for secure attachment. There is no doubt that the newborn baby at times needs periods of complete rest and that the requirements of their medical condition may make handling more difficult. However, when this is the case, it needs to be thought through carefully and constructively, and wherever and however possible, therapeutic touch should be employed.

The areas of attachment and bonding are important concepts in the establishment of this new parent-child relationship and both the parents and the baby have their own unique contribution to make. The terms attachment and bonding are sometimes confused; bonding is the term predominantly used to describe the drivers of the relationship from the parental side and attachment is the term used to describe what happens in the child, which will be elaborated on below. Humans are social animals and the relationships that they have with others can be subdivided into those that include features of attachment, close family relationships or friendships and those that consist of weak ties between individuals such as work colleagues who share a connection. Attachment is the first of these relationships that has a significant influence on the relationships that follow; a mother (and father) begins the process of attachment to their future child before birth and even before conception as they develop expectations based on their own mental wellbeing and unique life experiences. The aims of this early attachment relationship would seem to be to convey to the new baby the nature of the world in which they live i.e. are they able to trust and depend on those around them or should there be an element of heightened emotional vigilance? This concept of emotional attachment was proposed by John Bowlby, a psychoanalyst who believed that initial survival in many animal species was dependent on developing a close relationship with their mother (or permanent mother substitute) and not just on being fed. This concept was further developed by Mary Ainsworth. A further category of disorganised (fearful avoidant) has also been described (Naveed, Saboor, and Zeshan 2020). Both attachment theory and mindfulness are considered as humanistic psychological theories and the relationship between them may be even stronger (Snyder et al. 2012); mindfulness has been shown to increase emotional regulation and decrease anxiety, enhancing internal coping strategies to facilitate the transition to parenthood. This leads to the provision of an environment for secure attachment within the child and this secure attachment may facilitate the development of a mindful way of being. The importance of the persistence of attachment patterns of behaviour into adulthood must not be underestimated as the pattern of secure, insecure avoidant or insecure ambivalent are likely to persist within close personal adult relationships (McCarthy 1999; Chopik, Nuttall, and Oh 2022).

The family experience

The NICU physical environment and unique culture will be unfamiliar to many families and the location of most NICUs within a large hospital may also be associated with other unpleasant memories (including loss). It has been well documented that some families do not always feel welcome when visiting their baby on NICU and experience isolation and a feeling of being judged (Cleveland and Gill 2013; Hugill 2014). One of the reasons for this may be as an unintended consequence of staff both being, and appearing, busy with various tasks. This feeling of not being welcomed may contribute to families not being as physically present with their child on the NICU as expected.

Although families with a baby admitted to NICU may be subjected to similar processes and procedures, their interpretation of these will be unique to them, influenced by their own expectations and prior experiences. Their relationships with the neonatal staff will be influenced by their own personal 'fetal programming', early childhood experiences and attachment style as well as their experiences of healthcare and particularly their perinatal experiences. Families may also feel disempowered in this artificial environment with a loss of control. The construct of control has been extensively studied and can be simplified as the belief in an internal (this is happening because of me and I take full responsibility) or an external (this is being done to me and is not my responsibility) locus of control (Goddard 2012).

These two constructs combine in everyone to produce different results; a primarily internal locus of control has the advantage that the individual believes they have agency to change the outcome but they are accountable for that outcome while the external locus has the advantage that they do not hold themselves accountable but they may feel totally without agency regarding the situation in which they find themselves. The way in which clinical staff communicate with families during their NICU experience may unintentionally exacerbate this loss of control.

In writing this section it has become clear to us that when we talk to families we may frame our communication as to what we (the clinical staff) will do. Consider the example of a baby born extremely preterm (gestation less than 28 weeks). This baby has immature organ systems that are too underdeveloped to survive without various degrees of help immediately following birth including breathing support. Below is an example of initial communication that may occur prior to the birth of a preterm baby:

> *when your baby is born **we** will put them into a plastic bag to keep them warm, if possible **we** will let them have a bit of the blood from the placenta before starting resuscitation. Most babies at this gestation won't have the strength to cry, **we** will put a mask over your babies face and start them breathing. If they need, **we** will put a tube down into their lungs to give more support and medication to help their lungs work*

This description of resuscitation does not encompass the parents' role; staff use a shared language, with implied understanding and expectations which can further exacerbate the sense of isolation that families may feel. The resuscitation of a baby born extremely preterm is a team effort and the parents and wider family are part of that team which needs to be emphasised from the beginning.

The physical separation from an infant that has been admitted to the NICU may have a negative influence on the ability of parents to bond with their baby and may also interfere with the foundation of the baby's developing attachment. Many NICUs have a philosophy that explicitly promotes family-integrated or family-centred care with 24-hour visiting for parents, but there may be hidden or implicit barriers to this (which may have become more explicit during the restrictions of the Covid pandemic). These include the geographical location of the NICU (e.g. transport to and from the Hospital), its physical environment (e.g. locked entrance, lack of privacy) and the psychosocial culture (influenced by a wide variety of professionals with different roles, experience and opinions). The experience of having a baby admitted to NICU has also been shown to be associated with higher levels of anxiety, grieving for the loss of the 'normal' parenthood experiences and a feeling of failure as a parent (Fowler et al. 2019). Some parents experience a very real chance of their child dying multiple times during the NICU stay which can be a significant inhibitor to the consistent sensitive parenting required to allow the development of a secure attachment pattern. This can be further complicated by the complexity of the parent's previous and current life experiences, culture religion and race. These may include their own 'ghosts in the nursery', a term used to refer to the permanent subconscious effects of their own childhood experiences (Fraiberg, Adelson, and Shapiro 1974).

The significant psychosocial distress experienced by many parents because of the admission of their baby to NICU may lead to more instinctive or programmed patterns of behaviour (the opposite of mindful). This includes anxiety and anger which can pose further challenges for the development of a therapeutic relationship with staff.

One of the long-term consequences for families of having had a preterm baby admitted to NICU, is a greater potential for relationship breakdown as well as increased rates of addiction (drug and alcohol) and poor mental health (Grunberg et al. 2022). Attribution of to what extent these outcomes are due to the already challenging psychosocial environments that are more common in parents having preterm infants or to the adversity associated with a neonatal admission is very individual and complex.

Some personal stories

Framing

> She's so perfect, I can't believe it's all gone so well.

By many objective measures, this made no sense. Our pregnancy had been complicated by poor intrauterine growth, an episode of concern over blood pressure and a terrifying trip to the hospital with absent foetal movement. Even the birth process was complicated. An induction, delay in the second stage and foetal distress that led to an assisted delivery with the necessary cast of thousands. Yet my wife was glowing and happy with how well everything had gone.

> Well, what did you expect?.

On reflection, this question has a lot to do with my wife's enduring happiness with the birth of our daughter. My wife is medical and throughout the end of the pregnancy, there were weekly reminders in the form of ultrasounds that this was not a normal pregnancy. Her experience was framed by the knowledge of what can go wrong. From the context of a possible intrauterine demise, a permanently injured baby or a preterm birth our experience of a gentle instrumental with a calm and reassuring obstetrician, and a healthy baby girl was a great outcome. She had framed a successful birth in terms of having a healthy baby, and had expected that some medical intervention may be needed. From that frame of reference, the birth had gone very well.

Neonatal staff

> My job is to gamble well; to understand the odds, risks and payoffs. But my patients often appear to need certainty in the face of the unknowable. This makes me uncomfortable as it's dishonest in the first incidence and exposes me to the risk that a being wrong will be my fault.

There are a wide variety of professionals that contribute to the care of the babies admitted to NICU which includes those who provide the infrastructure, often unseen but essential. This list would include administrative staff, support staff, cleaners and volunteers and the clinical staff which includes nursing, medical and specialty staff such as dieticians, lactation consultants, pharmacists, psychologists, social workers and speech and language therapists. The perspectives of each of these clinical roles are different but complementary and all are essential in providing the collaborative process that aims to increase the probability of an optimal outcome for the baby and family. However, one of the challenges of healthcare is that these outcomes are often unpredictable and occasionally tragic which may or may not be preventable. How do we prepare new clinical staff for this trauma and prevent emotional, physical and cognitive exhaustion in our experienced staff?

The narrative *fallacy* is an important concept to understand in the psychology of trauma as it describes the human tendency to create a simple and flawed story out of events which can be influenced by selective recollection of those events. Simply said we may inappropriately blame ourselves for a tragic outcome and this is known as attribution error. Attribution error refers to a tendency to **under** attribute to context and **over** attribute to individual personal differences. These inherent cognitive biases can make the current situation appear a more likely outcome and lead us to believe that we could have seen this coming, and logically that we could have made choices along the way which would have changed the outcome. Our recall of an event risks unwarranted weighting to remembered factors and ignores chance and context. In doing so we are at risk of making ourselves responsible for all our patients' outcomes, even those that we had no opportunity to foresee or prevent. These personal cortical scars together with well-publicised national or international tragic events can affect future care; we may pay more attention to aspects that relate to our own cortical scars, or are interesting or unusual leading to a biasing of our human innate risk probability calculations.

Unfortunately, the physical and emotional challenges of a career in NICU are well documented and physician burnout is estimated to be around 20–30% (Tawfik and Profit 2020). Burnout was originally described by Freudenberger, a German-born psychologist and psychotherapist, and Christina Maslach, a social psychologist, later developed a psychometric test of burnout (the Maslach Burnout Inventory or MBI). The features of burnout include a combination of mental fatigue or emotional exhaustion, depersonalisation and a decrease in feelings of personal accomplishment. There is a well-established relationship between burnout and quality of patient care with higher rates of burnout being **associated** with worse patient outcomes, increased medical errors, increased unprofessional behaviour and staff turnover (McAlpine 2020). It should be noted the careful use of word association rather than causation as the factors driving high rates of burnout may not be independent from those factors that influence patient outcome. Within this context, causation is more complex and considered to be multifactorial. This includes personal factors (such as skill level, personality, trait anxiety (a person's self-talk) and task complexity) in combination with professional or organisational factors (overwork/lack of control or autonomy/sense of isolation/insufficient rewards/absence of fairness and values conflict). The recip-rocal component of burnout has been demonstrated in a study in Taiwan. Res-ident doctors who felt they had a more trusted by their patients reported lower rates of burnout (Huang et al. 2019).

Where we have got it right and where there is still work to do

NICU environment

There is huge variation in the design of NICUs internationally and much thought goes into the provision of spaces that provide the opportunities for efficient intensive care for those babies that are medically very unwell, as well as discrete family and baby pods that facilitate bonding and attachment. NICUs are often located within larger hospitals which have financial and healthcare delivery advantages but there is also an argument for the location of the less intensive areas (e.g. transitional care units) within birthing centres where there is less of a pathological focus. This is likely to be associated with families expe-riencing less anxiety and feeling enabled to be more involved. The challenge in these situations would be to ensure that any medical needs were met and that there was the ability for immediate transfer to an intensive care setting if required.

The modern NICU can be a place full of sensory experiences that can be un-pleasant for the preterm baby as well as their family. This often includes the need to be attached to monitoring equipment with sound alarms, a powerful visual and auditory reminder of their fragility. The developmental approaches such as NIDCAP (Neonatal Individualised Developmental Care) and FiCare (Family Integrated Care) have provided clear frameworks for the developmental support in these situations, particularly of preterm babies. However, the effective imple-mentation of these frameworks requires adequate human resourcing as well as prioritisation of opportunities for training and continued development of prac-tice. Staff leaders and managers also need to be aware of the complexity of mes-sages that parents and families receive; there may be multiple posters and leaflets regarding explicit intent but the implied or 'hidden' messages may conflict with these. It is important for us to be aware that this may have strong influences on family expectations and behaviour.

The importance of the physical environment is discussed at length in Chapter 8 in relation to parturition. However, many of the principles have an application that is grounded in a mindful approach in any healthcare setting in-cluding NICU.

Baby

It is important to remember that some of the earliest neonatal paediatricians such as Donald Winnicott, Lily Dubowitz and others, as well as those that trained the older ones amongst us often used approaches that could be considered mindful in their day-to-day practice. It was not uncommon to observe these inspiring clinicians sit quietly with a young baby observing their physiological status, neurological behaviour and response to interventions as they reflected on the underlying pathophysiology and what interventions would be helpful. Knowing a baby is sitting with them, holding them, watching their breathing and cues and learning their style of communication and there are many who continue to aim for this style of practice.

There is no doubt that the medical and scientific advances in neonatal care have continued to improve the chances of life as well as minimising long-term morbidity. However, as the medical interventions have become more complex and automated, the perceived need as well as available time to sit quietly at the side of an extreme preterm with their family has become less prioritised. This aspect of care needs to be re-emphasised. Our experience is that when this is practiced, even in a small way while adjusting ventilator settings, just sometimes the infant feels heard and responds.

Family

Before the birth of the baby, the family would normally have expected to be in a familiar environment with mostly predictable challenges, supported within their own social networks. They did not expect to be exposed to issues of life and death in an unfamiliar environment. The facilitation of conditions that will enable the development of the parent relationship with their baby must be prioritised, which includes normalising kangaroo care. These opportunities for quiet episodes of skin-to-skin contact with their baby have significant physiological, psychological and social benefits for both the baby and family. The challenge is for staff to be enabled to prioritise this vital intervention and for families to feel enabled to request it.

One of the remaining questions from a neonatal perspective is if NICU could do more to improve the psychosocial environments that babies will go home to. This process would mean a significant shift in much of the paradigm of neonatal care and consider the infants place in their family, their greater social and cultural network and their environment. As neonatologists we need to be mindful of our own cultural and social expectations and beliefs to engage collaboratively not paternalistically for positive change.

Staff

There is no doubting that the provision of 'care' is fundamental to all NICUs. NICU staff both feel empathy and express compassion, to the babies, families and to each other. The challenge is to feel empathy within the moment of an interaction so that it positively informs compassion but that staff are not burdened with the responsibility of these strong emotions beyond the patient and family interaction. This capacity together with the development of self-attunement and self-compassion (see Chapter 3) provide the foundation for an individual integrating mindfulness processes and ultimately developing their own mindfulness capacity and way of being.

The risk of burnout in healthcare is unfortunately increasing and there needs to be organisational as well as individual strategies to maintain a healthy workforce. Meta-analysis has shown that both organisational factors and individual approaches can improve provider stress and burnout (West et al. 2016; Panagioti et al. 2017). At an organisational level, the simplest operational factors would include the hours of work; as an example, junior medical staff in New Zealand have a maximal working week of 72 hours with at least eight hours off between shifts, which compares to a maximum working week of 48 hours with 11 hours off between shifts in the United Kingdom. There is a known association of fatigue-related errors and single vehicle road accidents with increased shift lengths. The importance of sufficient rest and sleep is increasingly recognised as important in preserving both physical and mental health and enabling resilience. Another organisational factor that is not as well studied in healthcare is that of educational support; what are the essential components of training that need to be provided to enable fulfilment of service commitments and how should staff be supported in their reflections? What are the roles of peer support, mentorship and coaching? At least one university in New Zealand has incorporated a component of mindfulness in their undergraduate medical curriculum for some years now with some resulting promising research (Fernando, Skinner, and Consedine 2017). This is something which could be considered in all healthcare programmes (see Chapter 15).

Incorporating mindfulness to continue to improve the neonatal care experience

The nature of all healing involves the development of a therapeutic relationship. This has been well studied in psychotherapy and while acknowledged in healthcare may not always be given the attention it deserves. This situation is more complex in the areas of paediatrics and neonatology; there is no doubt that the baby under NICU care is searching for the permanent adult with whom to form an attachment (primary relationship) but there will also be reciprocal relationships with nursing staff particularly. The professional relationships of staff with the family of the baby will be critical and are likely to have multiple therapeutic influences.

The conceptualisation of mindfulness as both a process and an outcome provides a framework to understand its applicability to healthcare including within NICU. Mindfulness practice is a *process* that involves holding others in high regard, being clear about one's intentions and cultivating sustained and concentrated attention. Mindfulness as an *outcome* suggests a way of being for the individual. The cultivation of sustained and concentrated attention and the incorporation of mindfulness as a way of being requires sustained practice. This can be considered as purposeful but informal practice, within both personal and professional interactions and formal practice using meditation.

It is important for healthcare staff to be aware that the hospital or NICU environment is their professional home and they are likely to instinctively feel comfortable in the familiarity of their physical surroundings. This is often in contrast to patients, families and visitors and even healthcare professionals working in other areas. All healthcare staff should share the responsibility of making others feel welcome and included. An attractive possibility would be to develop the capacity of staff to consider every potential interaction as an opportunity for a mindful connection, demanding their attention with a compassionate attitude. This process would require practice but could begin with an initial behavioural approach that includes offering a welcoming smile and greeting families when encountered in a corridor or when they arrive to visit their baby.

There are ways in which the stress of an NICU admission for families can be reduced in the short term and the risk of post-traumatic stress minimised in the long term. This includes encouraging realistic rather than idealistic expectations for all of us as we begin our parenting experiences, e.g., expectant families should be aware that there is a reasonable possibility of a temporary admission to NICU even when all will ultimately be well. It is not always possible to predict or prevent a short admission and with the correct support, this should not have any influence on the bonding of a parent to their baby or the attachment of the baby to them. In the antenatal period, there will be some families who have been identified as having a baby that is likely to require admission to NICU. There may be some unknowns and this can be a highly anxious time. These families need to be provided with relevant information and support and introduced to the environment of NICU. This may be a time when an introduction to mindfulness may be beneficial to help reduce anxiety and to learn some relaxation skills (see Chapter 7).

The NICU admission process itself can be overwhelming (McGrath 2008); there is a need to fully evaluate the baby's clinical condition, to implement treatment that is both immediately required to stabilise the baby and likely to be necessary to minimise heat loss and enable adequate hydration and nutrition. Parents often move to the periphery as silent observers, not wanting to interfere or distract from what they understand are important processes. This initial experience of NICU can be traumatic, even when accompanied by excellent communication and support from staff, especially for those families that were not expecting the need for any healthcare intervention. The admission process will also include a significant amount of communication and documentation; the parents may be asked multiple questions about this pregnancy and previous pregnancy experiences, as well as screening questions that may include those related to alcohol or drug intake and experiences of family violence. They will also be asked to confirm their address and contact numbers and asked how and when they wish to be contacted. In return, they will be given information which will include the health of their baby, the treatment, staff roles and visiting on the NICU. These initial processes have developed as the complexity of NICU has developed and it is likely would benefit from a complete redesign where the experiences of families should be sought to inform this process.

The evaluation of mindfulness strategies to reduce stress in parents in a variety of contexts within the NICU environment has been increasing over the last few years and this is an exciting area of development (Joseph, Wellings, and Votta 2019). In 2018 a randomised controlled pilot study looked at the effect of mindfulness-based neurodevelopmental care in parents of preterm infants and there was some evidence in stress reduction as well as reduced length of hospital stay for their infant (Petteys and Adoumie 2018). The feasibility of incorporating mindfulness-based training for parents of babies born less than 32 weeks gestation has also been studied which did show some evidence of stress reduction (Marshall et al. 2019). It is important not to look only at the short-term financial cost: benefit ratio of such interventions as any reduction in the emotional load felt by parents is of value and is likely to have long-term wellbeing consequences for them and their baby. The importance of skin-to-skin or kangaroo care has already been discussed but this essential component of neonatal care is often not maximised and one of the contributors to this may be parental anxiety. A recent paper where mindfulness coaching was used to provide parents with techniques to use during kangaroo care showed a reduction in anxiety, depression and stress (Landry et al. 2022). It is hoped that with the help of experienced psychologists, this intervention may be evaluated further over the next few years.

The trauma of an admission to NICU can disrupt the attachment process for a variety of reasons which include the limitations of healthcare as well as the family context. The use of counselling services during significant health traumas should be normalised for families and staff and psychologists should also consider the screening for trauma (Moreyra et al. 2021). However, there are opportunities within the NICU experience to enable the development of long-term relationships by minimising discomfort and stress and providing consistency and predictability. An admission to the NICU should also be considered as an opportunity to educate, support and grow a family at a time when they may have the time (parental leave) to engage in the process. Supported accommodation should be provided and therapists should be made available to work with families to develop their practical parenting skills and promote healthy and secure attachments. If applicable and families wish to engage it may also be possible to begin a process of working through previous and current psychological traumas. While it's not possible to undo the patterns, behaviours and trauma of the past, it's a very real opportunity to engage with skilled, caring and supportive professionals to make a better future for the family (see Chapter 4).

The experience of providing care within the NICU can be both physically and emotionally exhausting but can also be incredibly rewarding. The staff are human beings and an understanding of human factors (ergonomics), human psychology and behaviour are necessary when considering any work environment and the allocation of tasks; there is likely to be significant value to the baby, family and staff by automating or re-allocating mundane or repetitive tasks to give clinical staff time to watch, listen and interact with the baby and develop healthy therapeutic relationships with families and to partner with them in the practice of family centred, 'humanistic' care. This 'still' time needs to be valued by those that commission and pay for neonatal care. The continued professional development of staff needs to be extended beyond the cognitive (knowledge) and technical (skills). The non-technical and emotional skills need to be recognised and supported in the context of everyone's experience and culture to understand behaviour and biases and new staff need to be both mentored and counselled through this process.

Being in tune or attunement has been considered a precursor to compassion and the development of self attunement and self-compassion are likely to both enhance the therapeutic relationship with the families that we care for and also minimise our own emotional trauma see Chapter 3). Self-compassion should be actively developed. The importance of a professional debrief following a particularly challenging or tragic clinical situation together with ongoing support from a senior colleague or coach cannot be overstated. Although mindfulness-based practice has not been extensively studied in NICU, it is known to encourage the development of objectivity within personal reflection and to improve the quality of sleep and regulation of cortisol levels, both of which will facilitate a professionally calm demeanour. Is it time we started treating staff like elite athletes with technical coaches, performance psychologists, training plans that balance both development and recovery?

Conclusion

In this chapter, our aim has been to frame our thoughts around the importance of the concept of mindfulness both for the infant and family and for the healthcare professional involved in their care. There is increasing interest in the concept of mindfulness but it is also important to remember that the art of medicine has a long history. The ancient Greeks classified medicine as one of the original arts and in the 16th-century Paracelsus described medicine as:

> *not only a science; it is also an art. It does not consist of compounding pills and plasters; it deals with the very processes of life, which must be understood before they may be guided.*

Over the last 200 years, many eminent psychologists had their foundations in the science of medicine (Sigmund Freud, Carl Jung) and some advances in medicine have occurred because of important observational (intuitive) techniques (puerperal sepsis was proposed to be reduced by handwashing before there was any knowledge of infective organisms). In our own careers, we have experienced clinicians with a range of approaches, from the truly holistic and inclusive to the system focused scientific. We hope that we are now truly moving in a direction where our medications, machines, and experience can let us collaborate with infants in compassionate care.

We have also been struck in writing this chapter by the importance of understanding the concept of 'subconscious programming' within all humans and contrasting this with the 'conscious mindful' approach and the influence of both on communication and behaviour. Programming in this context refers to a set of subconscious routines, paradigms and automated cognitive processes that are often used to efficiently handle tasks or situations that are routine. These processes are rapid and require minimal conscious effort to evoke or monitor. They are formed and maintained because they are useful and accurate enough in most situations, most of the time. Daniel Kahneman explored these ideas in his book 'Thinking; fast and Slow' (Kahneman 2011). Mindfulness is in many ways the antithesis of these 'fast' programmed responses; it is slow, conscious and effortful. It is active, requires time and aims to increase accuracy by considering as many of the internal and external informational inputs as possible. Through mindful reflection on our beliefs, practices, culture and experiences we can prepare ourselves for effortful, 'slow' and compassionate communication and care. To truly deliver the best care, and the best outcomes, then clinicians and families need to understand, be mindful of, and be educated in how our mental models, experiences and interactions can have huge and lasting impacts on the lives under our care.

References

Alberman, E. et al. 2001. "Origins of neonatal intensive care in the United Kingdom." Welcome Institute for the History of Medicine.

Barker, D. J. 1995. "Fetal origins of coronary heart disease." *BMJ* 311 (6998): 171–174.

———. 2000. "In utero programming of cardiovascular disease." *Theriogenology* 53 (2): 555–574.

Bergman, N. J. 2014. "The neuroscience of birth—and the case for zero separation." *Curationis* 37 (2): e1–e4.

Bergman, N. J., R. J. Ludwig, B. Westrup, and M. G. Welch. 2019. "Nurturescience versus neuroscience: A case for rethinking perinatal mother-infant behaviors and relationship." *Birth Defects Res* 111 (15): 1110–1127.

Braun, D., E. Braun, V. Chiu, A. E. Burgos, M. Gupta, M. Volodarskiy, and D. Getahun. 2020. "Trends in neonatal intensive care unit utilization in a large integrated health care system." *JAMA Netw Open* 3 (6): e205239.

Campbell-Yeo, M., C. C. Johnston, B. Benoit, T. Disher, K. Caddell, M. Vincer, C. D. Walker, M. Latimer, D. L. Streiner, and D. Inglis. 2019. "Sustained efficacy of kangaroo care for repeated painful procedures over neonatal intensive care unit hospitalization: A single-blind randomized controlled trial." *Pain* 160 (11): 2580–2588.

Chopik, W. J., A. K. Nuttall, and J. Oh. 2022. "Relationship-specific satisfaction and adjustment in emerging adulthood: The moderating role of adult attachment orientation." *J Adult Dev* 29 (1): 40–52.

Cleveland, L. M., and S. L. Gill. 2013. ""Try not to judge": Mothers of substance exposed infants." *MCN Am J Matern Child Nurs* 38 (4): 200–205.

Coutts, S., A. Woldring, A. Pederson, J. De Salaberry, H. Osiovich, and L. A. Brotto. 2021. "What is stopping us? An implementation science study of kangaroo care in British Columbia's neonatal intensive care units." *BMC Pregnancy Childbirth* 21 (1): 52.

DeSocio, J. E. 2018. "Epigenetics, maternal prenatal psychosocial stress, and infant mental health." *Arch Psychiatr Nurs* 32 (6): 901–906.

Dickinson, C., V. Vangaveti, and A. Browne. 2022. "Psychological impact of neonatal intensive care unit admissions on parents: A regional perspective." *Aust J Rural Health* 30 (3): 373–384.

Fernando, A. T., K. Skinner, and N. S. Consedine. 2017. "Increasing compassion in medical decision-making: Can a brief mindfulness intervention help?" *Mindfulness* 8: 276–285. https://doi.org/10.1007/s12671-016-0598-5

Fowler, C., J. Green, D. Elliott, J. Petty, and L. Whiting. 2019. "The forgotten mothers of extremely preterm babies: A qualitative study." *J Clin Nurs* 28 (11–12): 2124–2134.

Fraiberg, Selma, Edna Adelson, and Vivian Shapiro. 1974. "A psychoanalytic approach to the problems of impaired infant-mother relationships." Boston Psychoanalytic Society and Institute, Boston.

Goddard, Nick. 2012. "Chapter 5- Psychology." In *Core Psychiatry (Third Edition)*, edited by Pádraig Wright, Julian Stern, and Michael Phelan, 63–82. Oxford: W.B. Saunders.

Grunberg, V. A., P. A. Geller, A. Bonacquisti, et al. 2019. "NICU infant health severity and family outcomes: A systematic review of assessments and findings in psychosocial research." *J Perinatol* 39: 156–172. https://doi.org/10.1038/s41372-018-0282-9

Huang, E. C., C. Pu, N. Huang, and Y. J. Chou. 2019. "Resident burnout in Taiwan hospitals-and its relation to physician felt trust from patients." *J Formos Med Assoc* 118 (10): 1438–1449.

Hugill, Kevin. 2014. "Father-staff relationships in a neonatal unit: Being judged and judging." *Infant* 10 (4): 128–131.

Joseph, R., A. Wellings, and G. Votta. 2019. "Mindfulness-based strategies: A cost-effective stress reduction method for parents in the NICU." *Neonatal Netw* 38 (3): 135–143.

Kahneman. D. 2011. *Thinking, Fast and Slow*. New York: Farrar, Straus and Giroux.

Landry, M. A., K. Kumaran, J. M. Tyebkhan, V. Levesque, and M. Spinella. 2022. "Mindful kangaroo care: Mindfulness intervention for mothers during skin-to-skin care: A randomized control pilot study." *BMC Pregnancy Childbirth* 22 (1): 35.

Liberty, K., M. Tarren-Sweeney, S. Macfarlane, A. Basu, and J. Reid. 2016. "Behavior problems and post-traumatic stress symptoms in children beginning school: A comparison of pre- and post-earthquake groups." *PLoS Curr* 8.

Lombardo, M. V., E. Ashwin, B. Auyeung, B. Chakrabarti, M. C. Lai, K. Taylor, G. Hackett, E. T. Bullmore, and S. Baron-Cohen. 2012. "Fetal programming effects of testosterone on the reward system and behavioral approach tendencies in humans." *Biol Psychiatry* 72 (10): 839–847.

Marshall, A., U. Guillen, A. Mackley, and W. Sturtz. 2019. "Mindfulness training among parents with preterm neonates in the neonatal intensive care unit: A pilot study." *Am J Perinatol* 36 (14): 1514–1520.

McAlpine, Suzi. 2020. *Burnout A New Zealand Guide*. New Zealand: Penguin Random House

McCarthy, G. 1999. "Attachment style and adult love relationships and friendships: A study of a group of women at risk of experiencing relationship difficulties." *Br J Med Psychol* 72 (Pt 3): 305–321.

McGrath, J. M. 2008. "Trauma and admission to the neonatal intensive care unit: What is excellent nursing care during the admission process?" *J Perinat Neonatal Nurs* 22 (1): 6–7.

Moreyra, A., L. L. Dowtin, M. Ocampo, E. Perez, T. C. Borkovi, E. Wharton, S. Simon, E. G. Armer, and R. J. Shaw. 2021. "Implementing a standardized screening protocol for parental depression, anxiety, and PTSD symptoms in the neonatal intensive care unit." *Early Hum Dev* 154: 105279.

Naveed, S., S. Saboor, and M. Zeshan. 2020. "An overview of attachment patterns: Psychology, neurobiology, and clinical implications." *J Psychosoc Nurs Ment Health Serv* 58 (8): 18–22.

Panagioti, M., E. Panagopoulou, P. Bower, G. Lewith, E. Kontopantelis, C. Chew-Graham, S. Dawson, H. van Marwijk, K. Geraghty, and A. Esmail. 2017. "Controlled interventions to reduce burnout in physicians: A systematic review and meta-analysis." *JAMA Intern Med* 177 (2): 195–205.

Pereira, P. K., L. A. Lima, L. F. Legay, J. F. de Cintra Santos, and G. M. Lovisi. 2012. "Maternal mental disorders in pregnancy and the puerperium and risks to infant health." *World J Clin Pediatr* 1 (4): 20–23.

Pesonen, A. K., K. Raikkonen, E. Kajantie, K. Heinonen, T. E. Strandberg, and A. L. Jarvenpaa. 2006. "Fetal programming of temperamental negative affectivity among children born healthy at term." *Dev Psychobiol* 48 (8): 633–643.

Petteys, A. R., and D. Adoumie. 2018. "Mindfulness-based neurodevelopmental care: Impact on NICU parent stress and infant length of stay; A randomized controlled pilot study." *Adv Neonatal Care* 18 (2): E12–E22.

Porter, E., A. J. Lewis, S. J. Watson, and M. Galbally. 2019. "Perinatal maternal mental health and infant socio-emotional development: A growth curve analysis using the MPEWS cohort." *Infant Behav Dev* 57: 101336.

Schon, Donald A. 1983. *The REflective Practitioner: How Professionals Think in Action.* New York: Basi Books Inc.

Shapiro, S. L. 2009. "The integration of mindfulness and psychology." *J Clin Psychol* 65 (6): 555–560.

Shapiro, Shauna L, and Linda E Carlson. 2009. *The Art and Science of Mindfulness: Integrating Mindfulness into Psychology and the Helping Professions.* Washington, DC: American Psychological Association.

Snyder, R., Shapiro, S. & Treleaven, D. 2012. "Attachment theory and mindfulness." *J Child Fam Stud* 21: 709–717.

Taleb, Nassim Nicholas. 2007. *The Black Swan.* Edited by The Black Swan: The Impact of the Highly Improbable. New York: Random House.

Tarren-Sweeney, M. 2018. "The mental health of adolescents residing in court-ordered foster care: Findings from a population survey." *Child Psychiatry Hum Dev* 49 (3): 443–451.

Tawfik, D. S., and J. Profit. 2020. "Provider burnout: Implications for our perinatal patients." *Semin Perinatol* 44 (4): 151243.

Tracy, S. K., M. B. Tracy, and E. Sullivan. 2007. "Admission of term infants to neonatal intensive care: A population-based study." *Birth* 34 (4): 301–317.

Weber, A. M., and T. M. Harrison. 2019. "Reducing toxic stress in the neonatal intensive care unit to improve infant outcomes." *Nursing Outlook* 67 (2): 169–189.

West, C. P., L. N. Dyrbye, P. J. Erwin, and T. D. Shanafelt. 2016. "Interventions to prevent and reduce physician burnout: A systematic review and meta-analysis." *Lancet* 388 (10057): 2272–2281.

13

BEING MINDFUL ABOUT MINDFULNESS AND PERINATAL MENTAL HEALTH – EVIDENCE, CRITIQUE, AND NEW DIRECTIONS

Aigli Raouna and Angus Macbeth

Introduction

This chapter explores the relevance of, and evidence for mindfulness-based interventions (MBIs) as a psychological intervention option for perinatal mental health both ante- and post-natally. There is increasing awareness of the importance of perinatal mental health as a global public health priority. We will briefly describe what MBIs are, identify the evidence for their effectiveness (and the limits of that evidence base), and conclude by contextualising this literature within the pivot to digital mental health which has been accelerated by the Covid pandemic. We wish to advocate for a critical appreciation of the potential usefulness of mindfulness in perinatal mental health. To do so requires acknowledgement of MBIs' intuitive appeal around flexibility of intervention delivery, potential for implementation at scale and points of contact with other maternal health interventions such as yoga in pregnancy. However, this needs to be balanced against an awareness that the evidence base for MBI is somewhat limited by low-quality trials, and there are ongoing challenges in defining what is and is not an MBI.

About the authors

Angus is an academic Clinical Psychologist, with an interest in perinatal mental health and its impact on infant (and parental) wellbeing. He is also interested in the development and evaluation of psychological approaches to mental health and how mental health is conceptualised and worked with in middle- and low-resource settings (the "Global South"). His interest in perinatal mental health arose from his doctoral thesis on attachment theory in mental health (which suggests that, as an infant, how we experience being parented when under stress is a core part of our social and emotional development) and also his experiences

DOI: 10.4324/9781003165200-13

of becoming a parent while completing his Clinical Psychology training. Originally a mindfulness sceptic, over time he has come to recognise its intuitive appeal as an accessible psychologically informed approach, that potentially has portability across cultures and populations. However, one of his concerns is that we are able to see mindfulness as a useful technique, but not a mental health 'cure-all,' and that in doing so we target access to mindfulness practice in the first 1000 days in a way that is ethical, equitable and evidenced.

Aigli is a mixed-methods Clinical Psychology PhD candidate at the University of Edinburgh, UK. Her research focuses on perinatal mental health and baby's emotional development, especially in the context of bipolar disorder. She has been involved in several projects aiming to close the gap between research and the public, advocating that research findings should be translatable and accessible to everyone. Working as a research assistant and evaluating early parenting intervention and prevention programmes ignited her passion in prevention during the perinatal period, conceptualising it as the 'perfect time machine', whereby acting now potentially forestalls future sub-optimal pathways. As such, she has come to consider mindfulness-based interventions during this period a promising and potentially de-stigmatised mechanism that could support the wellbeing of expectant and new mothers, fathers, and their children. However, the question 'what works for whom' is still one that needs to be explored, in order to confidently provide targeted and tailored support for everyone who would benefit from it.

Why mindfulness, mental health, and the perinatal period?

Pregnancy and the post-natal period form a component of the "First 1000 Days" which covers the period from conception to the infant's second birthday. This is a time of rapid and significant change in a woman's life (and that of their close family and supports), combining biological, cultural, social, and psychological changes. For many women, this is a time of positive change, but for a substantial proportion pregnancy and parenthood is accompanied by significant mental health impacts, most commonly depression/low mood and anxiety. Both anxiety and depression have accompanying risks for both mother and baby, with the association of *un- or undertreated* post-natal depression and both suicide and infanticide the starkest, albeit occurring relatively rarely. Indeed, maternal suicide is a major cause of mortality in the global north (Mangla et al., 2019), outranking haemorrhage and pre-eclampsia. This is also increasing in the global south (Fellmeth et al., 2021). However, anxiety, depression, and stress all increase the risks for suboptimal early outcomes including preterm birth (e.g., Dole et al., 2003; Glynn et al., 2008) and low birth weight, which are themselves linked to increased likelihood of longer-term suboptimal mental and physical health outcomes (Abel et al., 2010; Hoffman et al., 2017). This process may be a partially related to biological processes in-utero, the "Developmental Origins of Health and Disease" hypothesis, but also via interpersonal and psychological processes, such as the impact on parent–child interaction (O'Donnell & Meaney, 2017).

Importantly, paternal depression may also impact child mental health outcomes, although this is often indirectly, via relationship quality and parenting styles (e.g., Sweeney & MacBeth, 2016).

Globally, mental health in pregnancy remains under-recognised and under-treated, and women are increasingly highlighting the importance of offering a broader range of treatments than simply prescribing psychotropic medication (i.e., anti-depressants and anxiolytics), whilst acknowledging that medication remains a valuable tool for treating mental health difficulties. Furthermore, psychological interventions offer a number of advantages including the potential for delivery by non-specialists or peers (Vanobberghen et al., 2020) and also the capacity to roll interventions out at population level, i.e., not necessarily stratified by mental health risk status. Furthermore, as we will see in this chapter, psychological approaches can also be readily pivoted into the digital frame that the Covid-19 pandemic has forced upon societies in both high- and low-resource countries.

The contemporary evidence base for mindfulness and perinatal mental health

There is substantial evidence that MBIs such as Mindfulness-based stress reduction (MBSR; Kabat-Zinn, 2003) and Mindfulness-based cognitive therapy (MBCT; Segal et al., 2002) are effective in reducing depression and anxiety levels in both clinical and non-clinical populations and settings (Kuyken et al., 2015). We list the distinctive characteristics of each approach in Table 13.1.

There is also a significant body of work suggesting that MBIs could be effective across the perinatal period, particularly for depression and common mental health difficulties. A recent review identified 18 studies (seven randomised controlled trials (RCTs), two non-randomised controlled trials and nine treatment evaluations) and suggested that MBIs targeted towards improving mental health in pregnancy were acceptable to women (Shi & MacBeth, 2017). Indeed, maternal participation in an MBI was associated with reductions in perinatal anxiety of moderate to large magnitude. Results for the effectiveness of MBIs on maternal perinatal depression were more variable, with pre-post treatment reductions of moderate magnitude, but no significant differences in perinatal depression scores (both ante- and post-natally) when MBI was compared with a control group. Since 2017, we have also identified at least 26 further studies of MBIs, suggesting further evidence is accumulating. However, meta-analytic modelling (a quantitative approach to synthesising results across studies) of perinatal mental health studies suggested results for reductions in anxiety, depression and stress were more tentative when comparing MBIs to a control intervention (Taylor, Cavanagh & Strauss, 2016). That said, qualitative data confirmed that MBIs were viewed by participants as a beneficial and acceptable form of psychological intervention. One further unanswered question is around the *mechanisms* by which MBIs can affect change in mental health symptoms across the perinatal period.

TABLE 13.1 Examples of Mindfulness-Based Interventions (MBIs)

Generic Mindfulness Interventions	
Mindfulness-based stress reduction (MBSR, e.g., Kabat-Zinn, 2003)	• Intervention combines mindfulness meditation, body scanning and simple yoga • Uses a group format • Typically delivered over the course of 8 weekly sessions • Uses home-practice to reinforce mindfulness techniques
Mindfulness-based cognitive therapy (MBCT; Segal et al., 2002)	• Originally developed for psychological treatment of recurrent depression • Combines standard cognitive-behavioural techniques to restructure maladaptive thoughts and increase behavioural activation, alongside mindfulness techniques to encourage awareness of the present moment. • Uses a group format • Typically delivered over the course of 8 weekly sessions • Uses home-practice to reinforce mindfulness techniques
Mindfulness Programmes Adapted for Pregnancy	
Mindfulness-based awareness (Guardino et al., 2014)	• Focussed mainly on mindfulness practice, adapted to pregnancy, labour, and motherhood concerns • Uses a group format • Delivered over six session format • Uses home-practice to reinforce mindfulness techniques
Mind Baby Body (Woolhouse et al., 2014)	• Psychoeducational format on thoughts, emotions, behaviours combined with mindfulness practice • Uses a group format • Delivered over six weekly, two-hour long sessions • Uses home-practice to reinforce mindfulness techniques
Mindful motherhood (Vieten & Astin, 2008)	• Combines mindful awareness techniques, mindful yoga, and mindful acceptance • Adapted for pregnancy and delivered in groups • Delivered over the course of eight weekly sessions of two hours duration per week • Home practice included

---

Generic Mindfulness Interventions

Mindfulness-based childbirth and parenting programme (Bardacke, 2012)	• Similar techniques and content to MBSR and MBCT with incorporation of specific approaches for increasing bonding with baby and pain management in labour • Group format with 9 × 3-hour weekly sessions • Home practice included

---

N.B. This is not an exhaustive list, particularly in terms of pregnancy-adapted programmes techniques and approaches are often combined with differential emphasis given to mindfulness awareness, mediation, cognitive and pregnancy-related components.

In our earlier review, we identified some evidence that perinatal MBIs were associated with increased mindfulness, but that this data was at a preliminary stage (Shi & MacBeth, 2017). These initial points highlight some of the challenges in trying to draw conclusions across a methodologically and theoretically broad literature, which we will explore below.

First, there are questions of what constitutes an MBI. There is consensus in the literature that interventions based around a psychological approach to focussing on the 'here and now', using attentional techniques and breathing constitute as "Mindfulness" interventions. The extent to which these interventions also seek to work to address maladaptive thoughts or to foster more adaptive, compassionate thoughts and coping strategies (see also Chapter 3), i.e., using the techniques of Cognitive Behavioural Therapy) lead to some variations in the overall MBI package, e.g., Mindfulness-Based Stress Reduction (MBSR, Kabat-Zinn, 2003) or Mindfulness-Based Cognitive Therapy (Segal et al., 2002). However, beyond this, the parameters practitioners and researchers used to identify an intervention as "MBI" are more fluid, which, in turn, has implications for the evidence base used to guide clinical decision making.

For instance, our own 2017 review included yoga-based interventions within the studies reviewed, given the popularity of yoga in pregnancy globally (Shi & MacBeth, 2017). That said, we only included these studies if there was clear evidence from the intervention description that the intervention included several components consistent with integrated mindfulness practice (e.g., techniques to encourage a non-judgemental focus on sensation experienced in the current moment, meditation, breathing, body scan, deep relaxation), rather than simply a description of yoga practices per se. In contrast, other reviews (e.g., (e.g., Lever Taylor et al., 2016) only included MBSR and MBCT trials. A more recent review by Guo et al. (2021) broadened the MBI definition to include all "Mind-Body Interventions", comparing MBIs with CBT, relaxation, and yoga. Notably, in their review, MBIs emerged as having a similar impact to yoga interventions on antenatal stress, with greater effects than relaxation and CBT.

This leads us to a second point that hampers interpretation of this literature. Taking a further look at the Guo et al. (2021) review highlights two further issues that emerge when we try to evaluate across studies. Although MBIs have a similar effectiveness to yoga in their review, this finding is based on comparing twelve MBI Controlled trials of $n=691$ participants with two yoga trials of $n=158$ participants. So, the effectiveness of the yoga intervention is somewhat unstable based on sample size and number of trials. MBIs may be as effective as yoga in lowering antenatal stress, but more yoga trials are needed to strengthen our confidence in that specific result. A more substantial concern in trying to interpret synthesised data is the influence of individual studies on the overall estimate of how effective an intervention is. The Guo et al. (2021) review suggests that the effectiveness of MBIs against controls is equivalent to $d=-1.06$ (95%CI −1.68 to −0.44), or that MBIs are better at reducing antenatal stress to a large magnitude. However, one of the studies included in this analysis (Muthukrishnan et al., 2016), has a significantly large MBI effect against control ($d=-11.54$). In statistical terms, we would be concerned that this study is an *outlier* −i.e., a one-off result. Indeed, if we re-run Guo's analyses without this one study, the magnitude of the effectiveness of MBIs drops to $d=-0.62$ (95% CI = 0.99 to −0.25). As a consequence of the omission of this single study, MBIs are shown to be effective in reducing antenatal stress, although potentially *less so* than focussed CBT or relaxation. As noted above in our description of MBIs, there are also challenges around the overlap of interventions, as MBCT incorporates elements of CBT, and most MBIs incorporate techniques akin to relaxation.

A further issue encountered in interrogating these studies is that the composition of participants in these trials often varies substantially – a feature encountered in all three reviews we refer to in this chapter (Taylor et al., 2016; Shi & MacBeth, 2017; Guo et al., 2021). Some individual studies use general samples of women in pregnancy, some stratify by anxiety or depression, some target groups at elevated risk of stress due to socio-economic or ethnic disadvantage. None of these groups are problematic *per se* for testing the effectiveness of the intervention. Indeed, targeting by the latter criteria makes sense from the perspective of reducing health inequalities, social determinants of health and the effects of structural racism. However, it does create challenges when we try to synthesise across studies. General population studies may have selection biases and also the degree to which individuals already enter the intervention with the tools to maximise their engagement with the MBI. Alternatively, groups with greater baseline difficulties may actually derive greater benefit from the intervention than those who are under less stress. Either way, problems arise when we compare across samples as the differential impact of the intervention on each group tends to wash out the overall picture, and as yet there are insufficient trials of MBIs in pregnancy to really tackle this issue comprehensively.

So, do we conclude that MBIs in pregnancy are ineffective or that evaluations are not to be trusted? No – the evidence suggests that they do have some effectiveness in reducing stress, anxiety, and low mood. But the current state of the evidence states that there is more work to be done on establishing for whom MBIs would be most beneficial, whether they should be targeted at 'vulnerable' groups or offered universally. A second question is whether the explosion in digital health care, fuelled by the pandemic, offers an opportunity to improve our implementation and evaluation of MBIs in pregnancy. We will explore this question further in the remainder of the chapter.

Pivoting to digital – why now?

In contemporary societies, we often find ourselves in busy, rushed lifestyles. We may lack transportation or access to childcare; we may experience stigma; or shortage of mental health care providers; and there may be limited availability of perinatal and culturally mindful care services – especially in rural and middle to low-income settings. These are just a few of the identified barriers for expectant and new mothers when it comes to accessing perinatal mental health support (Webb et al., 2021). In addition, the Covid-19 pandemic has further amplified the accessibility challenges of in-person interventions, often with high or increasing demand colliding with low provision capacity. Data suggest that more than one-third of pregnant and post-partum women reported experiencing significant depressive symptoms during the pandemic (Cameron et al., 2020), occurring against a backdrop of shortages in the availability of mental health care providers (Li, 2020). However, we can also see that in the midst of chaos there are perhaps unanticipated opportunities – in the case of the pandemic opportunity came in the form of technology, with health care services globally, including mental health care, forced to rapidly pivot to remote delivery (Kola et al., 2021). This digital mental health pivot encompasses a broad range of digital or technology-mediated approaches to assessment, intervention, and monitoring, including text, tele-, and video enhanced remote delivery of care, app-based assessment and interventions, and use of data-driven approaches to fine-tune mental health care delivery.

The rapid advancement and widespread use of technology have provided an attractive and relatively stigma-free opportunity to breach distances and connect providers to clients who otherwise would have limited or no access to professionals and services. Of course, digital mental health interventions are not just the aftermath of a global pandemic. Prior to the pandemic, there had been a steady increase in research and clinical applications of smartphone and web-based interventions, with the aim of improving accessibility and addressing inclusivity barriers. Indeed, digital interventions may represent a particularly promising approach for pregnant women who report engaging regularly with digital health technology and are found to be willing to participate in web-supported perinatal interventions (Urrutia et al., 2015). However, the experience of the digital pivot to the rapid provision of mental health care and interventions at scale gives compelling support to the position that now is a sensible time to shift our attention towards identifying and providing safe, remotely delivered, low-cost, and effective perinatal mental health interventions, consistent with the prevailing trend in mental health care in general (Holmes et al., 2020).

Questioning the effectiveness of digital MBI programmes

At the point of writing, there are more than 20,000 mental health-related apps, with a considerable number of them claiming to offer mindfulness and meditating benefits. Most of these available apps, however, have not been scientifically investigated and their validity, treatment effect, and safety have been sparingly explored (Huckvale et al., 2020). Despite enthusiasm and in some situations targeted marketing of mental health apps, ethical complications arising from rapid technological developments include a lack of rigour in studies and publications within this area, as emphasised by many researchers (e.g., Martinez-Martin et al., 2020; Balcombe & De Leo, 2021). So, alongside the promise and potential of digital mental health interventions, urgent questions over the quality, consistency, and sustainability of the current evidence for digital mental health remain.

Focusing in on perinatal mental health, evidence for digital mindfulness-based programmes for pregnant and post-partum women is still sparse and at its preliminary stages of establishing its effectiveness. Preliminary findings of studies exploring the feasibility of digital MBI show acceptability of the intervention among women during the perinatal period (Yang et al., 2019; Avalos et al., 2020; Felder et al., 2020; Kubo et al., 2021). Furthermore, evidence on the efficacy and effectiveness of digital MBIs show significant improvements in pre–post-intervention scores for depression symptoms, anxiety, perceived stress, sleep disturbance, mindfulness, and positive affect, as well as medium between-group effect sizes (Avalos et al., 2020; Goetz et al., 2020; Kubo et al., 2021; Latendresse et al., 2021; Sun et al., 2021). However, synthesising and drawing conclusions from the digital MBI evidence, although extremely limited compared to the in-person MBI literature, appears to pose similar challenges to that broader literature.

Existing electronic mindfulness interventions have mostly, but not exclusively, focused on working with antenatal women experiencing the full spectrum of depressive symptoms. This range spans from 'at-risk' women (Felder et al., 2017; Sun et al., 2021; Latendresse et al., 2021), through mild to moderate symptoms (Krusche et al., 2018; Yang et al., 2019; Latendresse et al., 2021) through moderate to severe symptoms (Avalos et al., 2020; Kubo et al., 2021), to hospitalised high-risk pregnant women (Goetz et al., 2020). Studies consist of a mix of randomised control trials, single-arm, and open trials, with sample size and length of digital MBIs varying from 27 to 185 women and from six to eight weeks, respectively. An exception to the above delivery was a one-week rapid electronic intervention tailored to the needs of inpatient pregnant women (Goetz et al., 2020). Importantly, current evidence highlighted two main approaches for delivering digital mindfulness-based interventions: (1) group or individual synchronous web-based adaptations of traditional mindfulness-based interventions and (2) individual, self-paced, asynchronous mobile intervention apps (mHealth). This distinction is important with regards to the extent to which providers require prior knowledge of the intervention protocol and/or the delivery method for the intervention, as each approach places a slightly different emphasis on each element.

Looking more closely at these two distinct digital MBI approaches there are a number of unique strengths and limitations. Although the use of technology has the potential to reach many people without being limited by geographic boundaries, studies using web-based versions of the traditional MBIs in a webinar format with a facilitator can still be time and resource-intensive, with limits on the flexibility for expectant or new mothers who are required to attend weekly scheduled sessions. On the other hand, comparatively low retention rates in MBI studies using self-paced smartphone apps suggest that the absence of a facilitator and the accountability imposed by a synchronous session (i.e., "real-time") may counteract participants' motivation to complete the intervention. Therefore, a scalable hybrid approach of asynchronous brief mindfulness-based sessions (i.e., user can access material at their convenience), automatic reminders triggered by brief app inactivity, and personal communication in cases where participants are not engaging with the app for a longer time may offer a solution to the above limitations.

Stepping back from the specific interventions, there is a broader set of questions regarding whether a pivot to digital MBIs is the best answer to the challenge of increased care demand at a time of increased resource constraints. We are content that the existing evidence suggests that the complexities of treatment delivery, evaluation research and implementation requires complex, person-centred answers, taking us back to the ongoing debate of what works for whom. As the evidence base for digital MBIs increases and evolves, we suggest that providers, developers, and stakeholders should take into account the following key factors in relation to MBI implantation, illustrated in Figure 13.1.

As can be seen from the evidence presented in this chapter, MBIs in pregnancy and the perinatal period are acceptable to women, are reasonably well tolerated as interventions, and have evidence of effectiveness in alleviating stress, anxiety, and low mood. More recently, there is emergent evidence that they can be adapted into a digital format, either via online 'real-time', synchronous delivery, or in an asynchronous app-based format. Therefore, MBIs offer one solution to bridging the gap between increasing demand for mental health care in pregnancy and ongoing resource constraints. There is also an intuitive attractiveness in using MBIs as a psychological intervention offering in pregnancy and post-natally, given their adaptability in terms of who delivers the intervention (mental health, general health, maternity professionals, or peer-delivered), relation to other evidence-based interventions (e.g., CBT) and in the mode of delivery (online or face-to-face; group or individual). However, a number of questions remain which are important for all those with an interest in improving the implementation of MBIs in the perinatal period to keep in mind.

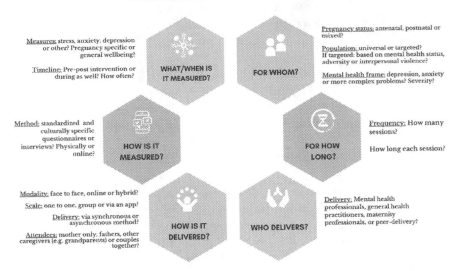

Key factors to consider when implementing and evaluating Mindfulness based interventions

Measures: stress, anxiety, depression or other? Pregnancy specific or general wellbeing?

Timeline: Pre-post intervention or during as well? How often?

WHAT/WHEN IS IT MEASURED?

Pregnancy status: antenatal, postnatal or mixed?

Population: universal or targeted? If targeted: based on mental health status, adversity or interpersonal violence?

FOR WHOM?

Mental health frame: depression, anxiety or more complex problems? Severity?

Method: standardized and culturally specific questionnaires or interviews? Physically or online?

HOW IS IT MEASURED?

Frequency: How many sessions?

How long each session?

FOR HOW LONG?

Modality: face to face, online or hybrid?
Scale: one to one, group or via an app?
Delivery: via synchronous or asynchronous method?
Attendees: mother only, fathers, other caregivers (e.g. grandparents) or couples together?

HOW IS IT DELIVERED?

Delivery: Mental health professionals, general health practitioners, maternity professionals, or peer-delivery?

WHO DELIVERS?

FIGURE 13.1   Key factors to consider when implementing and evaluating Mindfulness based interventions.

First, we still do not know which women we should target MBIs towards. This can be dissected in various ways – contrasting universal health MBI intervention protocols with targeted MBI interventions towards those most vulnerable in terms of mental health or adversity (such as experiences of multiple deprivation, interpersonal violence, conflict, or refugee status). Second, the choice of outcomes and measures makes a substantial difference to evaluating the effectiveness of MBI interventions. Providers should ensure measures for mental health are adapted for pregnancy/perinatal status such as using the two-item "Whooley" questions as a screen (Howard et al., 2018), with more detailed assessment if indicated using the Edinburgh Postnatal Depression Scale or Patient Health Questionnaire-9 (Levis et al., 2020). We also advocate that clear differentiation should be made between general mental health and pregnancy-specific symptoms, particularly anxiety. Third, the severity of mental health is often poorly captured across studies, with over-representation of mild levels of mood, anxiety, and stress in samples, and relatively few studies exploring more complex mental health presentations such as bipolar disorders, psychosis, and personality disorders. Relatedly, very few studies tap into social determinants of mental health such as previous adversity, experiences of interpersonal violence, socio-cultural appropriateness, and spiritual distress, which may themselves hold challenges for implementation of MBIs given the need for a feeling of 'safeness' required to benefit from these MBIs. Fourth, comparison between MBIs is hampered by the proliferation of delivery options – online, group, individual, guided, practitioner-led and more empirical examination is needed in this area too. There is a degree of inevitability here, as the flexibility and breadth of techniques involved in interventions labelled as MBIs create challenges for rigorous evaluation. Fifth, we still have relatively little qualitative material on participants and practitioners' experiences of engaging with perinatal MBIs, and this paucity of experiential exploration is needed. In addition, there is limited data on the cultural appropriateness of MBIs and what, if any, cultural adaptations would be needed to make them acceptable and accessible to a wider population. Finally, we note that MBIs are evolving in the context of Covid-related direct and indirect impacts, both in general and in relation to perinatal mental health (e.g. Smith et al., 2021; Zhang et al., 2021). We would therefore predict the growth in MBI digital delivery potentially offering new opportunities for developing MBIs in middle- and low-resource settings where resources are already even further constrained.

References

Abel, K. M., Wicks, S., Susser, E. S., Dalman, C., Pedersen, M. G., Mortensen, P. B., & Webb, R. T. (2010). Birth weight, schizophrenia, and adult mental disorder: Is risk confined to the smallest babies?. *Archives of General Psychiatry*, 67(9), 923–930.

Avalos, L. A., Aghaee, S., Kurtovich, E., Quesenberry Jr, C., Nkemere, L., McGinnis, M. K., & Kubo, A. (2020). A Mobile health mindfulness intervention for women with moderate to moderately severe postpartum depressive symptoms: Feasibility study. *JMIR Mental Health*, 7(11), e17405.

Balcombe, L., & De Leo, D. (2021). Digital mental health challenges and the horizon ahead for solutions. *JMIR Mental Health*, 8(3), e26811.

Bardacke, N. (2012). *Mindful birthing: Training the mind, body, and heart for childbirth and beyond*. Harper Collins.

Cameron, E. E., Joyce, K. M., Delaquis, C. P., Reynolds, K., Protudjer, J. L., & Roos, L. E. (2020). Maternal psychological distress & mental health service use during the COVID-19 pandemic. *Journal of Affective Disorders*, 276, 765–774.

Dole, N., Savitz, D. A., Hertz-Picciotto, I., Siega-Riz, A. M., McMahon, M. J., & Buekens, P. (2003). Maternal stress and preterm birth. *American Journal of Epidemiology*, 157(1), 14–24.

Felder, J. N., Epel, E. S., Neuhaus, J., Krystal, A. D., & Prather, A. A. (2020). Efficacy of digital cognitive behavioral therapy for the treatment of insomnia symptoms among pregnant women: A randomized clinical trial. *JAMA Psychiatry*, 77(5), 484–492. https://doi.org/10.1001/jamapsychiatry.2019.4491.

Felder, J. N., Segal, Z., Beck, A., Sherwood, N. E., Goodman, S. H., Boggs, J.,... & Dimidjian, S. (2017). An open trial of web-based mindfulness-based cognitive therapy for perinatal women at risk for depressive relapse. *Cognitive and Behavioral Practice*, 24(1), 26–37.

Fellmeth, G., Nosten, S., Khirikoekkong, N., Oo, M. M., Gilder, M. E., Plugge, E.,... & McGready, R. (2021). Suicidal ideation in the perinatal period: Findings from the Thailand–Myanmar border. *Journal of Public Health*.

Glynn, L. M., Schetter, C. D., Hobel, C. J., & Sandman, C. A. (2008). Pattern of perceived stress and anxiety in pregnancy predicts preterm birth. *Health Psychology*, 27(1), 43–51.

Goetz, M., Schiele, C., Müller, M., Matthies, L. M., Deutsch, T. M., Spano, C.,... & Wallwiener, S. (2020). Effects of a brief electronic mindfulness-based intervention on relieving prenatal depression and anxiety in hospitalized high-risk pregnant women: Exploratory pilot study. *Journal of Medical Internet Research*, 22(8), e17593.

Guardino, C., Dunkel Schetter, C., Bower, J., Lu, M., & Smalley, S. (2014). Randomised controlled pilot trial of mindfulness training for stress reduction during pregnancy. *Psychology and Health*, 29(3), 334–349. https://doi.org/10.1080/08870446.2013.852670

Guo, P., Zhang, X., Liu, N., Wang, J., Chen, D., Sun, W.,… & Zhang, W. (2021). Mind–body interventions on stress management in pregnant women: A systematic review and meta-analysis of randomized controlled trials. *Journal of Advanced Nursing*, 77(1), 125–146.

Hoffman, D. J., Reynolds, R. M. and Hardy, D. B. (2017). Developmental origins of health and disease: Current knowledge and potential mechanisms. *Nutrition Reviews*, 75(12), 951–970

Holmes, E. A., O'Connor, R. C., Perry, V. H., Tracey, I., Wessely, S., Arseneault, L., … & Bullmore, E. (2020). Multidisciplinary research priorities for the COVID-19 pandemic: A call for action for mental health science. *The Lancet Psychiatry*, 7(6), 547–560.

Howard, L. M., Ryan, E. G., Trevillion, K., Anderson, F., Bick, D., Bye, A.,… & Pickles, A. (2018). Accuracy of the Whooley questions and the Edinburgh Postnatal Depression Scale in identifying depression and other mental disorders in early pregnancy. *The British Journal of Psychiatry*, 212(1), 50–56.

Huckvale, K., Nicholas, J., Torous, J., & Larsen, M. E. (2020). Smartphone apps for the treatment of mental health conditions: Status and considerations. *Current Opinion in Psychology*, 36, 65–70.

Kabat-Zinn, J. (2003). Mindfulness-based interventions in context: Past, present, and future. *Clinical Psychology: Science and Practice*, 10(2), 144–156.

Kola, L., Kohrt, B. A., Hanlon, C., Naslund, J. A., Sikander, S., Balaji, M.,… & Patel, V. (2021). COVID-19 mental health impact and responses in low-income and middle-income countries: Reimagining global mental health. *The Lancet Psychiatry*, 8(6), 535–550.

Krusche, A., Dymond, M., Murphy, S. E., & Crane, C. (2018). Mindfulness for pregnancy: A randomised controlled study of online mindfulness during pregnancy. *Midwifery*, 65, 51–57.

Kubo, A., Aghaee, S., Kurtovich, E. M., Nkemere, L., Quesenberry, C. P., McGinnis, M. K., & Avalos, L. A. (2021). mHealth mindfulness intervention for women with moderate-to-moderately-severe antenatal depressive symptoms: A pilot study within an integrated health care system. *Mindfulness*, 12(6), 1387–1397.

Kuyken W, Hayes R, Barrett B, Byng R, Dalgleish T, Kessler D.,…& Byford S. 2015. Effectiveness and cost-effectiveness of mindfulness-based cognitive therapy compared with maintenance antidepressant treatment in the prevention of depressive relapse or recurrence (PREVENT): A randomised controlled trial. *Lancet*. Jul 4;386(9988):63–73. https://doi.org/10.1016/S0140-6736(14)62222-4. Epub 2015 Apr 20. Erratum for: Lancet. 2016 Oct 1;388(10052):1376. PMID: 25907157.

Latendresse, G., Bailey, E., Iacob, E., Murphy, H., Pentecost, R., Thompson, N., & Hogue, C. (2021). A group videoconference intervention for reducing perinatal depressive symptoms: A telehealth pilot study. *Journal of Midwifery & Women's Health*, 66(1), 70–77.

Lever Taylor, B., Cavanagh, K., & Strauss, C. (2016). The effectiveness of mindfulness-based interventions in the perinatal period: a systematic review and meta-analysis. *PloS one*, 11(5), e0155720.

Levis, B., Negeri, Z., Sun, Y., Benedetti, A., & Thombs, B. D. (2020). Accuracy of the Edinburgh Postnatal Depression Scale (EPDS) for screening to detect major depression among pregnant and postpartum women: Systematic review and meta-analysis of individual participant data. *bmj*, 371.

Li, L. (2020). Challenges and priorities in responding to COVID-19 in inpatient psychiatry. *Psychiatric Services*, 71(6), 624–626.

Mangla, K., Hoffman, M. C., Trumpff, C., O'Grady, S., & Monk, C. (2019). Maternal self-harm deaths: An unrecognized and preventable outcome. *American Journal of Obstetrics and Gynaecology*, 221(4), 295–303

Martinez-Martin, N., Dasgupta, I., Carter, A., Chandler, J. A., Kellmeyer, P., Kreitmair, K.,… & Cabrera, L. Y. (2020). Ethics of Digital Mental Health During COVID-19: Crisis and Opportunities. *JMIR Mental Health*, 7(12), e23776.

Muthukrishnan, S., Jain, R., Kohli, S., & Batra, S. (2016). Effect of mindfulness meditation on perceived stress scores and autonomic function tests of pregnant Indian women. *Journal of Clinical and Diagnostic Research: JCDR*, 10(4), CC05.

O'Donnell, Kieran J., and Michael J. Meaney. (2017). Fetal origins of mental health: the developmental origins of health and disease hypothesis. *American Journal of Psychiatry* 174(4): 319–328.

Segal, Z. V., Williams, J. M. G., & Teasdale, J. D. (2002). *Preventing depression: Mindfulness-based cognitive therapy*. New York: Guilford.

Shi, Z., & MacBeth, A. (2017). The effectiveness of mindfulness-based interventions on maternal perinatal mental health outcomes: A systematic review. *Mindfulness*, 8(4), 823–847.

Smith, R. B., Mahnert, N. D., Foote, J., Saunders, K. T., Mourad, J., & Huberty, J. (2021). Mindfulness effects in obstetric and gynecology patients during the coronavirus disease 2019 (COVID-19) pandemic: A randomized controlled trial. *Obstetrics and Gynecology*, 137(6), 1032–1040. https://doi.org/10.1097/AOG.0000000000004316

Sun, Y., Li, Y., Wang, J., Chen, Q., Bazzano, A. N., & Cao, F. (2021). Effectiveness of smartphone-based mindfulness training on maternal perinatal depression: Randomized controlled trial. *Journal of Medical Internet Research*, 23(1), e23410.

Sweeney, S., & MacBeth, A. (2016). The effects of paternal depression on child and adolescent outcomes: A systematic review. *Journal of Affective Disorders*, 205, 44–59.

Taylor, B. L., Cavanagh, K., & Strauss, C. (2016). The effectiveness of mindfulness-based interventions in the perinatal period: A systematic review and meta-analysis. *PloS One*, 11(5), e0155720.

Urrutia, R. P., Berger, A. A., Ivins, A. A., Urrutia, E. G., Beckham, A. J., Thorp Jr, J. M., & Nicholson, W. K. (2015). Internet use and access among pregnant women via computer and mobile phone: Implications for delivery of perinatal care. *JMIR mHealth and uHealth*, 3(1), e25.

Vanobbberghen, F., Weiss, H. A., Fuhr, D. C., Sikander, S., Afonso, E., Ahmad, I., … & Rahman, A. (2020). Effectiveness of the Thinking Healthy Programme for perinatal depression delivered through peers: Pooled analysis of two randomized controlled trials in India and Pakistan. *Journal of Affective Disorders*, 265, 660–668.

Vieten, C., & Astin, J. (2008). Effects of a mindfulness-based intervention during pregnancy on prenatal stress and mood: Results of a pilot study. *Archives of Women's Mental Health*, 11(1), 67–74. https://doi.org/10.1007/s00737-008-0214-3

Webb, R., Uddin, N., Ford, E., Easter, A., Shakespeare, J., Roberts, N.,… & Williams, L. R. (2021). Barriers and facilitators to implementing perinatal mental health care in health and social care settings: A systematic review. *The Lancet Psychiatry*, 8(6), 521–534.

Woolhouse, H., Mercuri, K., Judd, F., & Brown, S. J. (2014). Antenatal mindfulness intervention to reduce depression, anxiety, and stress: A pilot randomised controlled trial of the MindBabyBody program in an Australian tertiary maternity hospital. *BMC Pregnancy and Childbirth*, 14(1), 1–16.

Yang, M., Jia, G., Sun, S., Ye, C., Zhang, R., & Yu, X. (2019). Effects of an online mindfulness intervention focusing on attention monitoring and acceptance in pregnant women: A randomized controlled trial. *Journal of Midwifery & Women's Health*, 64(1), 68–77.

Zhang, H., Zhang, A., Liu, C., Xiao, J., & Wang, K. (2021). A brief online mindfulness-based group intervention for psychological distress among Chinese residents during COVID-19: A pilot randomized controlled trial. *Mindfulness*, 12(6), 1502–1512.

14

MINDFUL RESPONDING IN A CRISIS

Tracy Donegan

At some stage during our lives, we will all experience a crisis. In this chapter, I define crisis as an adverse or catastrophic event that is emotionally and/or physically stressful or traumatic. During times of crisis, effective solutions need to be found, coping resources accessed and sometimes difficult decisions are unavoidable. Navigating a crisis to minimize harm and optimize health, and in some cases for survival, demands clear rational thinking, focus and a calm balanced emotional state. However, in a crisis, the initial response is unlikely to be a calm focused mindset but one of overwhelm, stress and fear as the amygdala gets bombarded with stimuli (see Chapter 2). In this chapter, I will explore the benefits of mindfulness practices for parents and professionals during the unpredictable stressful events and emotions of a crisis around childbirth. The chapter begins by exploring the activity of the brain during an actual or perceived crisis.

The brain in crisis

When we experience what we perceive to be a catastrophic event, the perception of a threat (real or imagined) activates areas of the brain associated with survival. We enter a fight, flight or freeze response as a result of catecholamine[1] activation. In a crisis, the two hemispheres of the brain respond differently (Kunwar et al. 2015). The left part of the brain tries to make sense of what's happening by trying to find patterns and predictability about the events – even creating narratives that give the illusion of control. The left brain is responsible for retrieving facts, making plans and organizing lists, and has a very narrow view of what is happening in a broad context. The right brain communicates in imagery, is present, moment focused and considered the centre for emotions. The function of the right brain is to create meaning from experiences and it has a wider 'big picture' perspective (Corballis 2014; Niebauer 2019).

DOI: 10.4324/9781003165200-14

The brain has evolved to continuously scan the environment for threats (negativity bias[2]) but it can't determine whether the threat is external (being attacked in the street) or remembering the attack (an internal threat). Whether the threat is real or imagined, this survival mechanism can create additional mental and emotional chaos during a crisis.

There is an old Buddhist story of the second arrow:

> The Buddha once asked a student,
> "If a person is struck by an arrow (the initial crisis event) is it painful?"
> The student replied,
> "Yes of course as the first 'arrow' is unpredictable and uncontrollable."

Examples of 'arrows' certainly occur in a contemporary context, they might include, serious illness, a pandemic, divorce, death of a baby and birth trauma.

The student continued,

> "If the person is struck by a second arrow, is it even more painful?"

The Buddha explained that,

> In life, we cannot always control the first arrow (the crisis event). However, the second arrow is how we respond to the first and with this second arrow comes the possibility of choice.
> *Sallatha Sutta – translated by Thanissaro Bhikkhu (2013)*

However, this is not as simple as it may seem because sociocultural factors and even genetics influence the impact of the second arrow. We will therefore either feel more or less stress during a crisis according to how our brain habitually processes these events. This is where mindfulness training is key because as we become aware of the second arrow, our response to the crisis, we have the potential to choose how we respond, thereby influencing how crises impact us in the short and long term (Kang et al. 2012). Mindfulness training has been shown to change activity in the right amygdala, an area of the brain implicated in emotional processing, resulting in reduced stress (Kral et al. 2018). This effect has been demonstrated following only a week of mindfulness training in beginners (Taylor et al. 2011). Importantly, mindfulness training has a beneficial trait effect, vis-à-vis, the brain starts to function differently in ordinary daily life – not just when meditating. This changing trait effect means that the person practicing mindfulness becomes predisposed to react less intensely when a crisis occurs (Bränström et al. 2011).

There is a common misconception that mindfulness is simply a relaxation exercise. Although relaxation is beneficial in itself, one of the greatest benefits of mindfulness practice is an increase in insight into how our mind works and how much mental suffering we can avoid by investigating our habits of thought with curiosity and kindness (Feruglio et al. 2021; Hoffmann et al. 2016). During

stressful times we are more likely to be self-critical, therefore, developing awareness of our inner landscape is the beginning because we cannot change what we
are not aware of. Once we begin noticing unhelpful habits of thought we can
offer ourselves compassion, so that when we discover aspects of ourselves that we
do not like we can become intentionally kind to ourselves rather than reactive
and self-judging. Contrary to common misconceptions about meditative practices, mindfulness is not about having no thoughts but intentionally engaging
less with negative thoughts and emotions as they arise and leaving more room
for positive emotions. Negative ideas, fantasies and beliefs will always arise in the
mind – our lack of awareness that this is a tendency of the mind is the problem.
As with the arrow's analogy, we do have a choice not to react unquestioningly
and in a catastrophizing way to such negative thoughts and emotions. When we
are not aware of the mind's process, our state of a mind is freely wandering; in
times of stress, this can be debilitating.

Personally, I have experienced the positive effects of mindfulness in times
of stress. During the Covid-19 pandemic my mother developed a rare terminal
illness that necessitated leaving my family in the United States and moving back
to Ireland for several months at a time to coordinate care. Activation of the
default mode network (DMN), the normal state of a wandering mind, biases
the brain to focus on previous traumatic events and future worries (King et al.
2016). As the mind wanders throughout the day it is possible to overlook or
miss the ordinary, simple moments of our human experience, of being present
and connected in the moment with those dearest to us. My mindfulness and
self-compassion practices were reliable, nurturing and supportive during that
challenging time. Compassion practices such as the meditation focused 'Loving
Kindness', intentionally create psychological safety by activating the soothing-
affiliative system of the brain (Neff 2003 Gilbert 2019). By activating this brain
network the 'feel good' nurturing neurotransmitters oxytocin and endorphins
are released. These practices allowed me to be more present with my mother as
her health declined. They enabled me to make peace with her diagnosis, make
difficult decisions relating to her care and condition and endure the emotional
suffering that comes with a terminal illness, the care and ultimately the death of
a parent. As my mother's health deteriorated day by day, it would have been easy
to get stuck in automatic 'firefighting' mode because of the brain's evolutionary
negativity bias when confronted with threats and manifested worst-case scenarios in my mind. Kiken and Shook (2011) explain how mindfulness practices
reduce this negativity bias. Therefore, when the worst-case scenario is the reality
and circumstances cannot be changed, being present in the moment and accepting all emotions non-judgementally is a priceless gift we can give ourselves and
others during a time of stress and suffering.

Meditation and mindfulness provide us with the headspace to sit with difficult unwanted[3] emotions and circumstances with an attitude of curiosity and
acceptance as we return to the present moment again and again. By acknowledging that our thoughts and emotions are temporary passing mental events, we

can disengage from the internal drama that causes additional unnecessary stress during a crisis. As we become more mindful, we begin to recognize that just like these passing thoughts and challenging events, this crisis too shall pass. (For further information on self-compassion see Chapter 3.)

It is now established that mindfulness practice can alter brain functioning in everyday life and during times of crisis. Mindfulness practices offer us an opportunity to cultivate the necessary balanced emotional state required to access rational thought and focus during a crisis by engaging more of the right hemisphere of the brain which acts like a wide zoom lens so we can 'see' more (Schore 2014). Mindfulness may also act as a buffer against the damaging impact a crisis can have on mental health and psychological wellbeing (Behan 2020).

Different mindfulness and meditation practices affect different parts of the brain influencing behaviour (Böckler et al. 2018). There is generally agreement within the neuroscience community that mindfulness is associated with increased neural activity and structural changes in the insula, prefrontal and anterior cingulate cortices (Young et al. 2018). These are areas of the brain associated with emotional regulation, executive functioning, and pain. When we are locked into stress-based, left brain, unhelpful negative thinking we tend to become less kind and less altruistic (Jazaieri et al. 2015). Conversely, compassion practices are associated with distinct neural activity linked with increased social connection (Hutcherson et al. 2008). Therefore, in any crisis, we need clear thinking and additional compassion.

There are misconceptions around the use of mindfulness when our lives collide with crises. Mindfulness is not a 'technique' that solves everything if you just breathe or chant a mantra. According to Lazar et al. (2005) and Jha et al. (2007) mindfulness is a trainable skill that reduces activity in parts of the brain associated with reflexive, automatic behaviour including stressful rumination while increasing neural connections in parts of the brain associated with rational, clear thinking and top–down control. When we first experience a crisis, the fight/flight response is initiated and logical reasoning, planning and executive functioning are unavailable when we need them the most (Alexander et al. 2007; Arnsten 2009). Starting with a few mindful breaths we can bring that 'thinking' brain back on track and make decisions from a place of clear thinking. Evidence suggests that mindfulness training alters how the brain functions in our everyday interactions as well as in a crisis. Neuroplasticity, the brain's ability to change and adapt as a result of experience, means that we can intentionally train the brain to create measurable changes in brain functioning (Klimecki et al. 2013; Leung et al. 2012; McCall et al. 2014). Altering our own brain chemistry can bring a higher awareness of the self – as such, a central quality of mindfulness training is self-compassion.

Self-compassion

Linked with mindfulness practice is self-compassion, a trainable skill which involves elements of self-kindness, and recognition of our common humanity

(Neff and Germer 2013). A growing body of research demonstrates that self-compassion practices have significant benefits during times of difficulty and crisis. A key component of self-compassion is the absence of self-criticism, an early predictor of anxiety and depression (Blatt 1995). Moreover, the practice of self-compassion has been shown to activate the nurturing circuitry of the brain, the Vagus nerve, and the release of oxytocin (Gilbert 2019). Allen and Leary (2010) found that people who measure high in self-compassion are kinder toward themselves when experiencing negative events. Oxytocin has been coined the hormone of love and nurturing (Odent 2000). An increased presence of oxytocin due to Vagus nerve activation would therefore act to soothe the nervous system in a crisis.

One of my favourite self-compassion exercises is 'Compassionate Being' where I imagine the felt sense of my 'perfect nurturer'– a being that is non-judgemental, loving and kind and only a thought away. In my imagination, I sit in my safe place on a bench by the beach and everything feels okay. Responses from my compassionate being to my questions are always loving and kind (and sometimes humorous). I immediately feel stress melting away and have a sense of being held in limitless compassion. It feels like coming home. This compassionate focused imagery has been associated with a reduction in stress hormones and thought to be due to the activation of the soothing circuitry (oxytocin) of the brain (Rockliff et al. 2008). Experts often comment that compassion practices give us an opportunity to 're-parent' ourselves (Shonin and Van Gordon 2015). When I am working with people who have a difficult time with self-compassion and being kinder to themselves, I ask them to imagine being on a difficult hike in the mountains where they twist an ankle and feel very stressed. Which companion would you like to travel with – a companion who tells you how weak and pathetic you are, and that you need to 'suck it up and get on with it' – or would you prefer a companion who recognizes the pain you're in, and tells you 'I know this is really hard, but I'm here and we'll get through this together'? However, recognizing that we are worthy of our own kindness and care is the first step – this is the gift of self-compassion that can arise through mindfulness practices (for more detail on self-compassion see Chapter 3).

Types of crises

There are various types and severity of crisis situations. Situational crises are common and include events considered beyond human control such as earthquakes, hurricanes, famine and global pandemics. A personal crisis may include a divorce, injury, loss of employment or any unanticipated event that causes significant distress. In the maternity setting, the potential for personal crisis exists throughout the childbirth continuum. All crises, regardless of type and severity require a clear, centred, calm mindset to avoid escalation of the crisis and reduce distress and potential trauma.

Geopolitical effects, stress and mindfulness

A crisis of global magnitude has recently taught us a significant amount about the effects of stress in a crisis and will undoubtedly continue to do so for some time to come. In 2020, the world experienced the beginning of the public health crisis of the Covid-19 pandemic. As a result of the pandemic, how we lived our lives changed dramatically. Healthcare systems were overwhelmed, schools and businesses shut their doors, fear and anxiety became constant companions. As the virus spread and mutated, local and global recommendations changed regularly. The foundations of stability, employment, children's schooling and socializing with friends, all things we took for granted, were threatened albeit temporarily. This had significant consequences for many in terms of mental health and well-being. My personal mindfulness practice offered a reliable way to be with the emotion of fear without feeling completely overwhelmed; make important decisions and take intentional action from a place of calm instead of chaos. Mindfulness enabled me to notice any unhelpful spiralling of thoughts and negative emotions with gentle acknowledgement. This was achieved without me needing to engage in the drama that an 'unsupervised' mind can create when the default network of the wandering mind is given free reign.

As the Covid crisis continued we saw the publication of several studies supporting the efficacy of mindfulness practices during the pandemic (Antonova et al. 2021; Farris et al. 2021; Kam et al. 2021). Several articles linked mindfulness practices during the pandemic with improved mental health (Belen 2022; Dailey et al. 2022; Farewell et al. 2021). In 2020 an innovative study took place in a Madrid hospital to explore whether an on-site mindfulness-based crisis intervention designed for stress reduction for frontline staff could be implemented in a busy hospital during the pandemic. The intervention consisted of 5–10 min of mindfulness and self-compassion practices focused on the importance of self-care delivered twice daily. Over 3000 mindfulness sessions were delivered to staff. Staff found this short intervention helpful in reducing their stress with a mean rating of 8.4 on a scale from 0 to 10 (Rodriguez-Vega et al. 2020).

Likewise, war causes significant trauma and chronic stress. Mindfulness programs are now being facilitated in refugee camps taught by peers to alleviate some of the emotional suffering experienced by these vulnerable populations. Globally it's estimated that over 80 million people have been forcibly displaced from their homes during times of conflict. A unique mindfulness-based approach for refugees was found to be a safe and therapeutically transformative experience for vulnerable populations including survivors of torture, human trafficking, and former child soldiers. Studies demonstrated that there were significant reductions in mental health problems associated with their trauma. As the Ukrainian/Russian crisis unfolds at the time of writing, we can surmise that mindfulness interventions taught by peers in that region could act as a valuable buffer to the trauma of war and population displacement (Aizik-Reebs et al. 2021).

It is important to remember that amid geopolitical events, such as war and global health concerns like the Covid-19 pandemic, there are pregnant and birthing women and their families. As they navigate external crises, they are also coping with the additional stressors associated with bringing a new person into the world. However, what is perhaps a truism is that nothing remains the same, things always change with time.

Nothing stays the same

An important contemplation taken from the wisdom traditions such as Buddhism is the impermanence of the human experience. Everything in this world changes, nothing stays the same – even during the pandemic. However, during times of crisis many stressful emotions such as fear, confusion exist, and for some, physical pain can be experienced making it difficult to accept the inevitability of change. The components of mindfulness include an awareness of what is, knowing that you are not thinking clearly, and a non-judgemental attitude, not criticizing yourself for your response to the crisis. A kind acceptance of these elements can support the mitigation of difficult unhelpful emotions.

We tend to identify with our emotions and can attach huge importance to how we are feeling, which makes it almost impossible not to be consumed by our inner emotional landscape. With training, we can learn how to engage with emotions as well as thoughts by increasing the gap between the emotion and impulse to engage with it as well as reducing the intensity of conviction with which we engage. We can learn to 'hold' difficult emotions without identifying with those emotions and reduce their impact on our wellbeing. To accept both micro and macro changes in our lives that create challenges we need to employ awareness of what is and a non-judgemental attitude towards ourselves and others.

In the earlier phase of the Covid 19 pandemic, we had no vaccines, intensive care units were at capacity, and the future looked bleak. However, even with the unimaginable changes we have experienced, we have also appreciated glimpses of compassion, kindness and innovation as scientists and communities came together for the common good. The world in many regions continues to be in the grip of the pandemic yet the pandemic tide is turning and global events are now evolving into new crises – nothing stays the same.

Crisis in the birthsphere

Crisis from a midwifery perspective is generally speaking a highly individualized and subjective occurrence. These crises may include a diverse array of crisis such as fertility issues (see Chapter 6), obstetric events such as pregnancy complications, pregnancy loss, unplanned in-labour caesarean section and pre-existing medical conditions – all can trigger a crisis response. The postpartum period too can be a time of crisis as significant change and transition can culminate in poor perinatal mental health having deleterious influence on relationships leading to further crises (see Chapter 13).

Pregnancy – a predictable crisis

Joy at birth has been studied and shown to be central to the opening of possibilities initiating a reframing of childbirth experiences in all circumstances that encourages growth and human flourishing for all involved (Crowther 2021). As we become more familiar with the inner workings of our minds and subsequently reduce our interaction with negative thoughts and emotions, we create more space for joy. A midwife who adopts a salutogenic[4] approach to pregnancy, birth and postpartum may consider facilitating mindfulness and compassion training for parents to optimize health during pregnancy and help bring joy and positivity to the experience. Midwives strive to support parents to achieve the healthiest pregnancy possible, physically and mentally. This is ideally facilitated through resources shared with parents during antenatal appointments and as antenatal education. Although most midwives are not mental health specialists it is within our scope of practice to recommend evidence-based resources that support mental health. This can be a useful juncture to introduce the subject of mindfulness.

We recognize that pregnancy is not a commonly positive experience for everyone (Laney et al. 2015) and this makes it important for midwives and other health care professionals to have the knowledge and skills to enhance a woman's internal resilience[5]. This can be successfully achieved by recommending mindfulness practices. However, it is the author's opinion that these resources are rarely recommended due to potential midwifery regulatory body restrictions and a lack of midwifery knowledge. When discussing this aspect with midwifery colleagues their reasoning for not recommending a mindful approach is around the scope of practice and lack of mental health specialist training. Yet, as midwives, it is within our scope to recommend evidence-based practices that support emotional wellness throughout pregnancy, especially practices that have been proven to be protective of mental health. A bio-medical approach focuses on treating the symptoms of a crisis experience that has already happened instead of anticipating events that may result in a crisis for the individual woman and empowering people to be an active participant in the prevention of trauma in their lives. The inclusion of mindfulness in midwifery education is in its infancy and although some medical schools are including mindfulness within their curriculum, we have a long way to go in preparing practitioners to utilize these skills (see Chapter 15).

The reality is that for some women and their partners, pregnancy, childbirth, and the postpartum period will be viewed as a crisis. Practitioners in the birthsphere are tasked with the job of preparing new parents to step into their new roles in the healthiest way possible. Yet within our current system, parenting can be analogized to taking a boat out of the calm waters of the harbour having never sailed a boat before, not taking a life jacket or any instruments to navigate the way. Although midwives and others involved in care may understand that there is stormy weather coming for many parents, they are sent out in their metaphorical boats with relaxation exercises instead of the necessary mental skills to navigate their experiences optimally. In so doing, they are effectively set adrift to sink or swim. We cannot continue to ignore the growing body of evidence that mindfulness and compassion training can be a powerful resource for parents and professionals during times of significant emotional upheaval and crisis. During the recent pandemic, pregnant women diagnosed with Covid 19 were faced with additional distress as treatment recommendations continued to evolve. However, those who took part in a mindfulness-based program during that time experienced significantly reduced stress, fear and anxiety (Güney et al. 2022).

Mindful awareness of our emotional state is particularly helpful for decision-making during a crisis. It is a skill we can develop to reduce potential distress and build our capacity for resilience and compassionate clear thinking in the face of adversity. During pregnancy, women and their partners are expected to make many decisions, some of which will have significant ramifications. Below, Padayachy (2021) describes her experiences of working with the mindfulness resources in the GentleBirth App during her pregnancy.

Melissa's experience

> I was diagnosed with several spine and chronic pain issues in 2013 therefore my perception of pain was deep rooted and a daily challenge. I always said I would opt for a c section if I did get pregnant due to the fibromyalgia etc. and arthritis. Happy to say my Drs are shocked that my body has changed with improvements in my spine and wrists - no inflammation! The mind shift for me was huge.
>
> My birth was amazing I felt connected and empowered with no pain in fact while pushing. Birth was magical for me after years of physical pain my perception was altered profoundly.

Even after such a positive birth experience, Melissa Meshendri found the postpartum transition to parenthood difficult, but her mindfulness practices supported her to be kinder to herself and to recognize the additional difficulties of becoming a parent during lockdown.

Crisis within pregnancy and mindfulness

After the events of 9/11 researchers found a doubling of preterm birth and low birthweight babies over the next few years among women who were rescued, female recovery workers responding to the 9/11 crisis and women who resided below Canal Street in the World Trade Center's neighbourhood. It was apparent that women with the most intense exposures to the 9/11 crisis had poorer pregnancy outcomes. Moreover, these adverse outcomes persisted among infants conceived for up to three years following 9/11. Chronic maternal stress is known to be a contributor to preterm birth and low birth weight and other studies demonstrate that this is not just in extreme circumstances. Another example of similar outcomes was noted in the aftermath of the Christchurch earthquakes in New Zealand (Menclova and Stillman 2020). However, mindfulness-based interventions may mitigate these outcomes. An RCT from Thailand demonstrated a significant decrease in the onset of preterm labour in women who followed a hospital-based meditation program (Sriboonpimsuay 2011) and Chan (2014) demonstrated how mindfulness during pregnancy impacted infant behaviour.

Smalley and Winston (2010) describe mindfulness as a 'seat belt' for mental health, expanding the analogy perhaps compassion practice can be the airbag. Self-compassion is a predictor of trauma resilience and of reduced post-traumatic stress disorder (PTSD) (Braehler and Neff 2020). Research suggests that mindfulness is associated with a phenomenon known as posttraumatic growth. Posttraumatic growth (PTG) is a process of personal transformation following a traumatic life event (Shiyko et al. 2017) and recognized as an aspect in childbirth trauma research (Thomson and Downe 2012). When women and families have a mindset of suffering, for example, following a traumatic birth, self-compassion and mindfulness can offer a softer landing when crises suddenly crash into their lives. The practice of mindfulness at these crucial times may even be able to transform the experience into one of potential personal growth.

Short-duration antenatal classes that include MBIs (mindfulness-based interventions) as suggested in Sbrilli et al. (2020) may reduce perinatal mood disorders in women at risk of stress-related mental health disorders. This small RCT included long-term follow-up, but the results were limited by the enrolment of mostly healthy, white participants (also see Chapter 7). Antenatal depression (see Chapter 13) is estimated to affect approximately 15% of women (Petersen et al. 2018). However, rates of antenatal depression and stress are higher in minority ethnic groups living in high-income countries than in the rest of the population (Liu et al. 2016). Stigma can prevent women experiencing PMADs (Perinatal Mood and Anxiety Disorders) from seeking treatment. Attending an antenatal class with a focus on MBIs can be a sustainable and less threatening way to reach more parents. By encouraging parents to become more aware and present in their daily activities, they can take a positive step towards physical and emotional wellbeing in pregnancy and parenting. I contend that healthcare professionals are well positioned to educate parents on the benefits of mindfulness. Informal mindful awareness of mundane activities such as washing dishes, folding laundry, changing a nappy are simple practices for parents who may not have access to ongoing instruction (Donegan 2017).

Fear and mindfulness in the childbirth continuum

During a time of crisis, fear is one of the most intense emotions experienced. Cortisol is a steroid hormone that plays an important part in the stress response. Evidence suggests that the constant exposure to the chemical mediators of stress in a crisis such as cortisol is more damaging than the repeated exposure to the stressful event (McEwen 2000). Although most women will not be exposed to a major external crisis such as famine, the common anticipation of a negative labour experience is likely to increase cortisol levels (Çalik et al. 2018; Dahlen et al. 2021). Anggorowati et al. (2019) found that a mindfulness intervention reduced cortisol levels in first-time mothers. Both research evidence and anecdotal reports from midwives suggest that fear of labour and birth is associated with increased obstetric interventions and poor emotional and psychological health for women (Toohill et al. 2014).

Therefore, health workers in maternity would benefit from knowledge of the effect of mindfulness on reducing activity in the amygdala. Empirical data now supports this. MRI scans demonstrate that after an eight-week course of mindfulness practice, the brain's 'fight or flight' centre reduces in size (Kral et al. 2018). Moreover, pilot studies in pregnancy demonstrate a reported reduction in fear and stress with the practice of mindfulness (Byrne et al. 2013; Duncan et al. 2017). It is evident that the amygdala's' heightened activity can be mitigated in pregnant women by MBI.

The postnatal period too can be a time of crisis for many parents. The intensity of emotions, physical recovery, breastfeeding and lack of restorative sleep can all contribute to feelings of overwhelm. Shifting identities, brain plasticity, body image etc., make this one of the most intense transitions of adult life (Barba-Müller et al. 2018). MBI in this part of the childbirth experience can be useful in nurturing optimal transitions to parenthood and enhancing the changing relationships.

PART 2: Doing mindfulness

In the second part of this chapter, I am going to focus on application and ways of using mindfulness exercises within practice along with some physiological explanation about what is happening during the activities.

Mindfulness of the breath

When a crisis hits the most effective way to soothe the nervous system is to take a few mindful breaths. Even during the most difficult circumstances during a crisis, we can mindfully attend to the breath to regulate the powerful emotions we're experiencing. Breathing is the only system in the body that is both automatic and within our control. During times of crisis such as a sudden accident, hyperventilation is not uncommon leading to increased stress levels and deoxygenation of the body and brain. When we find ourselves in a crisis a state of shock is commonly followed by panic and fear.

HRV (heart rate variability) is the variation of the length of heartbeat intervals and indicates the adaptability of the heart to respond to internal (mental/emotional) and external events (Rajendra et al. 2006). High HRV has been found to be associated with reduced morbidity and mortality, as well as improved psychological well-being and quality of life. Slow mindful rhythmic breathing patterns are demonstrated to increase HRV with a substantial body of research indicating that anxiety and stress are all related to decreased HRV

(Kemp et al. 2010, 2012; Lehrer and Gevirtz 2014). Mindful compassion in-terventions are also shown to increase HRV (Petrocchi et al. 2016) and reduce blood cortisol levels. From this starting point of a simple pause to breathe, we can further bring the mind and body into a state of coherence by intentionally activating a positive emotional state.

Expanding on the simple 'pause' and slow rhythmic breathing mindful breathing involves noticing the breath as it moves through the body. Subse-quently when thoughts/feelings arise and the mind wanders and becomes cap-tivated by those thoughts we intentionally and gently return to the felt sense of the breath entering and leaving the body. Optimal breathing involves 'belly breathing' whereas many people breathe into the upper chest only which keeps the fight/flight response activated leading to heavier breathing.

In recent years researchers have concluded that nasal breathing (in and out of the nose) has significant benefits when compared to mouth breathing. Heart rate is reduced, nitric oxide reservoirs found in the nose dilate airways and blood ves-sels resulting in improved oxygen delivery throughout the body and brain and re-duced lactic acid in the muscles. So even when in a crisis whether physical, mental, war or a public health crisis mindful breathing can bring the mind and body back into a state of homeostasis. The ability to soothe the stress response quickly and bring ourselves to a calmer state during a crisis affords us the opportunity to build resiliency and confidence. Although the benefits of a regular mindfulness practice are well documented mindful breathing is a simple strategy for non-meditators during a crisis and can easily be learned with minimal instruction.

Mindfulness of the body

Traumatic experiences affect more than the mind. They also affect our body. The fight/flight/freeze response that protects and preserves us can also initiate recurring overwhelming sensations in the body long after the crisis has passed. The nervous system will always respond to a reminder of a past threat if the ra-tional 'thinking' part of the brain is offline (typically occurring during periods of stress). When executive functioning is offline the brain cannot determine if a memory is a real threat or just a memory.

Most of us spend our day living 'above the neck', caught up in negative thought loops, repetitive thinking, rumination, and mental time travelling. It can be difficult to stay in the present moment. In 2010, Harvard-based psycholo-gists Killingsworth and Gilbert demonstrated that we spend 47% of our waking moments worrying about the past or the future, leaving us chronically unhappy.

Every moment of every day the body is sending information to the brain. Based on expectations and previous experiences the brain then decides which signals are suggestive of a threat. However, by dropping down into the body we can experi-ence interoceptive awareness – a tuning into sensations into the sensations of the body with more awareness. The body is always in the present moment and when we drop into the body, we are activating the right hemisphere of the brain again.

Every emotion we experience is accompanied by physical sensations. During times of upset it's common to feel tightening in the body, sometimes an increase in temperature in the face. Anxiety leads to stomach churning and excitement is often described as 'butterflies'. But when we are not mindful of what is going on in our body, we can be driven by these sensations and engage in behaviours that do not serve us well. By learning how to pause and notice the sensations we have an opportunity to skilfully respond rather than react mindlessly. Staying present with these strong sensations such as panic, anxiety or pain is not easy. It is human nature to instinctively want to push away those difficult sensations or numb ourselves, so we don't feel them. We're conditioned to avoid unpleasant sensations and try to hold on to pleasant ones. This means we're continually trying to push away what we don't like and hold on tightly to things we like. Even when we hold onto the good, the satisfaction is temporary – we crave the next thing, so we keep postponing happiness – known as the 'Hedonic Treadmill'. Mindful attention to all sensations we perceive in the body we can keep ourselves grounded and present rather than allowing those sensations to hijack the brain during a crisis. This friendly kind curiosity allows us to simply notice what's happening without adding stories and judgements to these sensations. Mindful exploration and attention to the sensations of labour can reduce pain, body-centred practices are a key part of a mindfulness practice. When we start to notice feelings in the body, they can alert us when we are becoming stressed. When we notice those sensations, we can choose to be mindful in those moments which gives us an opportunity to respond skilfully rather than being hijacked by our emotions. One of the most widely used practices is the body scan meditation (BSM).

The BSM is a core part of Kabat-Zinn's MBSR program (Mindfulness-Based Stress Reduction). It has also been described as 'affectionate, openhearted [and] interested' attention to the body. Western culture sees the body and mind as separate however the brain is processing information from the body continuously whether we are consciously aware of that sensory input or not, this is known as non-duality in Buddhist traditions. "Sensations in the body are ground zero, the place where we directly experience the entire play of life" (Brach 2004).

Box 14.1 BSM

BSM can be practiced lying down or in an upright seated position. An upright seated position can be helpful if drowsy. It usually starts with the attention to the breath to settle the mind and body then we systematically move the spotlight of attention up over the feet, legs, torso arms to the top of the head. At each step of the way we pause and rest our attention on the sensations that we meet in the body, cultivating a sense of acceptance towards what we find there without judgement or criticism. We approach the sensations and any thoughts that are triggered by these sensations with kindness and curiosity.

Both the body scan and mindful breathing are considered practices that engage the interception circuitry of the brain and help to ground us in the present moment. Interoception is a core part of mindfulness. Also known as Interoceptive Awareness (IA) it is often defined as a 'moment-by-moment representation of the body's internal milieu' (Craig 2009). Another simple exercise I use frequently with clients is 'find your feet'. I invite the client to move their focus and attention to their feet, and with a curious kind attitude notice what's there – temperature, feeling of their shoes, connection points to the floor. This is a simple way to drop down from the storytelling mind that's generating stressful thoughts and move our attention down into the body. This is a simple effective way to turn down the stress response significantly during an unexpected crisis.

Potential adverse effects of mindfulness

Mindfulness has become evangelized as a panacea for a multitude of physical and psychological conditions and there seems to be a positivity bias in mindfulness research with limited reporting of potential risks (Britton 2019). There is an unspoken assumption that there are no adverse effects (Cebolla et al. 2017; Goldberg et al. 2021). In a crisis, the last thing we want to do is to add to someone's psychological burden.

Britton (2019) proposes that flashbacks, dissociation and increased anxiety may occur in individuals. Britton suggests that a personalized approach utilizing a combination of practices may reduce these effects. However, research has not yet defined what is considered a 'normative' meditation experience and 'psychopathology' (Lindahl et al. 2020). Interestingly, 2% of the staff participating in the intervention in the hospital in Madrid reported feeling dizzy and experienced an increase in stress after the intervention.

Mindfulness practices can be integrated into our lives easily, remembering to be mindful is often the biggest barrier. A mindful breath or 'find your feet' are simple exercises that require little to no training. But there are obvious benefits to starting and maintaining a formal mindfulness practice. Mindfulness provides us with a way of being with ourselves and others in a kinder, wiser more compassionate way. These practices give us the opportunity to hone effective skills and cultivate more resources to cope with any crisis we experience. Ultimately the application of these skills can empower all of us to do more than surviving a crisis. Mindfulness and compassion practices invite the possibility and potential to thrive, even during extraordinary circumstances.

Notes

1 Catecholamines are hormones produced by the brain, nerve tissues, and adrenal glands (the glands situated on top of the kidneys). In response to emotional or physical stress our bodies release catecholamines. Catecholamines are thus our physiological reaction to stress initiating a "fight-or-flight" response. There are different catecholamines called dopamine, adrenaline, and noradrenaline.

2 Negative bias is our tendency to fixate and overly focus on negative stimuli and situations.

3 Neurotransmitters are the chemical messengers of our body transmitting messages between neurons, or from neurons to muscles. This messaging or communication between two neurons happens in synaptic clefts - tiny gaps between the synapses of neurons. Oxytocin is a hormone neurotransmitter involved in childbirth and breast-feeding and is associated with empathy, trust, sexual activity, as well as feelings of love and relationship-building. Endorphins act as natural pain reliever produced in response to stress or/and discomfort.

4 Salutongenesis is defined by Downe (2010), see in reference list

5 Resilience in this instance refers to the ability to leverage positive emotions over negative (Reichet al. 2012), see reference list.

Behan, Caragh. 2020. "The benefits of meditation and mindfulness practices during times of crisis such as COVID-19." Irish journal of psychological medicine 37 (4):256-258.

Downe, Soo. 2010. "Towards salutogenic birth in the 21st century." In Essential midwifery practice: intrapartum care: 289–295. https://onlinelibrary.wiley.com/doi/10.1002/9781444317701.ch16

Odent, M. 2001. The scientification of love. London: Free Association Books.

Reich, John W, Alex J Zautra, and John Stuart Hall. 2010. Handbook of adult resilience: Guilford Press.

Thomson, G. 2011. "Abandonment of Being in Childbirth." In Qualitative research in midwifery and childbirth: Phenomenological approaches, edited by G. Thomson, F. Dykes and S. Downe, 133–152. London: Routledge.

References

Anggorowati, Anggorowati, Siti Munawaroh, and Meidiana Dwidiyanti. 2019. "Effects of 'STOP' Mindfulness on Decreasing Cortisol in Primigravida Mothers." Jurnal Keperawatan Soedirman 14, no. 3. https://doi.org/10.20884/1.jks.2019.14.3.893.

Aizik-Reebs, Anna, Kim Yuval, Yuval Hadash, Solomon Gebreyohans Gebremariam, and Amit Bernstein. 2021. "Mindfulness-Based Trauma Recovery for Refugees (MBTR-R): Randomized Waitlist-Control Evidence of Efficacy and Safety." Clinical Psychological Science 9, no. 6 (November): 1164–1184. https://doi.org/10.1177/2167702621998641.

Alexander, Jessica K., Ashleigh Hillier, Ryan M. Smith, Madalina E. Tivarus, and David Q. Beversdorf. 2007. "Beta-Adrenergic Modulation of Cognitive Flexibility during Stress." Journal of Cognitive Neuroscience, no. 3 (March): 468–478. https://doi.org/10.1162/jocn.2007.19.3.468.

Allen, A. B., and M. R. Leary. 2010. "Self-Compassion, Stress, and Coping." Social and Personality Psychology Compass, 4: 107–118. https://doi.org/10.1111/j.1751-9004.2009.00246.x.

Antonova, Elena, Karoly Schlosser, Rakesh Pandey, and Veena Kumari. 2021. "Coping With COVID-19: Mindfulness-Based Approaches for Mitigating Mental Health Crisis." Frontiers in Psychiatry, March. https://doi.org/10.3389/fpsyt.2021.563417.

Arnsten, Amy F. T. 2009. "Stress Signalling Pathways That Impair Prefrontal Cortex Structure and Function." Nature Reviews Neuroscience, no. 6 (June): 410–422. https://doi.org/10.1038/nrn2648.

Barba-Müller, Erika, Sinéad Craddock, Susanna Carmona, and Elseline Hoekzema. 2018. "Brain Plasticity in Pregnancy and the Postpartum Period: Links to Maternal Caregiving and Mental Health." Archives of Women's Mental Health, no. 2 (July): 289–299. https://doi.org/10.1007/s00737-018-0889-z.

Behan, Caragh. 2020. "The Benefits of Meditation and Mindfulness Practices during Times of Crisis Such as COVID-19." *Irish Journal of Psychological Medicine*, no. 4 (May): 256–258. https://doi.org/10.1017/ipm.2020.38.

Belen, H. 2002. "Fear of COVID-19 and Mental Health: The Role of Mindfulness in During Times of Crisis." *International Journal of Mental Health and Addiction*, 20: 607–618. https://doi.org/10.1007/s11469-020-00470-2.

Belsky, Jay, and Michael Rovine. 1990. "Patterns of Marital Change across the Transition to Parenthood: Pregnancy to Three Years Postpartum." *Journal of Marriage and the Family*, no. 1 (February): 5. https://doi.org/10.2307/352833.

Bhikkhu, Thanissaro. 2013. Sallatha Sutta: The Arrow. *Access to Insight* (BCBS Edition). http://www.accesstoinsight.org/tipitaka/sn/sn36/sn36.006.than.html.

Blatt, Sidney J. 1995. "The Destructiveness of Perfectionism: Implications for the Treatment of Depression." *American Psychologist*, no. 12 (December): 1003–1020. https://doi.org/10.1037/0003-066x.50.12.1003.

Böckler, Anne, Anita Tusche, Peter Schmidt, and Tania Singer. 2018. "Distinct Mental Trainings Differentially Affect Altruistically Motivated, Norm Motivated, and Self-Reported Prosocial Behaviour." *Scientific Reports*, no. 1 (September). https://doi.org/10.1038/s41598-018-31813-8.

Brach, Tara. 2004. *Radical Acceptance*. Bantam.

Braehler, Christine, and Kristin Neff. 2020. "Self-Compassion in PTSD." In *Emotion in Posttraumatic Stress Disorder*, edited by C. Braehler and K. Neff, Academic Press: Cambridge. 567–596.

Bränström, Richard, Larissa G. Duncan, and Judith Tedlie Moskowitz. 2011. "The Association between Dispositional Mindfulness, Psychological Well-Being, and Perceived Health in a Swedish Population-Based Sample." *British Journal of Health Psychology*, no. 2 (March): 300–316. https://doi.org/10.1348/135910710x501683.

Britton, Willoughby B. 2019. "Can Mindfulness Be Too Much of a Good Thing? The Value of a Middle Way." *Current Opinion in Psychology*, August, 159–165. https://doi.org/10.1016/j.copsyc.2018.12.011.

(Bud) Craig, A. D. 2009. "How Do You Feel — Now? The Anterior Insula and Human Awareness." *Nature Reviews Neuroscience*, no. 1 (January): 59–70. https://doi.org/10.1038/nrn2555.

Byrne, Jean, Yvonne Hauck, Colleen Fisher, Sara Bayes, and Robert Schutze. 2013. "Effectiveness of a Mindfulness-Based Childbirth Education Pilot Study on Maternal Self-Efficacy and Fear of Childbirth." *Journal of Midwifery & Women's Health*, no. 2 (December): 192–197. https://doi.org/10.1111/jmwh.12075.

Çalik, K.Y., Ö. Karabulutlu, and C. Yavuz. 2018. "First Do No Harm - Interventions during Labor and Maternal Satisfaction: A Descriptive Cross-Sectional Study." *BMC Pregnancy Childbirth* 18, 415 https://doi.org/10.1186/s12884-018-2054-0

Cebolla, Ausiàs, Marcelo Demarzo, Patricia Martins, Joaquim Soler, and Javier Garcia-Campayo. 2017. "Unwanted Effects: Is There a Negative Side of Meditation? A Multicentre Survey." *PLOS ONE*, no. 9 (September): e0183137. https://doi.org/10.1371/journal.pone.0183137.

Chan, Ka Po. 2014. "Prenatal Meditation Influences Infant Behaviors." *Infant Behavior and Development*, no. 4 (November): 556–561. https://doi.org/10.1016/j.infbeh.2014.06.011.

Corballis, Michael C. 2014 "Left Brain, Right Brain: Facts and Fantasies." *PLoS Biology* 12, 1 e1001767. doi:10.1371/journal.pbio.1001767

Crowther, Susan. 2021. *Joy at Birth: An Interpretive, Hermeneutic, Phenomenological Inquiry*. London: Routledge.

Dahlen, Hannah G., Charlene Thornton, Soo Downe, Ank de Jonge, Anna Seijmonsbergen-Schermers, Sally Tracy, Mark Tracy, Andrew Bisits, and Lilian Peters. 2021. "Intrapartum Interventions and Outcomes for Women and Children Following Induction of Labour at Term in Uncomplicated Pregnancies: A 16-Year Population-Based Linked Data Study." *BMJ Open*, no. 6 (May): e047040. https://doi.org/10.1136/bmjopen-2020-047040.

Dailey, Stephanie F., Maggie M. Parker, and Andrew Campbell. 2022. "Social Connectedness, Mindfulness, and Coping as Protective Factors During the COVID-19 Pandemic." *Journal of Counseling & Development*, 1–13. https://doi-org.op.idm.oclc.org/10.1002/jcad.12450 20

Donegan Tracy. *Mindful Pregnancy Meditation, Yoga, Hypnobirthing, Natural Remedies, and Nutrition - Trimester by Trimester*. Dorling Kindersley: London.

Duncan, Larissa G., Michael A. Cohn, Maria T. Chao, Joseph G. Cook, Jane Riccobono, and Nancy Bardacke. 2017. "Benefits of Preparing for Childbirth with Mindfulness Training: A Randomized Controlled Trial with Active Comparison." *BMC Pregnancy and Childbirth*, no. 1 (May). https://doi.org/10.1186/s12884-017-1319-3.

Downe, Soo. 2010. "Towards Salutogenic Birth in the 21st Century." In *Essential Midwifery Practice: Intrapartum Care*: 289–295. Wiley Blackwell: Hoboken New Jersey. https://onlinelibrary.wiley.com/doi/10.1002/9781444317701.ch16

Escott, Diane, Helen Spiby, Pauline Slade, and Robert B Fraser. 2004. "The Range of Coping Strategies Women Use to Manage Pain and Anxiety Prior to and during First Experience of Labour." *Midwifery*, no. 2 (June): 144–156. https://doi.org/10.1016/j.midw.2003.11.001.

Farewell, Charlotte V., Jessica Walls, Jamie N. Powers, Joanne Whalen, Meredith Shefferman, and Jenn A. Leiferman. 2021. "Feasibility of a Perinatal Mindfulness-Based Intervention Delivered Remotely Due to COVID-19." *OBM Integrative and Complementary Medicine*, 6, no. 3:17. https://doi.org/10.21926/obm.icm.2103028

Farris, Suzan R, Licia Grazzi, Miya Holley, Anna Dorsett, Kelly Xing, Charles R Pierce, Paige M Estave, Nathaniel O'Connell, and Rebecca Erwin Wells. 2021. "Online Mindfulness May Target Psychological Distress and Mental Health during COVID-19." *Global Advances in Health and Medicine*, January, 216495612110024. https://doi.org/10.1177/21649561211002461.

Feruglio, Susanna, Alessio Matiz, Giuseppe Pagnoni, Franco Fabbro, and Cristiano Crescentini. 2021. "The Impact of Mindfulness Meditation on the Wandering Mind: A Systematic Review." *Neuroscience & Biobehavioral Reviews*, December, 313–330. https://doi.org/10.1016/j.neubiorev.2021.09.032.

Gilbert, Paul. 2019. *The Compassionate Mind*. London: Robinson.

Goldberg, Simon B., Sin U. Lam, Willoughby B. Britton, and Richard J. Davidson. 2021. "Prevalence of Meditation-Related Adverse Effects in a Population-Based Sample in the United States." *Psychotherapy Research*, no. 3 (June): 291–305. https://doi.org/10.1080/10503307.2021.1933646.

Güney, Esra, Sıdıka Özlem Cengizhan, Esra Karataş Okyay, Zeynep Bal, and Tuba Uçar. 2022. "Effect of the Mindfulness-Based Stress Reduction Program on Stress, Anxiety, and Childbirth Fear in Pregnant Women Diagnosed with COVID-19." *Complementary Therapies in Clinical Practice*, May, 101566.

Hoffmann, Ferdinand, Christian Banzhaf, Philipp Kanske, Felix Bermpohl, and Tania Singer. 2016. "Where the Depressed Mind Wanders: Self-Generated Thought Patterns as Assessed through Experience Sampling as a State Marker of Depression." *Journal of Affective Disorders*, July, 127–134. https://doi.org/10.1016/j.jad.2016.03.005.

Hutcherson, Cendri A., Emma M. Seppala, and James J. Gross. 2008. "Loving-Kindness Meditation Increases Social Connectedness." *Emotion*, no. 5 (October): 720–724. https://doi.org/10.1037/a0013237.

Jazaieri, Hooria, Ihno A. Lee, Kelly McGonigal, Thupten Jinpa, James R. Doty, James J. Gross, and Philippe R. Goldin. 2015. "A Wandering Mind Is a Less Caring Mind: Daily Experience Sampling during Compassion Meditation Training." *The Journal of Positive Psychology*, no. 1 (March): 37–50. https://doi.org/10.1080/17439760.2015.1025418.

Jha, A. P., J. Krompinger, and M. J. Baime. 2007. "Mindfulness Training Modifies Subsystems of Attention." *Cognitive, Affective, & Behavioral Neuroscience*, no. 2 (June): 109–119. https://doi.org/10.3758/cabn.7.2.109.

Kam, Julia W. Y., Javeria Javed, Chelsie M. Hart, Jessica R. Andrews-Hanna, Lianne M. Tomfohr-Madsen, and Caitlin Mills. 2021. "Daily Mindfulness Training Reduces Negative Impact of COVID-19 News Exposure on Affective Well-Being." *Psychological Research*, June. https://doi.org/10.1007/s00426-021-01550-1.

Kang, Yoona, June Gruber, and Jeremy R. Gray. 2012. "Mindfulness and De-Automatization." *Emotion Review*, no. 2 (November): 192–201. https://doi.org/10.1177/1754073912451629.

Kemp, Andrew H., Daniel S. Quintana, Kim L. Felmingham, Slade Matthews, and Herbert F. Jelinek. 2012. "Depression, Comorbid Anxiety Disorders, and Heart Rate Variability in Physically Healthy, Unmedicated Patients: Implications for Cardiovascular Risk." *PLoS One* 7, no. 2: e30777. https://doi.org/10.1371/journal.pone.0030777. Epub 2012 Feb 15. PMID: 22355326; PMCID: PMC3280258.

Kemp, Andrew H., Daniel S. Quintana, Marcus A. Gray, Kim L. Felmingham, Kerri Brown, and Justine M. Gatt. 2010. "Impact of Depression and Antidepressant Treatment on Heart Rate Variability: A Review and Meta-Analysis." *Biological Psychiatry*, no. 11 (June): 1067–1074. https://doi.org/10.1016/j.biopsych.2009.12.012.

Kiken, Laura G., and Natalie J. Shook. "Looking Up: Mindfulness Increases Positive Judgments and Reduces Negativity Bias." *Social Psychological and Personality Science* 2, no. 4 (July 2011): 425–431. https://doi.org/10.1177/1948550610396585.

Killingsworth, Matthew A., and Daniel T. Gilbert. 2010. "A Wandering Mind Is an Unhappy Mind." *Science*, no. 6006 (November): 932–932. https://doi.org/10.1126/science.1192439.

King, Anthony P., Stefanie R. Block, Rebecca K. Sripada, Sheila Rauch, Nicholas Giardino, Todd Favorite, Michael Angstadt, Daniel Kessler, Robert Welsh, and Israel Liberzon. 2016. "Altered Default Mode Network (DMN) Resting State Functional Connectivity Following a Mindfulness-based Exposure Therapy for Posttraumatic Stress Disorder (PTSD) in Combat Veterans of Afghanistan and Iraq." *Depression and Anxiety*, no. 4 (April): 289–299. https://doi.org/10.1002/da.22481.

Klimecki, Olga M., Susanne Leiberg, Matthieu Ricard, and Tania Singer. 2013. "Differential Pattern of Functional Brain Plasticity after Compassion and Empathy Training." *Social Cognitive and Affective Neuroscience*, no. 6 (May): 873–879. https://doi.org/10.1093/scan/nst060.

Kral, Tammi R.A., Brianna S. Schuyler, Jeanette A. Mumford, Melissa A. Rosenkranz, Antoine Lutz, and Richard J. Davidson. 2018. "Impact of Short- and Long-Term Mindfulness Meditation Training on Amygdala Reactivity to Emotional Stimuli." *NeuroImage*, November, 301–313. https://doi.org/10.1016/j.neuroimage.2018.07.013.

Kunwar, Prabhat S., Moriel Zelikowsky, Ryan Remedios, Haijiang Cai, Melis Yilmaz, Markus Meister, and David J. Anderson. 2015. "Ventromedial Hypothalamic Neurons Control a Defensive Emotion State." *eLife*, 4:e06633.

Landry, Marc-Antoine, Kumar Kumaran, Juzer M. Tyebkhan, Valerie Levesque, and Marcello Spinella. 2022. "Mindful Kangaroo Care: Mindfulness Intervention for Mothers during Skin-to-Skin Care: A Randomized Control Pilot Study." *BMC Pregnancy and Childbirth*, no. 1 (January). https://doi.org/10.1186/s12884-021-04336-w.

Laney, Elizabeth K., M. Elizabeth Lewis Hall, Tamara L. Anderson, and Michele M. Willingham. 2015. "Becoming a Mother: The Influence of Motherhood on Women's Identity Development." *Identity*, no. 2 (April): 126–145. https://doi.org/10.1080/15283488.2015.1023440.

Lazar, Sara W., Catherine E. Kerr, Rachel H. Wasserman, Jeremy R. Gray, Douglas N. Greve, Michael T. Treadway, Metta McGarvey, et al. 2005. "Meditation Experience Is Associated with Increased Cortical Thickness." *NeuroReport*, no. 17 (November): 1893–1897. https://doi.org/10.1097/01.wnr.0000186598.66243.19.

Lehrer, Paul M., and Richard Gevirtz. 2014. "Heart Rate Variability Biofeedback: How and Why Does It Work?" *Frontiers in Psychology*, July. https://doi.org/10.3389/fpsyg.2014.00756.

Leung, Mei-Kei, Chetwyn C. H. Chan, Jing Yin, Chack-Fan Lee, Kwok-Fai So, and Tatia M. C. Lee. 2012. "Increased Gray Matter Volume in the Right Angular and Posterior Parahippocampal Gyri in Loving-Kindness Meditators." *Social Cognitive and Affective Neuroscience*, no. 1 (July): 34–39. https://doi.org/10.1093/scan/nss076.

Lindahl, Jared, David J. Cooper, Nathan E. Fisher, L. Kirmayer, and Willoughby B. Britton. 2020. "Progress or Pathology? Differential Diagnosis and Intervention Criteria for Meditation-Related Challenges: Perspectives from Buddhist Meditation Teachers and Practitioners." *Frontiers in Psychology* 11: 1905.

Little, Kathleen K., and Laura E. Sockol. 2020. "Romantic Relationship Satisfaction and Parent-Infant Bonding during the Transition to Parenthood: An Attachment-Based Perspective." *Frontiers in Psychology*, August. https://doi.org/10.3389/fpsyg.2020.02068.

Lothian, Judith A. 2012. "Risk, Safety, and Choice in Childbirth." *The Journal of Perinatal Education*, no. 1: 45–47. https://doi.org/10.1891/1058-1243.21.1.45.

Luce, Ann, Marilyn Cash, Vanora Hundley, Helen Cheyne, Edwin van Teijlingen, and Catherine Angell. 2016. "'Is It Realistic?' The Portrayal of Pregnancy and Childbirth in the Media." *BMC Pregnancy and Childbirth*, no. 1 (February). https://doi.org/10.1186/s12884-016-0827-x.

McCall, Cade, Nikolaus Steinbeis, Matthieu Ricard, and Tania Singer. 2014. "Compassion Meditators Show Less Anger, Less Punishment, and More Compensation of Victims in Response to Fairness Violations." *Frontiers in Behavioral Neuroscience*, December. https://doi.org/10.3389/fnbeh.2014.00424.

McEwen, Bruce S. 2000. "The Neurobiology of Stress: From Serendipity to Clinical Relevance11Published on the World Wide Web on 22 November 2000." *Brain Research*, no. 1–2 (December): 172–189. https://doi.org/10.1016/s0006-8993(00)02950-4.

Menclova, A.K. and Stillman, S. 2020. "Maternal Stress and Birth Outcomes: Evidence from an Unexpected Earthquake Swarm." *Health Economics*, 29: 1705–1720. https://doi.org/10.1002/hec.4162

Navarro-Gil, Mayte, Yolanda Lopez-del-Hoyo, Marta Modrego-Alarcón, Jesus Montero-Marin, William Van Gordon, Edo Shonin, and Javier Garcia-Campayo. 2018. "Effects of Attachment-Based Compassion Therapy (ABCT) on Self-Compassion and Attachment Style in Healthy People." *Mindfulness*, no. 1 (February): 51–62. https://doi.org/10.1007/s12671-018-0896-1.

Neff, Kirsten. 2003. "Self-Compassion: An Alternative Conceptualization of a Healthy Attitude Towards Oneself." *Self and Identity*, 2: 85–101.

Neff, Kirsten D., and Chris K. Germer. 2013. "A Pilot Study and Randomized Controlled Trial of the Mindful Self-Compassion Program." *Journal of Clinical Psychology*, 69: 28–44. https://doi.org/10.1002/jclp.21923.

Niebauer, Chris. 2019. *No Self, No Problem*. 1st ed. New York: Hierophant Publishing.

Odent, Michel. 2000. *The Scientification of Love*. London: Free Association Books.

Padayachy, Meshendri. 2021. Meshendri's life changing pregnancy and birth experience. *Gentlebirth*. https://www.blog.gentlebirth.com/home/first-time-perfect-birth

Perez-Blasco, Josefa, Paz Viguer, and Maria F. Rodrigo. 2013. "Effects of a Mindfulness-Based Intervention on Psychological Distress, Well-Being, and Maternal Self-Efficacy in Breast-Feeding Mothers: Results of a Pilot Study." *Archives of Women's Mental Health*, no. 3 (March): 227–236. https://doi.org/10.1007/s00737-013-0337-z.

Petersen, Irene, Tomi Peltola, Samuel Kaski, et al. 2018. "Depression, Depressive Symptoms and Treatments in Women Who Have Recently Given Birth: UK Cohort Study." *BMJ Open*, 8: e022152. https://doi.org/10.1136/bmjopen-2018-022152.

Petrocchi, Nicola, Cristina Ottaviani, and Alessandro Couyoumdjian. 2016. "Compassion at the Mirror: Exposure to a Mirror Increases the Efficacy of a Self-Compassion Manipulation in Enhancing Soothing Positive Affect and Heart Rate Variability." *The Journal of Positive Psychology*, no. 6 (July): 525–536. https://doi.org/10.1080/17439760.2016.1209544.

Rajendra Acharya, U., K. Paul Joseph, N. Kannathal, Choo Min Lim, and Jasjit S. Suri. 2006. "Heart Rate Variability: A Review." *Medical & Biological Engineering Computing* 44, no. 12 (November): 1031–1051. https://doi.org/10.1007/s11517-006-0119-0.

Rockliff, Helen, Paul Gilbert, Kirsten McEwan, Stafford Lightman, and David Glover. 2008. "A Pilot Exploration of Heart Rate Variability and Salivary Cortisol Responses to Compassion-Focused Imagery." *Clinical Neuropsychiatry: Journal of Treatment Evaluation*, 5(3): 132–139.

Rodriguez-Vega, Beatriz, Ángela Palao, Ainoa Muñoz-Sanjose, Marta Torrijos, Pablo Aguirre, Arancha Fernández, Blanca Amador, et al. 2020. "Implementation of a Mindfulness-Based Crisis Intervention for Frontline Healthcare Workers During the COVID-19 Outbreak in a Public General Hospital in Madrid, Spain." *Frontiers in Psychiatry*, October. https://doi.org/10.3389/fpsyt.2020.562578.

Sbrilli, M. D., L. G. Duncan, and H. K. Laurent. 2020. "Effects of Prenatal Mindfulness-Based Childbirth Education on Child-Bearers' Trajectories of Distress: A Randomized Control Trial." *BMC Pregnancy Childbirth* 20: 623. https://doi.org/10.1186/s12884-020-03318-8

Schore, Allan N. 2014. "The Right Brain Is Dominant in Psychotherapy." *Psychotherapy*, no. 3: 388–397. https://doi.org/10.1037/a0037083.

Shiyko, Mariya P., Sean Hallinan, and Tatsuhiko Naito. 2017. "Effects of Mindfulness Training on Posttraumatic Growth: A Systematic Review and Meta-Analysis." *Mindfulness*, no. 4 (March): 848–858. https://doi.org/10.1007/s12671-017-0684-3.

Shonin, Edo, and William Van Gordon. 2015. "Thupten Jingpa on Compassion and Mindfulness." *Mindfulness*, no. 1 (October): 279–283. https://doi.org/10.1007/s12671-015-0448-x.

Smalley, Susan L., and Diana Winston. 2010. *Fully Present*. Lebanon: Da Capo Lifelong Books.

Sriboonpimsuay, Wanlapa. 2011. "Meditation for Preterm Birth Prevention: A Randomized Controlled Trial in Udonthani, Thailand". *International Journal of Public Health Research* 1, no. 1: 31–39.

Taylor, Véronique A., Joshua Grant, Véronique Daneault, Geneviève Scavone, Estelle Breton, Sébastien Roffe-Vidal, Jérôme Courtemanche, Anaïs S. Lavarenne, and

Mario Beauregard. 2011. "Impact of Mindfulness on the Neural Responses to Emotional Pictures in Experienced and Beginner Meditators." *NeuroImage*, no. 4 (August): 1524–1533. https://doi.org/10.1016/j.neuroimage.2011.06.001.

Thomson, Gillian, and Soo Downe. 2012. "Changing the Future to Change the Past: Women's Experiences of a Positive Birth Following a Traumatic Birth Experience." *Journal of Reproductive and Infant Psychology*, 28: 102–112. https://doi.org/10.1080/02646830903295000

Toohill, Jocelyn, Jennifer Fenwick, Jenny Gamble, Debra K. Creedy, Anne Buist, Erika Turkstra, and Elsa-Lena Ryding. 2014. "A Randomized Controlled Trial of a Psycho-Education Intervention by Midwives in Reducing Childbirth Fear in Pregnant Women." *Birth*, no. 4 (October): 384–394. https://doi.org/10.1111/birt.12136.

Young, Katherine S., Anne Maj van der Velden, Michelle G. Craske, Karen Johanne Pallesen, Lone Fjorback, Andreas Roepstorff, and Christine E. Parsons. 2018. "The Impact of Mindfulness-Based Interventions on Brain Activity: A Systematic Review of Functional Magnetic Resonance Imaging Studies." *Neuroscience & Biobehavioral Reviews*, January, 424–433. https://doi.org/10.1016/j.neubiorev.2017.08.003.

15

EMBRACING MINDFULNESS IN MIDWIFERY EDUCATION

Lorna Davies, Melanie Welfare and Kathleen Maki

Introduction

The use of mindfulness as a tool in education has been garnering interest and awareness in a range of educational settings over recent years (Campbell 2014; Weare 2018). Perhaps understandably, this is particularly prevalent in programmes where health and well-being are the central focus (Raab 2014; Chmielewski 2021; Hassed 2021). We believe that this interest has been generated for a number of reasons. First, an understanding of the science behind the practice of mindfulness has improved significantly in recent years as outlined within the other chapters in the book. Second, there is a synergy between the fields of health and well-being and mindfulness when disciplines are using a biopsychosocial, and we would add cultural and spiritual approach, where the interconnection between biology, psychology, sociocultural and environmental factors is generally evident (Kakoschke et al. 2021). Third, mindfulness can provide a counterbalance to the stresses of contemporary life by introducing a way of switching the central nervous system from 'flight and fight' to 'rest and digest'. In demanding areas of employment such as healthcare, this is a key consideration (Alshak and Das 2021). Given these reasons, mindfulness can be understood as a life skill that health workers can benefit greatly from as carers (Chung et al. 2018).

In this chapter, we focus on the use of mindfulness within the context of midwifery education and will address how within the milieu of self-sustainability, the practice of mindfulness can be introduced, developed, and utilized as a valuable skill, not simply for practice but for life.

Stress and burnout in midwifery practice

Midwives like other caring professionals are all too familiar with the challenges that stress can create, and burnout is a universally recognized phenomenon in

DOI: 10.4324/9781003165200-15

the field (Henriksen and Lukasse 2016; Pezaro et al. 2016; Hunter et al. 2019; Callander et al. 2020; Clemons et al. 2020; Sidhu et al. 2020). The women and families that they work with are also susceptible to stress-related effects (see Chapters 2, 4, 7, 10 and 13). Mental health is recognized as a significant perinatal issue in maternity care with suicide being the major cause of maternal mortality in many OECD countries (WHO 2019). It is therefore imperative that strategies that help us to deal with the current complexity of life, such as self-compassion and mindfulness, are introduced to student midwives to enable them to utilize and apply such practice in both their working and personal lives. To begin our discussion, we present a personal case study.

A midwifery education case study

We (the authors of this chapter) are 'pracademics' who have worked in a variety of midwifery education settings over a long period of time. We also have long-standing interest in the field of mindfulness and have used the practice of mindfulness in our personal and clinical lives as well as within the educational setting. For several years we worked together on the Bachelor of Midwifery (BM) at Ara Institute of Canterbury in Christchurch, New Zealand, which is a three-year under-graduate programme delivered within a model of blended learning. The programme delivery constitutes a combination of face-to-face teaching, on-line tutorials, self-directed learning modules, and practice placements. These include community, primary and tertiary hospital settings, neonatal units, and lactation consultant placements. These and others serve to provide students with a wide range of experiences. For the past 12 years or so, the broad concept of sustainability has informed and shaped this BM programme as an underlying philosophical precept.

Sustainability is woven in as a thread throughout all three years of the programme and is a guiding principle within the strategic vision of the degree. Self-sustainability, which encompasses the concepts of mindfulness, self-compassion, self-care and resilience, has played a significant part in contributing to the sustainability literacy of student midwives within the programme. We were therefore confident that there were good foundations in place to enable the students to observe their own progress on the programme through a lens of self-sustainability.

Recognizing the importance of self-care and self-sustainability

There was little doubt that the students valued the inclusion of self-sustainability within the programme and saw the significance of a more mindful approach when caring for self and others. They expressed this very clearly in the findings of a 2019 study which set out to gather qualitative data about midwifery students' beliefs about sustainability as a concept within midwifery (Davies, Kara and Harre 2020).[1] Data were collected both before the students were introduced to the sustainability curriculum content and afterwards. This took place both in the first year and the third year of the programme. The study identified that the student's perspective on the concept of sustainability changed considerably over the three years. During the first year, the students were more focused on the environmental aspects of sustainability in practice. There was some elementary awareness of self-sustainability and self-care. However, by the second half of the first year following a sustainability workshop which incorporated some content on self-sustainability, there was a notable shift to comments that related to the importance of self-care in their own lives and in the midwifery profession. In relation to the question "What does the word sustainability convey to you generally? the students replied thus:

> *looking at making our own working environment sustainable and taking care of ourselves so women still have plenty of midwives about to work with.*
>
> Sally-Anne (Yr 1 Student)

> *We can role model. We need to protect our profession so that it is sustainable, and we need to look after ourselves.*
>
> Bethany (Yr 1 Student)

By the end of the third year of the programme, the majority of the comments relating to the question around how issues relating to sustainability were evident in practice, the respondents commented extensively on self-care and burn out.

> *Yes, especially as a third year I have continuous worries about how I can become a sustainable LMC [Lead Maternity carer] midwife so I don't burnout too quickly once in practice and so I can have a balance, work life balance.*
>
> Ali (Yr 3 Student)

> *If we don't practice in a sustainable way, we will likely face burnout like many others before us.*
>
> Sam (Yr 3 Student)

Some of the comments from the third years in the study suggested that although there was a relatively strong thread of self-sustainability throughout the programme, this was not enough to prepare them for practice. They described feeling inadequate in terms of what they could do to address this perceived reality, or worse feeling a sense of despair before they had even stepped into practice as a qualified midwife.

> *Yes, in terms of practice sustainability there have been times that I've noticed an impact on my own wellbeing due to the midwifery course and witnessing the impact of practicing in the community on midwives themselves.*
>
> Aroha (Year 3 Student)

We ourselves are only human and can only help the women we work with if we look after ourselves and our own families too!

Ali (Year 3 Student)

if we don't practice in a sustainable way, we will likely face burnout like many others before us. We do not have to be superhero midwives. And of course, things like less job satisfaction, resentment, women might be impacted by care. If, however we work sustainably we may be happier in our work, have better work relationships, have more time for ourselves and our family.

Zara (Year 3 Student)

It was clear that although we were acknowledging the importance of caring for self in the programme, we still had some work to do. The study had set out to explore how the inclusion of sustainability in the programme affected awareness of issues related to sustainability in its broadest sense including self-sustainability. We had included the perspectives of Year 1 and Year 3 students but had unwittingly neglected to consider how these two years were bridged by the second year of the programme. An elementary analysis of the content relating to the core concept of mindfulness within the programme, not surprisingly revealed this, as it became clear that although there was a reasonable inclusion of mindfulness in Year 1 of the programme, in Year 2, it was barely visible. It transpired that our assumption that mindfulness was embedded within the programme in the broad guise of sustainability was not borne out in reality. If mindfulness was to have an intrinsic value for the students, it had to be more evident throughout the whole of the programme.

Mindfulness and self-compassion

There is a good body of evidence that suggests that students in healthcare who are introduced to mindfulness within their programme of study have decreased levels of stress and anxiety and demonstrate higher levels of self-compassion (Chen et al. 2013; Erogul et al. 2014; Harwani 2014; Kelly 2017). The words of the global spiritual leader Thich Nhat Hanh, who is sometimes referred to as the father of mindfulness (Shenoy 2019), are worth considering in this context. Hahn states that "If we do not know how to take care of ourselves and love ourselves, we cannot take care of the people we love" (Thich Nhat Hanh 2011). These words should serve to be a powerful reminder of the importance of self-care. The 'oxygen analogy' has been sometimes used to demonstrate the importance of ensuring our own well-being before attending to the needs of those in our care. This alludes to the instructions given by cabin crew in the pre-flight safety briefing where functioning adults are advised that they should put their own oxygen mask in place before applying it on a child or other person requiring additional support. The parallel in midwifery practice is that if we do not take care of ourselves, we will be unable to fully serve the needs of the women and their families that we encounter in our working lives. It would seem that self-sustainability, which it could be argued should be the cornerstone of a sustainability model, had not been given the primacy that it deserves within the context of the programme.

Our next step was to unpack the element of self-sustainability in the programme more fully, so that we could identify the areas within the programme that needed strengthening and to consider how might be the best way to achieve this.

Creative ways of introducing mindfulness to student midwives

Mindfulness is introduced to the students within the first week of the programme during orientation where an introductory session on mindfulness is provided. This consists of some guided meditation and discussion around the principles of self-care and self-sustainability both within the programme and in the practice setting. For some of the students, this is the first exposure to mindfulness as a concept and for those who do have some experience or understanding of the practice, it is a segue into mindfulness within the context of healthcare. In addition, during this week the group are invited to participate in a session where they are invited to paint an image that represents their own philosophy of birth (see Box 15.1). This is based on the work of US Nurse-Midwife Pam England (1998). The activity creates a safe and supportive mindful space for the students to consider their own perspective around birth as a concept. By using art in a meditative environment, the students are able to access their own real and sometimes imagined/projected experiences to give insight into

---

Box 15.1 Birth art session

A mini meditation is introduced which leads into a visualization exercise where the students are invited to create an image of normal birth based on what that means to them. They are advised that they may visualize their own experience of giving birth or even of being born. Alternatively, their image may be based on a birth that they have attended or a representation from the media. They are asked to conjure in their minds where they are, who is present, what the light is like, what colours are there, what sounds they can hear and what the temperature of the environment is. Then they are invited to return to the room but are asked to retain the image in their minds eye and to stay with it. They are then taken into a room that is set up with painting materials and paper and invited to paint what they saw in their imagined birthing environment. Following the painting, they are invited to share their work and to discuss the experience and what they painted if they feel able.

their own thoughts around the birthing process. This is a profoundly reflective activity that offers insights that can change the way the students view the birthing sphere, and the responses are often emotionally charged. The students are invited to share their work with others if they wish in order to learn about themselves and others in the cohort.

Mindfulness is introduced in other ways within the first year of the programme. For example, a session of mindful eating is used as an introduction to nutrition (see Box 15.2). The students are taught to incorporate six seconds of deep breathing (see Box 15.3) as a means of altering their physiology to enable a calmer state of mind prior to starting an exam. They also receive a guided meditation session during the communication workshops that encourages/enables them to consider the importance of good communication.

Box 15.2 Mindful eating

Being present as we are eating and approaching what is happening in our mind and body as we eat with a non-judgmental, curious, and compassionate interest can positively influence our relationship with food. Whatever is happening for us at the table or anywhere that we choose to eat we can allow by simply being present (Bays 2009). A sensory exploration of the simple but complex act of eating a piece of fruit can have a profound effect. By contemplating how the grape/strawberry mandarin looks, feels, smells, tastes, and even sounds, encourages the students to spend time in the moment and have an appreciative moment in the presence of an item of food and encouraging them to view the fruit in a new and different ways.

Box 15.3 Resetting our physiology

An area clearly identified has been just prior to the start of exams where many students have high levels of anxiety and stress. For students who wish to participate, providing the opportunity for a mindful moment, a simple six-second reset helps to allay some of the stress and appears to enable several students to reduce their anxiety levels. They are simply guided to take a deep diaphragmatic breath in through the nose and out through the mouth and then to repeat the exercise. Students have reported back to the lecturers that this is a helpful inclusion at the start of their exams. It has also been noted that more lecturers are starting to naturally incorporate this into their exam rooms as they see others set an example.

Mātaraunga Māori

There is an indigenous perspective/worldview that informs the concept of self-sustainability in our country and this plays an important part throughout the programme, but particularly during Year 1. New Zealand/Aotearoa is a bi-cultural country with tango whenua and tangata Tiriti (please see Table 15.1 for translation). The articles and principles of Te Tiriti o Waitangi[2] are an integral part of curriculum development and delivery, and the Te Tiriti principles of Partnership, Protection and Participation are firmly embedded into the programme. Concepts from Mātaraunga Māori are used to strengthen and support the learning and teaching of cultural competence and cultural safety. Te Reo is incorporated into the programme documents and course delivery, with the use of terms such as Kaiako, ākonga and wānanga. Learners are also educated in the tikanga or deeper meanings behind these terms, for example ākonga is not just a group of learners and a kaiako, but it is a way of being within the group of sharing and respecting the transfer of knowledge between the participants. It is not only the way that Te Reo is embedded but the way in which things are done to ensure alignment with the kupu (words used).

This indigenous perspective represents a holistic worldview which although fundamentally focussed on the power of the collective in terms of whanau, hapu and iwi, there is also space for self-sustainability (see Chapter 3).

The introduction to mindfulness and the birth art activity discussed earlier takes place during a stay on a Marae where the students are immersed in tikanga and the concept of whanaungatanga (a relationship between shared experiences,

TABLE 15.1 Māori Words and Phrases – The Translation of the Te Reo Simplifies the Complex Constructs and Meaning behind the Words

Tangata Whenua	*People of the Land*
Te Tiriti o Waitangi	The Treaty of Waitangi
Mātaraunga Māori	Māori Knowledge
Te Reo	Māori language
Kaiako	Teacher
ākonga	Small learning group
wānanga	Face to face whole group learning
Hui	Meeting
Waiata	Song
Karakia	Blessing, say grace, rituals
whakapapa	Interconnection, lineage or descendent
mauri	Life force that can oscillate and become stronger or weaker
whakatauākī	Māori proverb
whanaungatanga	Relationship, kinship, sense of family connection
manaakitanga	Hospitality and support
Mana	Prestige, authority, ability to lead, can be enhanced or diminished
tangata Tiriti	"People of the Treaty", or New Zealanders of non-Maori origin

TABLE 15.2 Whakatauākī That Can Be Used at the Beginning of Sessions as a Mindfulness Practice

Whakatauākī	Translation
Ehara taku toa i te toa takitahi Engari, he toa takitini	My successes are not mine alone, they are ours – the greatest successes we will have are from working together
Poipoia te kakano Kia puawai	Nurture the seed and it will blossom
Karakia	**Translation**
Whakataka te hau ki te uru	The wind swings to the west
Whakataka te hau ki te tonga.	then turns southerly.
Kia mākinakina ki uta	making it prickly cold inland,
Kia mātaratara ki tai.	and piercingly cold on the coast.
E hī ake ana te atakura.	May the dawn rise red-tipped
He tio, he huka, he hauhū.	on ice, on snow, on frost.
Tihei Mauri Ora!	Join! Gather! Intertwine!

kinship, connection) is demonstrated from the outset of the programme. Therefore, when the students attend wānanga, they are welcomed with a whakatauākī such as those in Table 15.2 or a karakia. These traditions are used in the context of the midwifery programme to set up the space for learning, settle the students into the week and form connections between the student group and lecturers.

The use of Te Reo Māori and adhering to relevant tikanga and mātauranga Māori concepts within the programme, is a reminder that the construct of mindfulness aligns well with the holistic concepts of health and well-being within Te ao Māori and promotes the principles of te Tiriti o Waitangi and tikanga Māori. This is discussed at length in Chapter 4

The Māori worldview additionally informs the way in which the programme is structured. Ākonga provides an opportunity for students to debrief and share practice experience and establish whanaungatanga, under the watchful guidance of an experienced facilitator/kaiako. Most of the kaiako have incorporated an introductory component to their ākonga incorporating Māori principles of manaakitanga (hospitality and support), kaitiakitanga (guardianship) and whanaungatanga, as a means of reinforcing the interconnectedness within and around their learning. This then reminds students of the importance of staying connected with family and friends (whanau) and maintaining a balance between the programme and the other elements of their lives.

The use of ākonga has been incorporated within the blended programme since 2009 and is a critical point of contact for the students, provides whanaungatanga (a connection) between kaiako and students for debriefing, skill acquisition and is described as a 'community of enquiry' (Kensington et al. 2017, 43). Students meet in their small groups weekly and have a named lecturer (Kaiako) who is their point of contact throughout the year. This is especially important for supporting students who experience any unexpected outcomes within their practice placements or for those who need further pastoral care. The holistic nature of the learner/kaiako relationship and pedagogical underpinnings has been described by Stucki (2014) where the research supported this way of being within ākonga. Interestingly, students in a midwifery programme in the South of England were recruited into a qualitative study on mental well-being (Oates et al. 2020). The findings of this research corroborated with the findings of Kensington et al. (2017) as students identified that they needed to be "seen as an individual by at least one lecturer" (p. 1), connect with their peers, and have support that is consistent.

Year 2

Within the second year, the theme of mindfulness continues as a thread to some extent in ākonga but as previously identified it is not visible within the course content or during face-to-face teaching. This is largely due to the pressure that the students report on during Year 2. The students communicate that the pressure arises from courses that require increasingly complex levels of knowledge alongside a mounting number of practice-based placements in both the community and in hospital settings. It is also the point in the programme where 'worlds collide' or at least clash when the holistic nature of the first year of study is replaced with the mechanistic, atomistic, reductionist biomedical discourse of the complicated childbirth continuum. From programme and course evaluations, it is apparent that this is the year that students find the most challenging within the programme and where they would almost certainly benefit from a more mindful approach.

Year 3

The final year of the programme includes a course that focuses on sustainability in practice. One of the assignments for this course requires the students to produce a creative representation of their experiences during their practice placement (see Box 15.4).

The intention of including an arts-based focus within the programme was related to the desire to respect the art as well as the science of midwifery, thus promoting a holistic approach. However, this has achieved more than its original intent. By using an alternative modality to present their thoughts and feelings the students are able to tap into the limbic system which activates memory inputs from the anterior temporal lobe and the emotion of appreciation is evoked (Chakravarty 2012). By pulling on the power of the aesthetic the student can activate other ways of knowing and being from the more conventional academic approaches thus cultivating creativity through mindfulness (Hensley 2020).

Over the years it has been found that learners incorporate the concept of mindfulness within both assignments in different but equally valuable ways. The

---

Box 15.4 Creative representation

The students are required to develop a creative representation that embodies aspects of their practice placement. The piece may be presented in the form of a poster, pamphlet, art form, poem, or other aesthetic form. They are asked to critically reflect on the process of creating the piece and the under-lying meaning for them and to then present their work to their Kaiako and reflect on what the work represents, i.e., metaphors and symbolism. They are expected to utilise relevant literature to inform your presentation – this may relate more to a specific reflection on practice that arises out of what you create or why you created this representation.

---

arts assessment is very reflexive and autoethnographic, which calls on quite advanced levels of self-awareness and insight. The blueprint from sustainable practice requires the students to use a multi-focus approach to sustainability which incorporates self-care which frequently manifests in mindfulness or mediation practice. Although the students may not explicitly refer to this as mindfulness, although they sometimes do, it does suggest that they have taken on board the essence and significance of mindfulness during the programme implicitly. At this point in their learning, they can project how the concept of mindfulness will be useful in the practice setting once they enter the workforce. The programme ends with an activity that returns to the oxygen analogy, emphasizing the need for self-sustainability above all other considerations (see Box 15.5).

Our aspiration of creating a culture of mindful midwifery practice has been aided by engaging the expertise of a range of practitioners in this field. These include Robin Youngson, an NZ based anaesthetist who initiated the 'Hearts in Healthcare' movement in Aotearoa/New Zealand and Sheena Byrom and Soo Downe UK based midwifery academics who edited the seminal The Roar behind the Silence. In 2017 and 2018 "Hear the Roar Aotearoa" workshops were delivered for students and qualified midwives to attend. In these sessions, an introduction to the use of compassion within the practice setting and this is discussed further in Chapters 3 and 9). There have additionally been attempts to offer student and staff yoga and meditation sessions to access whilst at work or studying at Ara.

Revisiting mindfulness within the programme

We recognized that what we had achieved within the programme structure and content was encouraging, but also had to acknowledge that we still had a way to journey.

Box 15.5 Closing the circle

At the very end of the programme, the students and the lecturers form a circle. A bag containing semi-precious stones representing midwifery is passed around the circle and the students are invited to dip their hand into the bag and take a stone. They then re-introduce themselves to the group by identifying their name, their favourite animal, and their favourite place. After each person has done this, the stones are passed to the left. When each person has spoken in the circle, their original stone will have returned to its 'owner' complete with the energy of each person present. They are advised that this ritual has provided them with a touchstone for their midwifery journey ahead. With regard to their introduction, they are informed that their name represents the relationship with themselves, the animal represents their relationship with others and the favourite place represents their relationship with the earth. This serves to emphasise the importance of a mindful approach to practice and the importance of caring for themselves and how it will allow them then to care for others.

Having mapped the ways in which mindfulness was included within the programme, we were able to highlight the areas where further inclusion of mindfulness could be considered (Table 15.3). We felt this to be particularly important in the second year of the programme where we had identified that the busyness of the programme had ironically led to an omission of self-care strategies. Old Zen wisdom advises "you should sit in meditation for twenty minutes a day unless you are too busy and then should sit for an hour" and this resonated as we realized how we had unconsciously shied away from utilizing a mindful approach because of the busyness of the second year of study. A UK study by Oates et al. (2020) explored the 'roller-coaster' world of being a midwifery student and the effect this has on the mental-health and well-being of students. The findings from a group of 20 students in the Oates study identified that physical and mental well-being is impacted by the "relentless" pace of the programme and the conflicting pressures of study, clinical placement, home, and family life. Interestingly, mindfulness and self-care were encouraged by the lecturers in the Oates study. However, it would appear from their study that the ways in which students are affected by the demands of a midwifery programme are not taken into account when designing and planning programmes.

A profession in crisis

In NZ midwives are either community-based practitioners who are contracted by the Ministry of Health to provide primary care or they are employed within

TABLE 15.3 The Distribution of Mindfulness Content Within a Bachelor of Midwifery Curriculum

Year 1	Course	Area	Teaching/Assessment
	Ways of knowing	Birth philosophy	Visualisation and birth art
		Introduction to mindfulness	Guided meditation
	Bioscience	Neurohormonal system and influence of calm on mother and fetus	Online content Akonga discussion Exam
	Midwifery communication	Conflict resolution Selfcare in the stressed workplace	Workshop Online content
		Mindfulness–based reflective practice	Portfolio – Reflections
		Self-compassion	Journal
	Midwifery practice skills	Antenatal and postnatal modules	Online content. Akonga discussion
		Preparation for childbirth and parenting education	Online content Workshop
Year 2			
	Bioscience – reproductive health	Neurohormonal physiology in reproductive health	Online content Ākonga discussion Exam
	Research	Mindful inquiry	Online content
	Breastfeeding	Being mindfully present	Online content Case study Reflection
	Midwifery scope of practice	Supporting birth	Online content Ākonga discussion Portfolio reflection
	Collaborative practice	Maternal and infant mental health	Online content. Workshop
	Collaborative practice	Emergency situations – Six second physiological reset.	Ākonga discussion Wananga session
	Newborn health	Effects of stress on fetal health and well-being. Gentle birth.	Online content Ākonga discussion Wananga session

(*Continued*)

Year 1	Course	Area	Teaching/Assessment
Year 3			
	Ways of knowing	Evaluation of personal and professional development within the programme	Reflexive autoethnography
	Sustainability and midwifery practice	Self-care in practice	Module in online learning

Key

Actively incorporated in course	Not included in course currently	Incorporated but not explicitly related to mindfulness and self-care

a variety of healthcare settings as what are commonly referred to as 'core' midwives. Although the community-based midwives have a considerable amount of autonomy in their practice, they are under significant stress at times for several reasons. These include the requirements of the Ministry of Health which are considerable; the increasing complexity that women are presenting with in pregnancy, from medical and obstetric conditions and also in the shape of psychosocial challenges. These factors, in conjunction with a sense of ever-increasing uncertainty in the world, impact on both workload and well-being of midwives (Davies 2017; Bealing 2020). There is a perception that midwives despite their love for their work, are tired and this has had the effect of creating a profession that sometimes expresses dissatisfaction and a feeling of disenfranchisement (Welfare 2018). This has potentially far-reaching consequences for the midwifery profession in terms of retention in the workforce. Globally, the recruitment, retention and the resilience of the midwifery workforce are viewed as concerning and a consistent theme to emerge is that midwifery, on a global level, is a workforce under duress (Lancet 2020).

This perceived state of uncertainty in midwifery is perhaps understandably reflected in the mood of the student body at times and anecdotally at least, it is not unusual to hear Year 3 students stating that they are in a 'state of burnout' before they have even entered the workforce. Many new graduates move directly into part-time work or soon after qualifying and some make the decision to not even practice (Harvie et al. 2019). In their 2019 study, Eaves and Payne concluded that the "stress of midwifery training is linked to burnout and that both stress and reduced resilience are linked to intention to quit" (p. 189). They advocate that more research is needed to explore strategies for developing resilience in nascent practitioners if we are to improve retention rates and prevent burnout. Clohessy et al.'s (2019) concept analysis explored resilience within both the midwifery workforce and the student population in the UK. Their analysis revealed that some midwives and students possessed what appeared to be a natural ability to demonstrate resilience, whereas others needed to learn these skills. The building of self-efficacy as a coping mechanism for students can lead to an increased ability to manage stressful and complex situations within the placement environment. Self-efficacy also helps to establish effective coping mechanisms and leads to increased mental well-being. The authors conclude with the recommendation that this process should be "embedded into midwifery education programmes" (Clohessy et al. 2019).

The practice of midwifery is described as both art and science. In midwifery education, students are equipped with knowledge and skills that embrace both the art and science of practice. Some of these are considered to be 'hard' determinate skills that rely on cognitive proficiency, whilst others are seen as more intuitive and indeterminate 'soft skills' and would include things like communication and possibly mindfulness. Traditionally it has been harder to justify spending time on soft skills within midwifery programmes chiefly because they are harder to measure and therefore less tangible (Murphy 2021). Additionally, just as the introduction of the concept of mindfulness within midwifery practice can be challenging in a pressured environment with a stressed workforce and poor staffing levels, the 'buy in' of students to a less concrete domain of learning can be problematic. The inclusion of what could be viewed by some as gratuitous content in a heavily laden curriculum alongside a multitude of other demands on student midwives means that additional calls on their time need to be handled with due care and sensitivity. However, if students are introduced to mindfulness as a holistic paradigm that aligns with both the art and science of healthcare, they can value the benefits for themselves as well as the women and families that they serve in their role. Mindfulness has the capacity to bridge the divide as both a science and an art. In an editorial in the Lancet in 2014, Richard Horton warns that the art of mindfulness does not offer a pick and mix approach where we can select simply to use the scientific benefits of mindfulness as a tool to support our current sociopolitical values and beliefs. Rather, the values and the belief systems that brought mindfulness into being must be acknowledged and incorporated into any use of the concept. As Horton wisely surmises,

> The "armour of mindfulness" may offer us protections that can be measured by the standards of western science. But a fuller understanding of mindfulness will not be gained by randomisation or systematic review alone. The poverty of our own (scientific) culture is revealed by our belief in such simplicities.

(Horton 2014)

Conclusion

The World Health Organization (WHO) estimates that there will be a global shortfall of 9 million midwives and nurses by 2030 and we need to find practical ways of addressing this potentially catastrophic occurrence. We recognize that mindfulness cannot be used as a panacea for all ills and cannot save the world alone. There are factors operating at a systemic level that conspire to generate challenges such as technocratic, risk focused and litigious healthcare systems. We believe that midwifery education programmes need to commit to educating future midwives so that they are able to understand the socioeconomic and economic forces at play that impact on both their personal and professional lives. This includes investment in professional development to prepare lecturers to design and deliver a curriculum that incorporates a mindful philosophical approach (Chapman 2021). Self-sustainability is an important element in the broader construct of sustainability and to return to the oxygen analogy of starting with self, self-sustainability provides a platform on which to build and expand a greater understanding of the broader existential elements of sustainability (Noble and Powietrzynska 2021). Mindfulness as a tool and as a discipline within the context of midwifery education provides a means of working towards achieving this and by integrating the principles of mindfulness into every corner of the curriculum we believe that it can truly become a central and core value of a midwifery education programme.

Notes

1 The project was titled "The outcomes of using a values based approach to sustainability literacy in a Bachelor of Midwifery Programme" Approval from Ara Institute of Technology Ethics Research Committee was granted in August 2018.
2 The Treaty of Waitangi or Te Tiriti o Waitangi is the founding document of Aotearoa/New Zealand.

References

Alshak, Mark N., and Das, Joe M. 2021. *Neuroanatomy, Sympathetic Nervous System*. Stat Pearls Publishing. https://www.ncbi.nlm.nih.gov/books/NBK542195

Bays, Jan Chozen. 2009. *Mindful Eating: A Guide to Rediscovering a Healthy and Joyful Relationship with Food*. United States: Shambhala.

Bealing, Michael. 2020. Sustainable midwifery supporting improved wellbeing and greater equity. *NZ Institute of Economic Research Report to New Zealand College of Midwives*. NZIER.

Callander, Emily, Sidebotham, Mary, Gamble, Jenny, and Lindsay, Daniel. 2020. The future of the Australian midwifery workforce – Impacts of ageing and workforce exit. *Women and Birth* 34(1), 56–60.

Campbell, Emily. 2014. Mindfulness in education research highlights. *Greater Good Magazine*. https://greatergood.berkeley.edu/article/item/mindfulness_in_education_research_highlights. Accessed 3rd July 2021.

Chakravarty, Ambar. 2012. The neural circuitry of visual artistic production and appreciation: A proposition. *Annals of Indian Academy of Neurology* 15(2), 71–75. https://doi.org/10.4103/0972-2327.94986

Chapman, Laura Roche. 2021. Contemplative pedagogy: Creating mindful educators and classrooms. *Perspectives of the ASHA Special Interest Groups* 6(6), 1540–1553.

Chen, Yu, Yang, Xueling, Wang, Liyuan, and Zhang, Xiaoyuan. 2013. A randomized controlled trial of the effects of brief mindfulness meditation on anxiety symptoms and systolic blood pressure in Chinese nursing students. *Nurse Education Today* 33(10), 1166–1172. https://doi.org/10.1016/j.nedt.2012.11.014

Chmielewski, Jacek, Łoś, Kacper, and Łuczyński, Wlodzimierz. 2021. Mindfulness in healthcare professionals and medical education. *International Journal of Occupational Medicine and Environmental Health* 7:34(1), 1–14. https://doi.org/10.13075/ijomeh.1896.01542. Epub 2020 Nov 12. PMID: 33223537.

Chung, Arlene S., Smart, Jon, Zdradzinski, Michael, Roth, Sarah, and Gende, Alecia. 2018. "Educator toolkits on second victim syndrome, mindfulness and meditation, and positive psychology". The 2017 Resident Wellness Consensus Summit. *The Western Journal of Emergency Medicine* 19(2), 327–331. https://doi.org/10.5811/cpcem.2017.11.36179

Clemons, Janine H., Gilkison, Andrea, Mhrarpara, Tago L., Dixon, Lesley, and McAra-Couper, Judith. 2020. Midwifery job autonomy in New Zealand: I do it all the time. *Women and Birth* 34(1), 30–37 https://doi.org/10.1016/j.wombi.2020.09.004

Clohessy, Nicole, McKeller, Lois, and Fleet, Julie. 2019. Understanding resilience in the context of midwifery: A concept analysis. *Evidence Based Midwifery* 17(1), 10–18.

Davies, Lorna, Kara, Kelly, and Harre, Nicci. 2020. A values-based approach to sustainability literacy in a Bachelor of Midwifery programme. In L. Davies, R. Daellenbach and M. Kensington (Eds.), *Sustainability, Midwifery and Birth*. London. Routledge.

Eaves, Jane L. and Payne, Nicola. 2019. Resilience, stress and burnout in student midwives. *Nurse Education Today* 08(79), 188–193. https://doi.org/10.1016/j.nedt.2019.05.012.

England, P. and Horwitz, R. 1998. *Birthing from Within: An Extra-Ordinary Guide to Childbirth Preparation*. Albuquerque: Partera Press.

Erogul, Mert, Singer, Gary, McIntyre, Thomas, and Stefanov, Dimitre G. 2014. Abridged mindfulness intervention to support wellness in first-year medical students. *Teaching and Learning in Medicine* 26(4), 350–356. https://doi.org/10.1080/10401334.2014.945025

Harvie, K., Sidebotham, Mary, and Fenwick, Jenny. 2019. Australian midwives' intentions to leave the profession and the reasons why. *Women and Birth* 32(6), e584–e593.

Harwani, Neha, Motz, Kevin, Graves, Kristi, Amri H., Harazduk, Nancy, and Haramati, Aviad. 2014. Impact of changes in mindfulness on perceived stress and empathic concern in medical students. *Journal of Alternative and Complementary Medicine* 20(5), A7. https://doi.org/10.1089/acm.2014.5016.abstract

Hassed, Craig. 2021. The art of introducing mindfulness into medical and allied health curricula. *Mindfulness* 12, 1909–1919. https://doi.org/10.1007/s12671-021-01647-z

Henriksen, Lina, and Lukasse, Mirjam. 2016. Burnout among Norwegian midwives and the contribution of personal and work-related factors: A cross-sectional study. *Sexual & Reproductive Healthcare* 9, 42– 47.

Hensley, N. 2020. Educating for sustainable development: Cultivating creativity through mindfulness. *Journal of Cleaner Production* 243, 118542.

Horton, Richard. 2014. Offline: Mindfulness – Evidence, out of place. *The Lancet* 383(9919), 768. https://doi.org/10.1016/S0140-6736(14)60271-3

Hunter, Billie, Fenwick, Jenny, Sidebotham, Mary, and Henley, Josie. 2019. Levels of burnout, depression, anxiety and stress and associated predictors. *Midwifery* 79, 102526. https://doi.org/10.1016/j.midw.2019.08.008

Kakoschke, Naomi, Hassed, Craig, Chambers, Richard, and Lee, Kevin. 2021. The importance of formal versus informal mindfulness practice for enhancing psychological wellbeing and study engagement in a medical student cohort with a 5-week mindfulness-based lifestyle program. *PLoS One* 16(10), e0258999. https://doi.org/10.1371/journal.pone.0258999

Kelly, M. 2017. Does Mindfulness practice improve the mental health and wellbeing of healthcare students? *Journal of Psychiatric-Mental Health Nurses* 24, 84–89. https://doi.org/10.1111/jpm.12348

Kensington, Mary, Davies, Lorna, Daellenbach, Rea, Deery, Ruth and Richards, Julie. 2017. Using small tutorial groups within a blended Bachelor of Midwifery programme: Bridging the theory-practice divide. *New Zealand College of Midwives Journal* 53, 38–44.

Lancet. 2020. The status of nursing and midwifery in the world

Murphy. H. 2021. The importance of "Soft" skills in nursing & healthcare professions. https://evolve.elsevier.com/education/expertise/faculty-development/the-importance-of-soft-skills-in-healthcare-professions/

Noble, L. and Powietrzynska, M. 2021. Bushwhacking a path forward: Contemplative pedagogy for wellbeing in higher education. In Narelle Lemon (Ed.), *Creating a Place for Self-care and Wellbeing in Higher Education: Finding Meaning across Academia*, pp 147–158. London: Routledge.

Oates, J., Topping, A., Watts, K., Charles, P., Hunter, C., and Arias, T. 2020. The rollercoaster: A qualitative study of midwifery students' experiences affecting their mental wellbeing. *Midwifery* 88, 102735. https://doi.org/10.1016/j.midw.2020.102735

Pezaro, Sally, Clyne, Wendy, Turner, Andrew, Fulton, Emily A., and Gerada, Clare. 2016. 'Midwives Overboard!' Inside their hearts are breaking, their makeup may be flaking but their smile still stays on. *Women and Birth* 29(3), e59–66.

Raab, Kelley. 2014. Mindfulness, self-compassion, and empathy among health care professionals: A review of the literature. *Journal of Health Care Chaplaincy* 20(3), 95–108.

Shenoy, Rupa. 2019. The "father of mindfulness" prepares for the next life. The World Religion. January 2019. https://theworld.org/stories/2019-01-30/father-mindfulness-prepares-next-life. Accessed 17th May 2021.

Sidhu, Rawel, Su, Bowen, Shapiro, Kate, and Stoll, Kathrin. 2020. Prevalence of and factors associated with burnout in Midwifery: A scoping review. *European Journal of Midwifery* 4 (February), 4. https://doi.org/10.18332/ejm/115983

Stucki, Paora. 2014. A Māori Pedagogy: weaving the strands together. *Kairaranga* 13(1), 7–15.

Thich Nhat Hanh. 2011. *Your True Home.* Shambhala Publications, ISBN: 9780834827684.

Weare, Katherine. 2018. The evidence or mindfulness in schools or children and young people. Semantic Scholar https://www.semanticscholar.org/paper/the-evidence-for-mindfulness-in-schools-for-and-weare/491d5bd27fb615b2674ae-3ba46b703ef1be5e4d7. Accessed 4th June 2021.

Welfare, Melanie. 2018. *The good, the bad and the ugly: The experiences of midwives who transition work settings: A qualitative descriptive study.* Wellington: Victoria University of Wellington.

World Health Organization. 2019. Nursing and midwifery. [Cited 2020 Apr 29]. Available from: https://www.who.int/news-room/fact-sheets/detail/nursing-and-midwifery. Accessed 30th May 2021.

16

NURTURING HUMANITY IN MIDWIFERY

Compassionate, mindful leadership

Sheena Byrom

This chapter is a reflexive account of my journey as a nurse, midwife and leader where I pave the theory of compassionate, mindful leadership into the continuum of the path on which I travel. As such the chapter is a work of mindful self-inquiry rooted deeply in my own experiential encounter with mindfulness, compassionate care and leadership. Such an inquiry attunes to the "mindful self" – a practice associated with positive changes in attitudes towards the self that can promote well-being and self-development (Xiao et al. 2017).

Situating myself and my journey to mindfulness

I am a midwife consultant and the co-director of an organisation which provides educational and supportive resources for midwives, student midwives and other birth workers. My conscious interest in leadership theory in health care came by chance. Undertaking a master's degree and working in various senior midwifery positions afforded me a deeper understanding of my own leadership traits. I have a natural affiliation to kindness and compassion in both my personal and professional life mainly from the connection I had with my mother, but also the consequence of life events. By providing examples of my lived experience I hope to inspire readers to recognise their own leadership capabilities through a compassionate, mindful lens. As Youngson (2012) contends, we are, by our very existence as human beings, hard wired to be compassionate. Moreover, West (2021) suggests that it is crucial for the future of our health, and for generations to come, to lead compassionately so that wisdom, humanity and presence are sustained.

Mindful self-inquiry has been shown to provide inspiration and meaning in periods of personal challenge; especially when there is existential threat (Azarova 2019). We may always feel the consequences of the COVID-19 pandemic. When the world stopped and all was quiet, I spent time in isolation due to a health

DOI: 10.4324/9781003165200-16

vulnerability, apart from a permitted daily walk. During those strolls in my locality I breathed cleaner air, I paused to absorb the sight of trees and hills that I'd previously rushed past and not really noticed at all. After ten years of hopping from country to country to deliver lectures and workshops as a midwife, I stayed home and soaked up the benefits of rest, repose and reset. During the summer I tended to flowers. There was no pressure to do anything, no fear of missing out, nowhere to go. The noise that usually infiltrated our home from two busy roads was gone. Although I had read about the concept of mindfulness it was only during this time that I really appreciated what it meant to be intently appreciative of what was around me. From a quiet and reflective vantage point, I felt gratitude for the wonderful acts of compassion which gave me some respite from the absolute fear of dying that the virus had imposed on me. I was aware of my fortunate position to do this when the media poured out horrific detail of suffering and death. At the same time, I was overwhelmed with emotion as I saw extraordinary acts of kindness and of compassion within communities. For a time, due to the need to support survival, individuals and groups of people went out of their way to help others in need. As humans, it is in our nature to be altruistic (West 2021), yet in our fast-paced consumer-driven world, we are often too busy to stop, to think and to reach out. These events were remarkable.

My work as a midwife continued remotely from a tiny room in our garden. I was encouraged and felt nurtured by the loving relationships of my colleagues, friends and family. With those basic needs met I spent hours considering my life and my career as a midwife – I wrote my feelings down in a notebook and I've drawn upon some of those reflections and considerations when writing this chapter.

What does this have to do with leadership? With mindful leadership? I actually think the natural pause afforded by COVID-19 and my writing during that time, gave me the opportunity to review my career as first a nurse and then midwife. My career to date has been heavily influenced by situational factors and by those I have worked alongside or observed from a distance. I had time to consider the colleagues and leaders who nearly broke me, as well as the ones who lifted me higher than their shoulders, giving me self-belief through opportunity and support. It has been an interesting and pleasurable experience for me to do this. There have been many revealing moments as I've connected my life experiences with the knowledge I now have of the evidence and theory relating to both mindful and compassionate leadership. So, in this chapter, I will reflect on some of the individuals who moulded and shaped me, that I shall name 'the glorious ones'. I will attempt to isolate the individual personality traits of these glorious ones in order to distil the essence of their leadership skills. In so doing, I hope to stimulate and provoke interest, inspiration and instil hope for the future.

Mindfully compassionate and leading others

As I prepared this chapter, I began to fully recognise the synergy between mindfulness and compassion. Compassion is a core human value, a desire and motivation to help others who are suffering. I often use this Paul Gilbert (2016) quote when articulating the power of compassion:

> *Compassion is not just about kindness or 'softness' and it is certainly not a weakness. It is one of the most important declarations of strength and courage known to humanity. It is difficult and powerful, infectious and influential. And crucially, is perhaps the only universally recognised language with the ability to change the world.*

Mindfulness has been defined as '*the basic human ability to be fully present, aware of where we are and what we're doing, and not overly reactive or overwhelmed by what's going on around us*' (Mindful.org 2020). It could be suggested therefore that mindfulness helps us to activate our compassionate selves – to be present and have clarity to act with meaning and consideration. In Chapter 3, Diane and Jenny present their research findings which highlight the importance of compassion and mindfulness in maternity care and how they are interwoven in reference to childbirth trauma. Compassion is core to being human – and evidence demonstrates that the protective factor of nurturing relationships and connection is remarkable, resulting in improved health outcomes and experience of care or support (West 2021). There are benefits for carers too. Youngson (2012) and West (2021) share studies which demonstrate less burnout in clinicians and carers who are compassionate, and they highlight the importance and advantages of staff caring for each other too. Craig and Richard in Chapter 2 explore the mindful practitioner in relation to mitigating burnout, workload stress and mental health concerns in the practitioner. They suggest that mindful leadership is crucial for employee engagement and optimal organisational performance. Compassionate working environments that are able to sustain staff need compassionate leaders who can role model behaviours that influence the culture of the shift, the department, and the whole organisation. This shift in culture requires attuning to inclusiveness so that all can contribute in their own unique way and inclusiveness is therefore a crucial aspect of compassionate leadership. Compassionate leaders celebrate diversity valuing all team members, supporting them to contribute creatively and with enthusiasm to team and organisational goals (West 2021).

Michael West is a professor of organisational psychology and has published widely on compassionate care and leadership for health and social care services. Building on previous chapters, I now draw on West's work to further highlight the benefits of compassionate leadership as a solution for improving maternity care. West (2021) describes four behaviours for compassionate leadership:

Attending: this involves being present with others, and yourself, and 'listening with fascination' (Kline 2002) to the needs and challenges presented. West suggests that listening with fascination is probably the most important trait of a compassionate leader.

Understanding: taking time to properly explore and understand the situation people are struggling with. This involves trying to appreciate without imposing own understanding through dialogue.

Empathising: caring for those we lead, empathising with them without being consumed by the issues.

Helping: taking action to help and support if able. It is this behaviour that differentiates empathy from compassion – the empathetic stage mobilises the action.

The inclusive nature of compassionate leadership permeates these four behaviours. Being compassionate promotes trust through understanding and without judgement; it means to include and be alongside others, encouraging a sense of belonging and mutual support (West 2021). Mindful and compassionate leaders are self-reflective, checking in on their personal preferences and biases continually and seeking to improve. The connection between mindful and compassionate leadership is summed up in this sentence '*A mindful leader is someone who embodies leadership presence by cultivating focus, clarity, creativity and compassion in the service of others'* (Marturano 2013).

This quality of leadership is more difficult if we are continually pulled away, distracted through competing demands and conflicting situations. In the busyness and often chaotic episodes of working life mixed with juggling complex home situations – we all need time to still our minds so that we can reflect, refocus and recharge. We need to time to listen and to be heard. Mindful, compassionate leaders are aware of their own abilities and limitations to create work places where staff can thrive and innovate and they pursue opportunities for personal growth (Pipe et al. 2016). It is important to acknowledge the synergy of mindful compassionate leadership and the body of work concerning servant leadership linked to ethical and value-based leadership (Pawar et al. 2020) and the transformational leadership being evidenced in midwifery research (Turner et al. 2021). See Table 16.1 for a summary of the different types of leadership discussed in this chapter.

I have recently engaged in a programme which has helped me enormously. 'One Thought' helps individuals to comprehend the function of 'thought' and how our understanding of thought can help improve clarity of mind (Turner 2020). Rather than trying to relinquish thoughts as with mindfulness, participants learn to acknowledge how thought influences the state of mind and body. This is not a 'technique' but an understanding that enables a new way of being, and as I become more aware of the benefits, I am learning to respond rather than react. In her book, Jan Smith (2021) shares insights into the importance of considering our own mental and physical wellness as we care for others. The book includes tips for individuals to consider at work and in their personal lives, and mindfulness is encouraged as a protective factor against stress and burnout. As West (2021) emphasises compassionate leaders facilitate the well-being of their staff as they recognise the need for a healthy and happy workforce. Kristin

TABLE 16.1 Types of Leadership

Types of Leadership Considered in this Chapter	
Transformative leadership	Transformative leaders encourage and inspire colleagues to grow and innovate, through personal support, role modelling and facilitating self-efficacy. Well-being of staff is a key focus.
Collaborative leadership	There is a focus on working with others towards a common goal, as opposed to a top-down approach historically used in healthcare. Collaborative leaders listen to the views and opinions of others and encourage transparency at all levels.
Compassionate leadership	Compassionate leaders focus on relationships through careful listening to, understanding, empathising with, and supporting individuals so that they feel valued, respected and cared for. The aim is to enable followers to do the best for themselves and their organisation.
Servant leadership	Servant leadership focuses on the growth and well-being of those they lead. Instead of a hierarchical top-down leadership style, the servant-leader shares power, puts the needs of others first helping them to develop and perform as highly as possible.
Relational leadership	Relational leaders, as the name implies, focus on building relationships with followers to enable growth and development. Inclusiveness is important and they consider everyone's viewpoint and experiences when making decisions. The leader may ultimately make the final decision, but perspectives are carefully considered.
Mindful leadership	Mindful leaders consciously develop their ability to be present, open-minded, and compassionate when interacting with others – and they show the same care and consideration to themselves. Well-being of staff is a key focus.

Neff (2022) is a major proponent of self-compassion, and her website includes a free-to-access self-assessment questionnaire measuring self-kindness and self-judgement. Neff shares resources on 'mindful self-compassion' as a means of supporting individual well-being, which is useful for leaders to use with their teams. Indeed, mindfulness is increasingly suggested as a tool for personal resilience within working adults (Rupprecht et al. 2019).

In the beginning

I felt the impact of authentic, positive leadership before I understood what it was. I am a seasoned midwife of more than four decades and have experiences of being in both subordinate and leadership roles. My early career was a baptism of fire where I was plunged into hierarchical cultures within the National Health Service. As a student nurse at the tender age of 18, my senses were challenged. I was consistently directed not to be emotional, to detach myself from the people I was caring for. This was particularly hard for me as an 'empath', a term not yet discovered, in that I cried almost as much as I laughed and was chastised for it – and because of this I believed I would be doomed as a nurse. I vividly recall a time as a student nurse seeing a distressed relative weeping loudly over their loved one who had died. I did not know what to do so just stood close by, with my hand gently touching the relative. It was almost impossible for me to hold back the tears and the ward sister caught sight of me and chastised me later. How could I block human emotion? It seemed that I had to try.

During those formative years, I was an incessant observer, quiet in my approach to learn from the 'good' nurses. They were the ones who looked the part, smart, clean, used gentle language and connected with patients in a way I related to. I sought out role models who embodied what I believed a nurse should be and I think the backdrop to that was my childhood and my mother's influence. Kathleen (my mother) was the kindest human being I ever met; she oozed compassion yet had a strong air of dignity and she commanded respect. My mum was a leader – she was unaware that her mothering represented a feminist viewpoint. I am the youngest of five girls so she had a significant task! I had no idea there was a gender imbalance in the world – we five girls thought we ruled it!

One of my sisters was a nurse and my aunt a midwife and they shared their principles of professionalism and caring values in their everyday communication with me. So all in all I had a blueprint of how I wanted to practice. The reality, however, was somewhat different.

After qualifying as a nurse I trained to be a midwife. My affinity to a holistic approach in midwifery care, supporting and promoting undisturbed birth, was sparked early in my career whilst working in a maternity home. Bramley Meade was a community hospital where midwives provided intrapartum care and only called the family doctor if needed. This was in direct contrast to my midwifery training which took place in a district general hospital during the 1970s, when medical interventions were growing at pace and seen as progressive. I rarely witnessed normal physiological childbirth and was induced with my first two children during this time for no medical reason. So when I witnessed birth for the first time at the maternity home it was an epiphany for me; it was revealing, exciting and transformative – from then on I learned to be a midwife. I gave birth to two more children in this environment supported by Carla Gazzola, my midwife and my colleague, who was naturally quiet when I was in labour and gave birth – but always present. This midwife was one of my role models, I aspired to be like Carla. Carla took time to think situations through and always, at the beginning of each shift, listened carefully to the needs of each woman/person she was caring for. She went out of her way to help, rallying support from us, even when a solution seemed almost impossible. When considering Carla's approach to her work, I can see that she was a mindful midwifery practitioner

(Plested 2014), and a mindful leader – influencing compassionately and involving others. I worked for eight years with Carla, in this nurturing yet often challenging environment, until the establishment closed in 1989.

From then on my preference was to practice in 'low-tech' community settings and I loved supporting and facilitating home birth. When working in the hospital environment, I was the midwife who generally stayed in birthing rooms and practised 'watchful waiting' (de Jonge et al. 2021). This practice of attending to and focusing on the person we are caring for, whilst being both physically and mindfully present, is a fundamental element of woman or person-centred care that can optimise the physiological and psycho-emotional outcomes for mothers and babies. I would contend that the midwifery practice of 'watchful waiting' is certainly a form of mindfulness in the birthing room which is hugely beneficial (see Chapters 3 and 8).

I loved connecting with women and families using all my senses. 'Being with' was where I wanted to be, although I wasn't aware of either of these terms at this stage – it was just how I was reinforced by Carla's influence. I was drawn to others who practised this way. On reflection, I think this is mindful midwifery practice at its most pure.

Aspiring to be this kind of midwife was a constant challenge. I felt the growing fear and tension in maternity services as technology and medical interventions advanced. I witnessed first-hand the explosion of the 'risk agenda' and I experienced the consequences – the suffocation that still exists. I experienced bullying at every level, as did many of my peers and I look back in dismay that it was never challenged. Bullying is a toxic yet common denominator running through maternity (and other health care) services (Farrell and Shafiei 2012) and affects midwifery students (Capper 2021). In my early career, it was deemed a 'rite of passage' to survive the tyrants. Bullying is both a symptom and consequence of negative culture and poor leadership. I have felt the impact of leaders who took pleasure in disempowering others using tactics such as 'divide and rule', criticising others to gain power. Others withheld information on opportunities or knowledge of changes in practice. These were the quietly coercive leaders; their actions often unspoken about or even unnoticed. Then there was the autocratic, destructive leaders who ridiculed me and others publicly, whilst their 'favourites' chimed 'they don't mean it'. I remember their names and faces clearly. They almost broke me.

As I grew as a midwife and an experienced practitioner, I tried to use the negative experiences to enhance my practice and I vowed to be different, to be kind, respectful and compassionate. I held on to the images and experiences of working with midwives who inspired me and I tried to emulate them. I was always drawn towards the quiet, reflective practitioners.

A catalytic episode took place when I first became a manager. It was a Community Midwife Manager position and I found it incredibly alien at first. I regretted the move I'd made as I missed being in direct contact with women and families. Then slowly I started to approach my work as I had done as a clinical midwife – that is, using the tenets of woman-centred care. I used a partnership approach (just as I would as a midwife with those I cared for) to manage and work alongside staff, avoiding hierarchical terminology and communication. I endeavoured to support and promote self-confidence in colleagues by listening to their concerns and needs and trying to help them if I could. As a consequence my job satisfaction improved considerably.

During this time I began studying for a Master's degree where I explored the possible connections between 'good' midwifery and 'good' leadership (Byrom and Downe 2010). Participants in my master's dissertation described the midwifery knowledge and skills of both the midwife and leader, as being integral and necessary. In addition, the study found that the quality which made both the midwife and the leader 'good' was their emotional capability. This research stimulated my interest in transformational leadership theory, and the crucial benefits of compassionate maternity care. Since then, my work has focused on the need to humanise childbirth at every level as a critical importance – from governments to those in direct contact with childbearing women, people and families. Relational, woman-centred care enhances both the woman's experience and health outcomes for her and her baby (Sandall et al. 2016).

Fast-forward: the challenges we face

Maternity services globally have become increasingly risk-averse, technology-driven environments where fear drives the actions of practitioners and the decisions service users make (Byrom and Byrom 2020; Crowther et al. 2020; Dahlen et al. 2020). The COVID-19 pandemic, and the consequences of warfare in some parts of the world, has had a devastating effect on childbearing women, people and families (Bashour et al. 2021; Davis-Floyd and Gutschow 2021).

Midwives have been at the sharp end of delivering services in these crisis situations and have felt the impact personally and professionally. The undervaluing and oppression of midwives globally have already been highlighted (Renfrew et al. 2014) despite the phenomenal impact of midwifery contributions (UNFPA 2021). Even before the COVID-19 pandemic midwives in the UK and other countries reported burnout and over-burdening pressure (Creedy et al. 2017; Hunter et al. 2019). The pandemic has intensified the issues making work life intolerable for many and midwives are leaving the profession or report the intention of leaving (Royal College of Midwives 2021). Under-resourced and pressured working environments are not only psychologically unsafe for staff but they are more likely to be unsafe for the people using the service (Crowther et al. 2020).

The resulting workplace culture due to internal and external stressors on maternity care providers and users can lead to relationships being devoid of meaning and nurturing in which human connection often remains elusive. This, together with overburdening workloads, lack of human resources and pressures within professional practice is the perfect breeding ground for staff burnout, moral distress and compassion fatigue (Smith 2021). In the UK, some of these factors have been highlighted in a recent report of a failing maternity service (Independent Maternity Review 2022). The Ockenden Report details devastating, and heart-breaking accounts of harm caused to families who used maternity services at the Shrewsbury and Telford NHS Trust. Highlighted within the report is detail of the toxic culture, lack of collaborative working and respectful relationships, and compassion. It is imperative that the recommendations for improvements are actioned; this is an invitation to engage mindfully and embrace the opportunity to engage with the issues with compassion and courage. Safety guru Suzette Woodward, in her paper on improving maternity safety (2020), is clear that influencing the culture and the way individuals behave towards each other is the solution. Woodward refers to behaviours that are helpful including compassionate leadership, listening, respect, kindness and gratitude.

Mindful, compassionate leadership is needed more now, then ever. The pandemic has brought a sense of helplessness and despair to staff in maternity services (Schmitt et al. 2021; Smith 2021). As well as addressing the need for more human and financial resources, we must strive to ensure that staff feel safe and valued so that they can give their full attention to those they serve from a position of strength and self-belief (West 2021). Caring for each other, small acts of kindness and other behaviours (see below) help to sustain the giver and the receiver and can positively influence working environments. Without a proactive mindful leadership response to these challenges the 'watchful waiting' midwife in the birthing space, as previously mentioned, is unlikely to flourish leaving care in childbirth as yet another wounded event in human life.

Compassionate leadership in action

I was privileged the opportunity of working as one of the UK's first consultant midwives, giving me the freedom to lead by example and to use my newly sourced knowledge to influence and push boundaries. The connection between midwifery practice and leading others was a deep one and I had learned to apply this phenomenon which enabled me to share my experiences with others. For example, whilst I hadn't conceptualised mindful or compassionate leadership, I spent hours creating spaces for women and families to recall their traumatic birth stories. I listened intently, sat silently with them, reflecting, empathising and then offering support. Their words were used to challenge maternity staff through drama and voice recordings, all within a safe space where nurturing was a priority. Being open and honest with my colleagues about the potential impact of their actions and words was crucial as they equally needed time to explore the trauma-based scenarios. Listening to staff is as important as listening to women and they needed the space to reflect, to work through solutions and to be valued.

The focus of my work as consultant midwife was 'public health' – and through effective negotiating and successful grant applications – I built up a team of specialist midwives who were able to work together to reduce health inequalities by leading transformation of services. It was one of the most successful achievements in my career and it was down to the fact that I was given the freedom to explore positive approaches to leading using my expanding knowledge of transformational and collaborative leadership approaches (see Table 16.1). I was able to nurture and support each team member by being present and open-minded, reflecting on my personality traits and capabilities as I practised emotionally intelligent communication. Our small team grew in numbers and in confidence – we were a highly performing and contented team. As part of the work I engaged with public health practitioners and voluntary agencies, I learned about community development approaches to influencing negative behaviour and focused on transforming the negative culture. This included a whole new dimension in acknowledging and adopting respectful and inclusive language. I was not aware of the term 'compassionate leadership' at that time, but now I recognise some of the elements of this model were engrained in how we all functioned as a team. Both transformational and compassionate leaders use facilitative approaches to engage with staff inclusively, to encourage and support others to grow through collaboration and role modelling positive behaviours.

Quietly confident – mindfully leading

To return to the theme of my glorious ones, I need to mention Sue Henry, a midwife who was a member of the team that I directly managed. Sue was described as 'quietly confident', and would concur that this was an appropriate description of her comportment. I learnt first-hand from her how to respond effectively to crises, dilemmas and conflicts. Sue was an infant feeding coordinator, and her role was challenging. She had to influence and negotiate with medical teams and midwifery staff as she took the service through the Baby Friendly Initiative (BFI)[1] accreditation with resounding success. I watched her as she moved through the postnatal wards, her presence quietly supportive and gentle. I read email responses where those against the BFI programme criticised her work and objectives. Yet Sue never faltered in her commitment. She was respectful and calm – always reflective and strong. Sue's leadership style was authentic and demonstrated integrity – both traits recognised within mindful leadership literature (Pipe et al. 2016). I was in awe of her leadership style, and impressed with her achievements, and I still, many years later, think of her when faced with a challenge or difference.

Compassionate, courageous action

West (2021) points out and dispels some of the myths around compassionate leadership. The compassionate leadership approach is often mistaken as 'soft and fluffy' rendering leaders unable to challenge the status quo or to make difficult decisions relating to performance management. However, West assures us that compassionate leaders are compelled to take action when needed, which includes having 'courageous conversations'. Courageous conversations can be used for addressing bullying behaviours as identified earlier in the section above, speaking up for more resources, or addressing poor practice. If staff have a compassionate leader who regularly engages with and cares for them, they are potentially more likely to accept challenging feedback (Hougaard, Carter, and Hobson 2020). Likewise, midwives often find themselves in conflict when caring for women who choose pathways of care that fall outside of maternity guidelines. When a woman describes her reasons for choosing a particular option the midwife feels compassionate and recognises the professional, ethical, and legal obligation to ensure women's birthing choices are supported and respected (NMC 2019), through informed decision-making (Birthrights 2021). However, midwives (and doctors), employed by institutions, report being afraid of recrimination and therefore feel unable or unwilling to appropriately support 'out of guideline' choices for women or other birthing people make (Feeley et al. 2019). This can lead to women feeling dissatisfied with their birth experience or even traumatised and be a reason for them choosing to birth outside the system without medical and/or midwifery assistance (Baranowska et al. 2019; Dahlen et al. 2020; Plested and Kirkham 2016).

In addition to the appropriate clinical skills, midwives and doctors need courage and commitment, and the right organisational support to enable them to provide personalised, safe, and meaningful care that is physically and psychologically safe. Feeley (2022) revealed influencing factors that played a part in supporting midwives to facilitate alternative choices safely and confidently. Feeley developed a mnemonic 'ASSET' to highlight that midwives are the 'asset' which enable women to get their needs met and it presents what midwives need to do for this to happen, both personally and through to organisational level. See Figure 16.1. I wasn't surprised to see empathy and compassion there (for both women and from colleagues) as well as trusting relationships, with women, colleagues, and employers.

Then there are situations where we need to find courage through compassion for our colleagues, and ourselves. I frequently find myself in situations where injustice prevails – either for me personally or someone I know. Whilst some of these instances have been intolerable, they have also given me hope and faith in the willingness of others to be compassionate AND courageous; two human values which, I believe, go hand I hand. In the following section, I describe two glorious ones and their outstanding examples of compassion and courage in leadership – the first in the UK context and the second in the Indian context.

When Cathy Warwick CBE was serving as the CEO of the Royal College of Midwives (UK), she listened carefully to serious concerns I had about specific, worrying situations, occurring over a period of several years. Cathy was courageous in her effort to stand alongside me, supporting me and others to resolve a troubling conflict which involved two student midwives, on separate issues. The ability for Cathy to listen, empathise and then act, deeply affected me and I feel that in a roundabout way, her actions potentially optimised safer maternity care.

- Autonomy
- Access, assess, & apply evidence-based information to individual women

- Skills- physiological birth experience and skills in a range of settings
- Skill development- ongoing CPD

- Systems approach that supports woman-centred care/full-scope midwifery
- Support (accessible, timely, restorative ~psychological safety)

- Empathy and compassion (for women and from colleagues)

- Trusting relationships; with women, colleagues, employers

FIGURE 16.1 'The ASSET model (first printed in Feeley 2019, published Feeley 2022 – permissions granted.').

In 2018 I was invited to India by Dr Evita Fernandez, a highly respected obstetrician to deliver workshops on compassionate, respectful maternity care. Evita is the owner of a group of maternity hospitals and is a passionate protector of human rights. I observed Evita working within her environment and in other establishments, and I witnessed the positive and humbling influence she has on others. I saw Evita walking through various departments, acknowledging each of her employees by name, stopping, taking time to ask how they were, their families. This included everyone from lift porters to senior clinicians. Evita's actions embodied compassion. One day Evita took me to a public hospital, and we witnessed blatant disrespectful care. It was shocking for me to see, and I reacted by asking Evita if we could leave. Evita quietly and confidently asked one of the doctors present why this situation was happening – the response of the doctor was inappropriate, and Evita challenged further. How Evita spoke was clear and to the point but respectful and considered. I'll never know whether the doctor paid attention to Evita's feedback; I hope she did. Evita's compassion for the woman whose naked body was exposed for all to see, gave her the courage to act and confront disrespectful abusive care in the actual moment it was occurring. We can all learn from this.

Creating virtuous cycles – a ripple effect

When I relay stories of positive leadership during workshops or presentations, the response is frequently 'we don't have leaders like this in our organisation'. I understand that comment. However, whilst organisational culture can be perceived as being a barrier to person–centred care, West suggests that each health service worker is responsible for the culture in the workplace, every word we speak and interaction we have (West 2021). Nonetheless, West adds that leaders can role model the way through example. When managers display compassionate and person-centred behaviours, staff are more likely to care for clients compassionately (Crowther et al. 2020). I agree with this, even in the most threatening and challenging times where we feel drawn into vicious circles of despair and hopelessness, we can create opportunities and shift perspectives by the way we are.

In the early 2000s, I was fortunate to be part of a programme of influence within the organisation where I worked. Led by a consultant nurse, the 'Being with Patients' programme was developed and rolled out to facilitate the 'reconnection of purpose' for hospital staff (Reid 2006). Part of the content of the programme focused on the power of authentic positive feedback; *authentic* being the important element. I have personally used this with consultant obstetricians, cleaners and in my personal life and the ripple effect is considerable.

Sometimes a ripple can be initiated by a simple observation and comment:

> *I saw the way you spoke to the relative on the corridor yesterday, It made me smile and I'm sure the person appreciated it too.*

Just imagine if you were given this kind of feedback on a regular basis instead of the constant negative comments and scrutiny. Retired Anaesthetist, Robin Youngson (2014) takes this a step further, using the mnemonic ACT (with Compassion). Youngson encourages us to:

*   **Appreciate** – tell the person why you appreciate what they did,
*   **Commend** – share the positive action with others, publicly if possible (i.e. at the nurses/midwives station or office) – then ask them to
*   **Teach** others.

If leaders (and others) practice this ACT authentically and mindfully they will positively influence the atmosphere of the workplace. In addition, they will make the environment safer as staff are more likely to report mistakes or ask for help if the leader works this way.

A midwife (Sarah) recently told me she used this in practice. She heard a student midwife (Sian) giving a woman who was being discharged, details of what she needed to do and to look out for. Sarah was at the other side of the screen and was impressed by the approach of Sian, the respectful language she used and generally how she delivered important information with diligence and kindness. Subsequently, Sarah approached Sian as she stood with colleagues completing paperwork at the desk. Sarah complimented Sian on her practice (acknowledged), detailing the specifics of what she'd overheard. Sian was surprised but delighted (if a little embarrassed) when Sarah addressed the others, letting them know why she was impressed (commended). Sarah suggested to the others that they observe Sian next time she discharged someone in her care – therefore sharing good practice (teaching).

When I have used ACT in my practice I have noticed the ripple effect. Individuals receiving positive authentic feedback feel valued and it supports their growth. They are more likely to do the same to others, which potentially improves working relationships, cultivates a positive working environment which, in turn, promotes safe practice. I would contend ACT is one of the hallmarks of mindful practitioner behaviour – a simple practice within our everyday working environment that can proactively foster and positively transform collegiality and affirming relationships.

Relationships matter and relational leadership

Workloads and pressures within maternity services are influenced by the need to monitor performance, targets and safety checks. These activities, in addition to ensuring evidence-based practices for safe and responsive maternity care, must not encourage us to overlook the crucial importance of relationships at all levels. The positive relationships we cultivate with each other, our leaders and our teams will hopefully infiltrate through to those we serve. We have seen in this chapter that the role of a good leader is to model attitudes and behaviour to the people in the organisation, so that others feel the urge and ability to follow – this requires mindfulness.

A call to action for a better future

In summation, if we are to optimise the childbirth experience and health outcomes for all women and their families, we must find a way to connect with the fundamental human emotion of love. Science is crucial for us to progress through learning and evidence, but it is love that roots us to the core meaning of life, enabling us and those we serve to flourish. Being mindful and gentle on ourselves, recognising when we need help and support and seeking it, increases our resilience and ability to nurture others and to be recipients of the same attention, in return.

This chapter is a call to action for midwives and midwifery leaders to nurture compassion within and for themselves and in the departments and organisations in which they work to cultivate a healthier, happier working environment. To do this we must challenge ourselves to have the authenticity and courage to mindfully lead in this way to nurture and sustain midwifery practice with an aim to promote safe maternity care now and in the future.

Note

1 The Baby Friendly Hospital Initiative (BFHI) is an international programme launched in 1991 by the World Health Organization (WHO) and the United Nations Children's Fund (UNICEF). The aims of the initiative are to ensure that all maternity services become centres of breastfeeding support worldwide and where healthcare

environments ensure breastfeeding is the norm by promoting optimal baby feeding practices through education and independent institutional accreditation.

References

Azarova, T., 2019. A mindful inquiry into the meaning of individual inspiration in a period of personal challenge (Doctoral dissertation, Fielding Graduate University).

Baranowska, B. 2019. The quality of childbirth in the light of research the new guidelines of the World Health Organization and Polish perinatal care standards. *Journal of Mother and Child* 23(1): 54–59. https://doi.org/10.34763/devperiodmed.20192301.5459

Bashour, H., Kharouf, M. and de Jong, J., 2021. Childbirth experiences and delivery care during times of war: Testimonies of Syrian women and doctors. *Frontier Global Women's Health* 2: 1–7.

Birthrights. 2021. *Birthrights and GMC – what does informed consent mean in maternity care?* https://www.birthrights.org.uk/2021/09/17/birthrights-and-gmc-what-does-informed-consent-mean-in-maternity-care/

Byrom, S. and Byrom, A., 2020. Shifting tides—from storm to salvation. In Gutteridge, K. (Ed.), *Understanding Anxiety Worry and Fear in Childbearing: A Resource for Midwives and Clinicians.* Cham: Springer.

Byrom, S. and Downe, S., 2010. 'She sort of shines': Midwives' accounts of 'good' midwifery and 'good' leadership. *Midwifery* 26: 126–137.

Capper, T., 2021. Social culture and the bullying of midwifery students whilst on clinical placement: a qualitative descriptive exploration. *Nurse Education in Practice* 52 (Online).

Creedy, D.K., Sidebotham, M., Gamble, J. Pallant, J. and Fenwick, J., 2017. Prevalence of burnout, depression, anxiety and stress in Australian midwives: A cross-sectional survey *BMC Pregnancy Childbirth* 17: 13.

Crowther, S., Cary, L., Meechan, F. and Ashkanasy, N.M., 2020. The role of emotion, empathy, and compassion in organisations. In Downe, S. and Byrom, S. (Eds.), *Squaring the Circle: Researching Normal Birth in a Technological Age.* London: Pinter and Martin.

Dahlen, H., Kumar-Hazard, B. and Schmied, V., 2020. *Birthing Outside the System: The Canary in the Coalmine.* London: Routledge Research in Nursing and Midwifery.

Dahlen, H., Teate, A., Ormsby, S. and Schmied, V., 2020. Working with worry and inspiring hope: Relationships with anxious and fearful women. In: Gutteridge, K. (Ed.), *Understanding Anxiety Worry and Fear in Childbearing: A Resource for Midwives and Clinicians.* Cham: Springer.

Davis-Floyd, R. and Gutschow, K., 2021. Editorial: The global impacts of COVID-19 on maternity care practices and childbearing experiences. *Frontiers in Sociology* 6: 721782. doi: 10.3389/fsoc.2021.721782. eCollection 2021.

de Jonge, A., Dahlen, H. and Downe, S., 2021. 'Watchful attendance' during labour and birth. *Sexual & Reproductive Healthcare* Jun. 28: 100617.

Farrell, G.A. and Shafiei, T. 2012. Workplace aggression, including bullying in nursing and midwifery: A descriptive survey (the SWAB study) *International Journal of Nursing Studies* 49: 1423–1431.

Feeley, C. 2019. 'Practising outside of the box, whilst within the system': A feminist narrative inquiry of NHS midwives supporting and facilitating women's alternative physiological birthing choices'. Doctoral Thesis. University of Central Lancashire. http://clok.uclan.ac.uk/30680/?fbclid=IwAR2oZ4x0NcVBjMBr0olaX-nliuN5Y9z8y2j4C-izwEMObvwwh-P_c-AJats

Feeley, C. 2022. The asset model: What midwives need to support alternative physiological births (outwith guidelines). *The Practising Midwife* 25(2) (Online).

Feeley, C., Thomson, G. and Downe, S. 2019. Caring for women making unconventional birth choices: A meta-ethnography exploring the views, attitudes, and experiences of midwives. *Midwifery* 72: 50–59.

Gilbert, P., 2016. *Compassion: Universally Misunderstood*. https://www.huffingtonpost.co.uk/-professor-paul-gilbert-obe/compassion-universally-misunderstood_b_8028276.html Accessed on 17.11.21.

Hougaard, R., Carter, J. and Hobson, N. 2020. Compassionate leadership is necessary—but not sufficient. *Harvard Business Review*. https://hbr.org/2020/12/compassionate-leadership-is-necessary-but-not-sufficient

Hunter, B., Fenwick, J., Sidebotham, M. and Henley, J., 2019. Midwives in the United Kingdom: Levels of burnout, depression, anxiety and stress and associated predictors. *Midwifery* 79 (Online).

Independent Maternity Review. 2022. *Ockenden Report – Final: Findings, Conclusions, and Essential Actions from the Independent Review of Maternity Services at the Shrewsbury and Telford Hospital NHS Trust (HC 1219)*. Crown.

Kline, N., 2002. *Time to Think: Listening to Ignite the Human Mind*. London: Cassell.

Marturano, J., 2013. What is a mindful leader? *Institute for Mindful Leadership*. https://instituteformindfulleadership.org/mindful-leader/ Accessed on 10.1.22.

Mindful.org. 2020. What is mindfulness? *Mindful, Healthy Mind, Healthy Life*. https://www.mindful.org/what-is-mindfulness/ Accessed on 8.3.22.

Neff, K., 2022. *Self compassion*. https://self-compassion.org

Nursing and Midwifery Council. 2019. *Future midwife: Standards of proficiency for midwives*. https://www.nmc.org.uk/globalassets/sitedocuments/standards/standards-of-proficiency-for-midwives.pdf

Nursing and Midwifery Council (NMC). 2019. *Future midwife: Standards of proficiency for midwives*. https://www.nmc.org.uk/globalassets/sitedocuments/midwifery/future-midwife-consultation/draft-standards-of-proficiency-for-midwives.pdf

Pawar, A., Sudan, K., Satini, S. and Sunarsi, D. 2020. Organizational servant leadership. *International Journal of Educational Administration, Management, and Leadership* 1(2): 63–76.

Pipe, T., FitzPatrick, K., Doucette, J., Cotton, A. and Arnow, D., 2016. The mindful nurse leader: Improving processes and outcomes; restoring joy to nursing. *Feature: Executive Extra Series, Part 1. Nursing Management*. 47(9): 44–48.

Plested, M., 2014. Mindful midwifery: A phenomenological paradigm. *The Practising Midwife* 17(11): 18–20.

Plested, Mariaamni and Kirkham, Mavis. 2016. Risk and fear in the lived experience of birth without a midwife. *Midwifery* 38: 29–34.

Reid, B., 2006. "Being With Patients" – Evaluating the Impact on Patients' Experiences of Care. *Foundation of Nursing Studies Dissemination Series* 4(1). https://www.fons.org/Resources/Documents/DissSeriesVol4No1.pdf

Renfrew, M., McFadden, A., Bastos, M., Campbell, J., Channon, A., Cheung, N., et al., 2014. Midwifery and quality care: Findings from a new evidence-informed framework for maternal and newborn care. *The Lancet* 384(9948): 1129–1145.

Royal College of Midwives. 2021. RCM warns of midwife exodus as maternity staffing crisis grows. *Members Experience Survey*. https://www.rcm.org.uk/media-releases/2021/september/rcm-warns-of-midwife-exodus-as-maternity-staffing-crisis-grows/

Rupprecht, S., Koole, W., Chaskalson, M., Tamdjidi, C. and West, M., 2019. Running too far ahead? Towards a broader understanding of mindfulness in organisations *Current Opinion in Psychology* 28: 32–36.

Sandall, J., Coxon, K., Mackintosh, N., Rayment-Jones, H., Locock, L. and Page, L., 2016. *Relationships: The Pathway to Safe, High-Quality Maternity Care: Sheila Kitzinger Symposium at Green Templeton College, Oxford: Summary Report.* https://www.gtc.ox.ac.uk/wp-content/uploads/2018/12/skp_report.pdf

Schmitt, N., Mattern, E., Cignacco, E., Seliger, G., Konig-Bachmann, M., Striebich, S. and Ayele, G.M., 2021. Effects of the Covid-19 pandemic on maternity staff in 2020 – a scoping review. *BMC Health Service Research* 27;21(1): 1364.

Smith, J., 2021. *Nurturing Maternity Staff: How to Tackle Trauma, Stress and Burnout to Create a Positive Working Culture in the NHS.* London: Pinter and Martin.

Turner, A., 2020. *One Thought.* https://onethought.com

Turner, S., Crowther, S. and Lau, A., 2021. A grounded theory study on midwifery managers' views and experiences of implementing and sustaining continuity of carer models within the UK maternity system. *Women and Birth* 35(5): e421–e431.

UNFPA, 2021. *The State of the World's Midwifery.* https://www.unfpa.org/publications/sowmy-2021

Youngson, R., 2014. *ACT with Compassion Coaching Model.* https://www.youtube.com/watch?v=pwQ6czxFIFw

Youngson, R., 2012. *Time to Care: How to Love your Patients and Your Job.* Auckland: Create Space Independent Publishing Platform.

West, M., 2021. *Compassionate Leadership: Sustaining Wisdom, Humanity and Presence in Health and Social Care.* London: Swirling Leaf Press.

Woodward, S., 2020. *Maternity Safety.* https://suzettewoodward.org/2020/10/04/maternity-safety/

Xiao, Q., Yue, C., He, W. and Yu, J.Y., 2017. The mindful self: A mindfulness-enlightened self-view. *Frontiers in Psychology* 8: 1752.

17

THE FINAL GONG

Being a mindful practitioner

Susan Crowther and Lorna Davies

When one attends a formal meditation and mindfulness practice retreat/
workshop it has a beginning and an end – the retreat/workshop often contains
multiple sessions of practice with some formal instruction and a series of contemplative exercises, such as walking meditations and housekeeping tasks conducted
often in silence. In many ways, such workshops and retreats are easier than maintaining a mindful approach to life beyond the retreat. In a similar way to a formal
retreat, each of the authors has provided written information and shared personal
insights and proffered some ideas on how to put these ideas into practice. With
any activity there is always a start and an end, likewise in the mindfulness retreat
the time arrives when the last session begins, and the final gong sounds the end.
This marks a time of completing a purposeful withdrawal from everyday busy
life and the next phase when one transitions back into the noise of society.

For me (Susan) in the early days of my own practice this final session was usually a moment when I said to myself – *'okay, this is it, now is the time to coalesce all
I have learnt and practiced and make this the best practice session ever!'* Then the gong
sounds, I make my farewells to other workshop participants, search for my car
keys or search my bus ticket and venture out gingerly with a degree of confidence
and good intentions to make good of what I have learnt and experienced. Yet,
to re-engage mindfully and lovingly and re-encounter the contextual complex
world can feel like an overwhelm of stimuli! As you have learnt in these pages,
mindfulness and being mindful is not purely a formal practice sat on a meditation
pillow far away from society. It can be, but as you have read in previous chapters
mindfulness is about a process of moment-to-moment awareness, of noticing
what you are doing, how you doing what you do, and naming what you are doing and how you are doing; the idea that reading the final chapter of a book will
provide the final absolute conclusion – is just that, another idea in a moment-to-
moment experience of life. Personally (SC), the final gong, signals to me, a time

DOI: 10.4324/9781003165200-17

to let go of persistent unhelpful fears in my life and imprisoning anxieties about what comes next – these are just mind games, thoughts transitioning across the mental plate – instead, the invitation is to breathe and allow the final gong to simply mark a transition from one moment to the next. There is no final destination, as Rumi reminds us:

> Keep walking, though there's no place to get to.
> Don't try to see through the distances.
> That's not for human beings. Move within,
> but don't move the way fear makes you move.
>
> *(Mawlana Jalal-al-Din Rumi, 13th Century)*

It is fitting that the final section of this book is focussed on governance and leadership across the childbirth sphere in relation to the central theme of mindfulness. In many ways, this brings us into an ever-moving iterative related holistic appreciation of how the grassroots actions and sense-making occurring in the birthing room are interdependent on the organisational and institutional structures that 'contain' 21st-century childbirth. Likewise, childbirth is one of historicity – it is built upon and informed by professional, organisational, management, research and educational historical contexts. All childbirth experiences, for all concerned, are always somehow constituted of significant nuanced psychosocial, cultural, spiritual and emotional wellbeing as interrelated dynamic parts in an ecological interplay. These parts do not stand alone but come together in what I have named an 'Ecology of Birth' (Crowther 2020) (see Figure 17.1). We would contend that bringing this awareness and openness across the childbirth sphere requires a mindful approach to care. In this final chapter, Lorna and I revisit the core insightful messages the authors have gifted to our thinking which can inform our actions in the birthing world. The ecology of birth will provide the template for revisiting these insights and learnings. Although Figure 17.1 specifies 'a moment of birth' – that is a misnomer because each moment is on a continuum of history through to the present and always onwards into possible futures – it does not imply a single moment separated out of our moment-to-moment coming into being. In each moment we are gifted the possibility of noticing our past meeting our future in every moment being lived. The potential released to us in this simple noticing allows some ordinary yet miraculous opportunity to encounter life anew. The authors of this book have revealed that this is no less true than how and what we do across the childbirth sphere.

Context

The constituents of context of childbirth, historic, contemporary and futural, as well as culture and socio-political are threaded through all the chapters. What is evident is how these constituent parts manifest in the personal, relational and collective and gather in the birthing room and thread through the entire childbirth

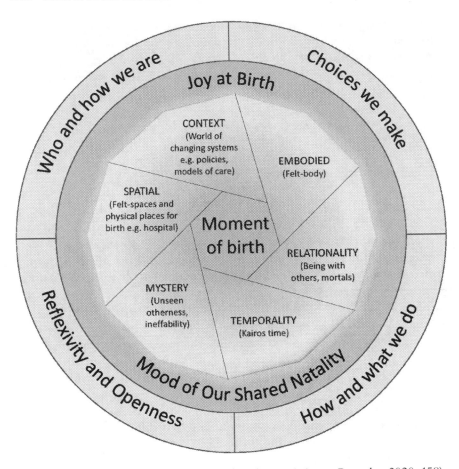

FIGURE 17.1 Ecology of birth (reproduced with permission – Crowther 2020: 159).

year. Childbirth cannot be extracted from human life and examined in a laboratory, childbirth is our shared natal experience and is the weave that holds the tapestry of life together and constantly propels us into possibilities yet to be discovered (Arendt 1958). This is beautifully illustrated in a number of chapters.

In Chapter 4, Miriama draws us close to Mātauranga Māori (Māori way of being and engaging in the world) she begins the chapter with a renowned whakatauki (Māori proverb) – 'Ko au te awa, ko te awa ko au' I am the river, and the river is me. With grace and cultural aligned insights Miriama invites us into a journey of thinking about the contextual significance of indigenous birthing in the modern world through a culturally specific mindfulness lens. This deeply personal chapter of historical trauma, historical and contemporary colonised birthing reflects a way of being in the world that is profoundly connected to context. This is mirrored in many ways again in Valerie's chapter. Valerie's mindful inquiry in Chapter 5 gifts us detailed autobiographical accounts of her own experiences as a fourth-generation German Lutheran in Milwaukee becoming a single mother and the experiences of William Hart becoming a parent as a gay man. Examining these experiences through the cornerstones of mindful inquiry: phenomenology, hermeneutics, critical theory and Buddhism Valerie aptly foregrounds the primacy of childbirth context with a startling immediacy that can be confronting and stirring.

When we consider the insights glimpsed through Valerie's words, we are goaded towards a moment of contemplation on the socio-political structures that situate childbirth care globally. As we contemplate the implications, we can see how much of childbirth has been colonised into a Eurocentric biomedical focussed institutionalised human experience. When we begin to mindfully consider the contemporary culture permeating childbirth, it is evident that in the pursuit of safety, lowering risk and saving lives we have covered over something of enormous significance. This is not to imply technology is not essential and a welcomed contribution to childbirth when used judiciously; it is a call to change our relationship with technology and begin the work of proactively decolonising by reimagining how care is delivered. For this, we also need to be concerned about how the prevalent and normative childbirth narratives and discourses influence women (Kay et al. 2017). Globally we have a plethora of approaches to childbirth care, yet models of care and organisational structures are abstract ideas and tell us little of the experience itself. To enable optimal affirming experiences in these models and structures a certain style of leadership is required to mindfully navigate and guide these constructed contexts.

Sheena's work on leadership in Chapter 16 speaks eloquently from the personal perspective about mindful leadership and how this must always be contextual, always about relationships, always enthused with compassion and positive shared vision. To change systems and approaches to care, well-attuned leadership is required that works mindfully in co-operative ways with others. This is concerned with truly caring for the maternity workforce not just so they can be resilient and keep turning up to work regardless of the context – but about nurturing working environments that enable others to flourish and find a sense of eudemonia – being well whilst doing good.

As Western concepts and ideas about childbirth create ever new whole systems of care, we see an unmindful unfolding of a global colonised homogenisation of the Earth's birthing culture with only small pockets of regional idiosyncratic projects to counteract this unrelenting trend. However, there is hope. As Miriama suggests mindfulness could help indigenous peoples everywhere who work to correct colonial injustices across the childbirth sphere. We see this as a call to do something concrete and suggest that we all need to inquire mindfully into reimagining the 21st-century childbirth context. This style of inquiry necessitates a close mindful examination of the social ontology of birth in which birth is understood as socially and culturally embedded within a historical narrative. This is urgent work that we can all engage proactively.

Spatial (spaces and places)

Birth environments are important to consider in the ecology of birth. Yet there is a distinction between the physical places of births, e.g., hospital birthing room, US clinic rooms, home, antenatal clinic and the experience of childbirth spaces that are not only the material physical structures and locations but also the felt-into spaces. Doreen and Maralyn's Chapter 8 'Disrupting the status quo to create the Mindful Birth Space – spaces that 'sing'!' provides valuable understandings about the significance of felt-spaces for childbirth. They highlight the importance of designing spaces in birthing environments that respect, promote and celebrate the esoteric aspects of birth as well as the tangible, visceral, physical aspects weaving webs of connection that honour and preserve the ecology of birth.

Likewise in Mo and Tracy's Chapter 9, further insights into how the space in and around birth can be influenced by the introduction of a programme of education that teaches midwives and student midwives about mindfulness and relaxation techniques. They describe the impact of emotional contagion on the birthing space and the need to be mindful of this influence on the birthing process. They contend that meditation can create a mental space for those in the birthing space to consciously respond instead of conditioned reactions and suggest that mindfulness practices be taught in undergraduate courses. Following on from this, Susan and Christine in Chapter 7 report on an aspect of an evaluation on Calmbirth and the use of mindfulness. Both chapters confer and suggest that effective change in the birthing space has to include all those there – not just the birthing women and her support but the healthcare professions too. Susan and Christine found that despite women and their partners evaluating the classes as worthwhile and acceptable, they also discovered that any learnt practices were more impactful on the childbirth experience when supported by care providers sharing a similar appreciation of the ethos of Calmbirth in birthing environments. Mo and Tracy's chapter highlights how culture of the birthing environment, and the practices of those working in them, play a significant role in birthing spaces and need to be a focus for mindfulness interventions to have maximum impact – as one of their study participants said, the midwife can be the 'game changer'.

Following on from the insights of Chapters 7 and 9, Lorna, Melanie and Kathleen share their work on the use of mindfulness in midwifery education in Chapter 15. They illustrate what can be achieved when students are introduced to mindfulness as a holistic paradigm that aligns with both the art and science of midwifery practice. Embedding a philosophy of mindfulness into programmes and courses at the nascent practitioner level embraces the power of change and transformation. Mindfulness becomes a central and core value which has the potential to influence a paradigm shift of magnitude. Similarly, in Chapter 12 Maggie and Dan explore how incorporating mindfulness education might help to improve the experience in the demanding environment of neonatal intensive care. Again, the importance of education as a vehicle for change is introduced.

Maggie and Dan consider ways in which mindfulness could be introduced within a multidisciplinary setting in order to support optimal team working and initiate better care that attunes to the needs of the unwell neonate and their families. The potential of developing mindful practices in clinical environments awakens the potential for a space to open that is self-sustaining, welcoming and affirming.

Embodied (felt-body)

Closely interconnected, or within the interiority of one another are embodied and spatial experiences. The distinction in experiential terms of felt space and felt body in our everyday dealings in the world is impossible because they are always and already coexistent – they are only conceived separately in order to articulate in language. Merleau–Ponty (1962/2002) suggested that the body is the medium of all perception and van Manen (1990) explains this as "...we are always bodily in the world" (p. 103). To have an embodied experience is both the material body and the living experiencing body that acts and feels in spaces. That is to say the body–space experience is an inseparable one. The experiences across the birth sphere are not merely determined by sensorial experiences alone e.g., seeing the first scan result, tears of joy at the birth and skin-to-skin contact at the first breastfeed. That is not to deny these physical sensorial experiences but to suggest that it is those experiences and much more. Many chapter authors gesture directly to this felt-body experience.

Craig and Richard's Chapter 2 on neuroscience and the mindful practitioner applies a therapeutic lens to discuss the physiological changes and mindfulness practices. They highlight how mindfulness can affect our experiences and mitigate adverse physiological concerns, such as burnout and improve the mental health of the maternity care provider. Craig and Richard give us valuable insights to operationalising mindfulness in the workplace through detailed examples. Their chapter outlines how clinical performance and decision-making can be influenced positively by mindfulness reducing clinical errors and practitioner fatigue.

Janetti's Chapter 6 on fertility and preconceptual care explores the very real felt-body experiences inherent in reproductive health. Janetti provides context to the fertility experience reminding us of the precarious nature of fertility for many. Her work emphasises how mindfulness can help mitigate emotional and psychological stressors often connected with fertility treatments and processes and how mindfulness can lessen depressive symptoms and self-depreciating idea-tion such as shame, entrapment and defeat. Mindfulness in the infertility context has the power to turn this around and promote self-compassion and acceptance. Janetti reminds us that infertility is both a medical condition and a psycho-social experience and she ends by providing a detailed description of embodied mind-fulness practices related to the infertility experience.

Pain is unarguably a bodily and emotional experience and for many an important aspect of childbirth. In Chapter 10, Liz, Laura and Lester examine the paradigm of pain in relation to mindfulness. In their chapter they describe how pain is an embodied multi-sensorial experience in response to threat, stress, injury and fear, serving as an alert that signals us to protect and perhaps take flight. In childbirth, pain is understood as a normal physiological experience, although it can also indicate pathology. Liz, Laura and Lester take us on a journey into the definitions and causes of pain perception and present to us the complex neurohormonal processes occurring in childbirth and how these need to be in the optimal balance. They discuss the biomedical approaches to pain relief and the debates around these interventions and how pain can be aggravated by some practices and how some pharmacological pain relief may actually cause iatrogenic harm.

Liz, Laura and Lester summarise the literature and present a reimagining of pain as physiological and functional and emphasise the importance of working with pain rather than against it. They unpack the evidence related to mindfulness and pain and show how mindfulness techniques can support and influence the hormonal responses in labour and birth. They conclude that mindfulness can quiet the neocortex and enable focused attention on the present moment assisting women to cope positively with the intensity of the birthing experience.

Several authors indicate and point to empirical works that show how taught mindfulness practices in the antenatal period have an impact in several ways on emotional and physical wellbeing, for example, mitigating poor mental health, reducing fear and anxiety, increasing self-efficacy, enhancing a sense of empowerment and altering perception and experience of pain. Taught antenatal mindfulness programmes are showing promise as a credible, acceptable and useful intervention that deserve further exploration.

Perinatal mental health is a crucial part of maternity care. It has been established that perinatal mental health has a major impact on childbirth experiences of parenting and infant(s). In Chapter 13, Aigli and Angus explore mindfulness approaches in perinatal mental health and highlight the emerging evidence of mindfulness-based interventions (MBI) in pregnancy and the perinatal period. The body-mind connection is a central aspect of the MBI psychological interventions explored. They show how such mindfulness interventions including techniques such as body scanning, are well tolerated and acceptable to many.

Interestingly, Aigli and Angus point out, that despite the obvious embodied and contextual experiences of perinatal mental health there remains a paucity of qualitative research on women's and practitioners' experiences who engage with perinatal mindfulness as well as limited amount of work on the cultural appropriateness of MBIs. Although mindfulness appears to show promise as an effective intervention to mitigate poor perinatal mental health this comes with cautionary advice that more empirical work in this area is required including further work in the way such interventions are delivered. They detail how further robust examination is required across various areas of this domain, specifically, the influence of social determinates of health and the impact on the most vulnerable; what variables need examining for good evaluation of such programmes; and closer scrutiny of the acuity and severity of perinatal mental health conditions when examining outcomes. Without doubt, the importance of poor perinatal mental health is surfacing as a major concern in many centres globally, particularly when we consider the disturbing rates of maternity suicide now being reported. There is emerging evidence that MBIs may be a valuable tool in the arsenal to counteract this trend.

Anna and Ira in Chapter 11 provide an account of breastfeeding as the ultimate mindful practice that illustrates vividly the embodied experience beyond the obvious skin-to-skin and suckling sensorial experiences. The profundity of Anna and Ira's chapter give us pause to consider how we care for newborns across the contextual, spatial and embodied experiences. Their chapter gives us pause to reflect on how we welcome the next generation amongst us and the quality of parenting. This reminds us of the insightful and moving work of Jean Liedloff (1975) and the continuum concept and the importance of mindful parenting:

> Without waiting to change society at all, we can behave correctly towards our infants and give them a sound personal base from which to deal with whatever situations they meet. Instead of depriving them so that they have only one hand with which to cope with the outside world, while the other is busy with inner conflicts, we can set them on their feet with both hands ready to take on the outside challenges
>
> *(p. 159)*

This profoundly speaks to our collective responsibility and accountability towards natal and parenting experiences and the significance of connectedness and relationships.

Relationality (with others)

Childbirth has the extraordinary capacity to gather others. As the birth approaches the intensity of such gathering can increase reaching a sense of crescendo at the moment when a baby is born. This gathering brings others near into a shared spatial and embodied experience bringing others nearer – not just physically but emotionally and spiritually, those alive and those departed and even those to come. Childbirth can be a uniting experience for many and may uncover conflicts and challenges within family and friendship relationships.

Childbirth is always in some way relational. Relationality is not just about physical proximity with others but cultural, emotional and social nearness. For example, the phone call to a grandfather after the birth of a baby brings the grandfather into nearness with the occasion, a birthing mother may think of her deceased mother who died the year before welcoming the presence of her mother into the gathering. Birth is a moment of profound significance that draws us near; it is something we all feel that often awakens tenderness, love, compassion and empathy.

Diane and Jenny's Chapter 3 gifts us valuable insights into their collective work on mindfulness and compassion in relation to birth trauma. They contend that individualised, attentive, reflective and mindful care is the core of midwifery practice, and that mindful self-compassion enables the delivery of safe acceptable care. Their focus on birth trauma powerfully illuminates the significance of compassionate mindful care embedded in relationality. The phrase 'Women needed compassion when they felt frightened, vulnerable and disempowered' in Diane's section is a potent reminder of the importance of health care provider comportment in childbirth and how the need for sensitive mindful care to help mitigate the experience of childbirth trauma. A significant part of this was listening, body language and tone of voice. The being-with, central to midwifery practice and philosophy, goes beyond the rhetoric and is strongly evident in their work. Jenny and Diane contend that developing a culture of mindful compassion in midwifery promotes connection (with self and others) and nurtures trust-based relationships that can reduce fear, increase safety and hold the possibility to improve psychological and physical outcomes.

The significance of quality relationships in maternity cannot be overstated. As Hunter et al. (2008) describe is it relationships that are the hidden threads that hold together the tapestry of maternity care. Relationships reflect the interpersonal spaces where humanising care unfolds. Yet there can be a separation in which professional knowledge and skills can become professionally narcissistic or overly objective and detached from the living moments of interpersonal interactions on the feeling human level. As Buber (2012) suggests, to be fully human is to be wary of being overly personal or overly impersonal – the aim is to be relatable across the personal and impersonal by dwelling in the interpersonal space. This interpersonal space brings an aliveness to practice and enlightens the environments in which childbirth occurs. This takes mindful self-awareness and understanding that can be disrupted by internal and external stimuli and stressors.

Craig and Richard, Chapter 2, examine how professional stress disrupts relationships in the birth settings and how mindfulness can lesson stress. The dehumanising effect of maternity services can create stressors that result in further alienation from one another and lead to compassion fatigue. Craig and Richard explain how this fatigue can lead to distancing from women and families by maternity care providers and hinder human connection. They suggest mindfulness can provide a more affirming adaptive alternative to this situation. They outline the importance of empathic listening which starts with mindful listening practice and how through a noticing practice we can mediate how we speak and respond. The resulting culture can improve teamwork with greater healthy connections between staff resulting in greater resilience in an environment where staff can flourish. Although they suggest that mindfulness practices have positive applications for women and families using the maternity services, they also caution not to impose mindfulness on people – this has to be offered as a choice.

Emotional and psychological challenges across the birth sphere can adversely impact relationships. This impact is often exacerbated when there are perinatal mental health concerns. As Aigli and Angus in Chapter 13 highlight poor perinatal mental health, including the advent of paternal depression, are often associated with deleterious consequences on interpersonal relationships. Aigli and Angus describe the primacy of the body-mind context connections in perinatal mental health and explain how this dyadic relationship between parent and infant can be severely interrupted in the context of poor mental health. However, as stated previously, they provide some encouraging insights into the effectiveness of MBIs in the area of perinatal mental health.

Another area posing significant stress on relationships for all involved is when a baby is unwell requiring care in a neonatal intensive care unit (NICU). In Chapter 12 Maggie and Dan introduce the notion of mindfulness in the NICU. They highlight the highly stressful environment of NICU and recognise the emotional and moral exhaustion in what they describe as a highly emotionally charged and intense medical environment. Maggie and Dan raise our awareness about the importance of nurturing relationships through organisational and individual mindfulness. They consider the experiences of the unwell neonate on NICU and the families as well as the health care providers navigating the psycho-social and emotional milieu of daily NICU life. It is easy to conceive from their explorations that the influence of ongoing daily stress responses experienced by NICU staff has a deleterious effect on communications, ability to connect, empathise and build supportive relationships. Maggie and Dan critique the literature in this domain and suggest that although there remains a paucity of relevant literature, they are encouraged by the growing appreciation that developing objectivity through personal reflection helps improve the quality of sleep and regulation of cortisol levels which facilitate a calm professional demeanour. They argue that clinicians, as well as families need to be mindful of how interactions impact on the lives of neonates. Moreover, they suggest that mindful reflection on beliefs, practices, culture and experiences would help NICU staff provide compassionate care and improve communication whilst simultaneously providing self-care for themselves. For this to occur focus on the wellbeing of NICU staff is crucial through good leadership. As Maggie and Dan contend it is '… time we started treating staff like elite athletes with technical coaches, performance psychologists, training plans that balance both development and recovery'. Their hope is that attending to these needs would enhance compassionate care for neonates. Attuning to the needs of staff requires proactive solutions led by compassionate leadership, as described by Sheena Byrom in Chapter 16. Sheena overtly privileges relationships through a compassionate leadership style that attunes to empathy for staff. It is evident that a compassionate relational and mindful approach to leadership is essential for the wellbeing of all working in maternity and neonatal care organisations.

When we ponder compassion, we are always already in relationship with self and others. Compassion is a noble human quality that affirms our humanity and speaks to social justice, honesty and integrity. It is about caring for our neighbours in professional and personal life in the most profound way.

Compassion means justice.
And compassion is just
to the extent that
it gives to each person what is his or hers.

(Meister Eckhart, c 1290)

Temporality (time)

Time across the childbirth sphere may appear lineal and clock or Chronos focussed. Our models of westernised childbirth care are highly structured around
timing of tests, screening, appointments, estimated dates of deliveries, time for
antenatal classes, time when fetal movement begin to be 'normal' and length of
pregnancy and labour. It is always curious to us that one of the first acts of a midwife when a baby is born is to note the clock time. These are examples of measurable and ordered time not a felt-time, a time which does not pass like clock
time in which it may stop, go slow or speed up. This is not to say the significance
of measurable time is less important. As Heidegger (1927/1962) reminds us, we
are not confined to the present but always projecting towards the future from
our pasts. Throughout this book, authors have discussed Chronos time and also
gestured to felt-time.

For example, in Chapter 14 Tracy draws our attention to times when we are
living through crises and trauma. Her work highlights how in stressful times
we become more self-critical and have disordered or wandering thinking that
can be debilitating and the need to be self-aware becomes important. In the
experience of felt-time in these scenarios sense of time can be disorientating and
even disconnected to the 'normal' lived time of others around us. In such stress
times our capacity to connect with others diminishes and feelings of separation
and isolation can occur. Tracy describes how mindfulness practices can help us
traverse stressful times, such as the Covid-19 pandemic, although the reality
and circumstances cannot be changed in many situations. Tracy describes how
mindfulness can provide significant benefits during times of difficulty and crisis
and provide solace in difficult times because it helps us accept arising emotional
states non-judgementally and helps nurture self-compassion. Felt-time is different to clock time in that it can move faster, slower and even feel like it has
stopped or in some way suspended us in an experience. Tracy reminds us that
despite current challenges in any moment – nothing stays the same; even if we
cannot contemplate the suffering and overwhelming emotions we may be experiencing in any given moment. Without doubt, crises can alter our perception of
time. Tracy concludes that mindfulness can provide us with a way of being with
ourselves and others. The practice of mindfulness can give us the opportunity
to cultivate effective skills and resources to manage any crisis we experience.
Mindfulness can provide us with the potential to thrive, even during extraordinary and challenging times. Moreover, there are times across the childbirth
sphere when we become overstimulated and overwhelmed and lose perspective.

Yet, something extraordinary may also be unfolding that we are unaware of and fail to notice.

When we reflect back on Miriama's Chapter 4, we are reminded that each person is one link in a chain of generations that extends back to an unknown beginning whilst stretching into future generations across times and cultures. For Miriama, protecting future progeny is important and how we do that is crucial because this influences the connections and relationships of future generations. I suspect her words resonate with us all. To bring mindful awareness to time across the childbirth sphere ignites the noticing of something that hitherto may be eluded and missed in the hectic functioning of our current maternity health systems and structures.

Mystery

When we consider time across the childbirth sphere it is evident that there is Chronos time and felt-time – however, there is another quality of felt-time, an elusive enchanting quality of time in the birth sphere alluded to by many chapter authors. This quality of time is when all notions of time; Chronos and Kairos, past present and future all converge in transformative felt moments. This quality of felt-time may reach beyond human understandings of temporality providing glimpses of Kairos time, a critical and powerful liminal experience (Crowther, Smythe, and Spence 2015; Kazenshe 2004). The liminality of childbirth experiences has been explored by numerous writers over the years and gestures to something mysterious often not brought to language. Mystery is situated last in the list of parts of the ecology of birth not as an indication of its lesser importance but a reminder of how all the preceding constitutive parts coalesce into a wholeness that is ungraspable. This felt mystery dwells in Kairos and is difficult to define because of its inter and intra-subjective idiosyncratic quality. Childbirth experiences, for all involved, are unique. Such experiences may be spiritual in nature, connected with a religious encounter or they may be experienced in a purely secular way – what is significant is that all experiences are valid and special, perhaps even sacred.

Each chapter illustrates how mindfulness practice can provoke a noticing where we can glimpse other possibilities in a moment of conscious awareness. This is a valuable insight that needs further unpacking. As Bartlett (2001) warns us if we only give priority to "safety" over "sacred" we risk reducing the experience of childbirth to something secular. There is certainly the need to provide safe care but there is also something ineffable about childbirth that affects us collectively and individually. This ineffable quality can inspire an awakening of compassion, empathy, connectedness, kindness, tenderness, profound reverence and awe with accompanying feelings of love. These qualities in turn can evince a provision of care that positively authenticates others and ourselves. Conversely in our pursuit of risk reduction and standardised safety practices this special quality of relational, temporal and embodied experience can be covered over and ignored, perhaps even forgotten in unmindful encounters with childbirth. We need to be mindful to avoid falling into these tendencies so that an awakening of something wondrous in the birth sphere can occur. The beautiful paradox of mindfulness is that it can nourish us on many levels – whilst being mindful in practice improves safety it can also open our hearts and minds, individually and collectively, to something more.

Becoming a mindful practitioner

Finally, the outer cycle of the ecology of birth brings our focus onto who and how we are, the choices we make, the how and what we do as well as well as our reflexiveness and openness – all tenets of a mindful practitioner! However, we acknowledge barriers and challenges to this aspiration. For a start we need to work towards better organisations where we can shake off the shackles of continuous multitasking, a skill seemingly taken primacy in contemporary practice and deemed a celebrated skill in midwifery. Mindfulness would teach us that multitasking is simply an idea. In reality, we live moment-to-moment, darting from one thing to the next is actually what we are doing when we multitask, albeit at great speed so as not to notice! – as you can imagine that is exhausting and unsustainable long term, it is certainly the antitheses of a mindful practitioner. Also, we need to appreciate birth in its wholeness and not a fragmentary phenomenon separated into unrelated parts that can be considered in a hierarchical way that may deny, ignore or lesson any of the parts of the ecology of birth. Maintaining any contrived separation of parts in the ecology is by itself exhausting and uninspiring.

> This artificial separation leaves the whole to fend for itself in the hope that somehow the parts will coalesce into an effective and acceptable whole that flourishes and sustains. This approach denies the inter-relational world of childbirth and risks losing something precious that could surface if the whole of and parts were understood together
>
> *(Crowther 2020: 156)*

We are fully cognizant that being mindful is an art that maybe difficult to observe in a busy environment with constant demands coming at you left and right – being a mindful practitioner takes effort that requires practice. But as you have read in this book there are rewards to this endeavour including improved energy and inspiration, increased self-awareness, an expansion of existential self-understanding, emotional self-regulation and growth in healthy psychosocial resilience. If these benefits were not enough, being mindful across the birth sphere also opens us to a special gift, an awakening of an enigmatic joyful mood. Being mindful can bring a renewed appreciation of our lives as we enjoy the celebration of our ultimate creativity, an extraordinary level of intimacy and tenderness and a feeling of coming into being at each birth. Being a mindful practitioner is to actively participate in the restoration and re-imagining of childbirth care and contribute to a global renaissance of birth culture. When we are mindful, we come more aware of our humanness and shared natal experience and are able to enjoy the bountiful meanings overflowing across the birth sphere.

Conclusion

The final gong signals a time when you put this book aside and enter the world with an increased orientation to mindfulness, to self-inquiry, hopefully a higher degree of loving kindness to yourself and others and a reinvigorated encouragement to embrace mindful action within your spheres of influence across the childbirth year. You owe this to yourself, to your colleagues and to all families, both present and in the future. The ecology of childbirth is threatened — yet solutions are available to you right now. The contents of this book provide many possible solutions to the threatened ecology of birth. The challenges and barriers that will be encountered in re-imagining an interconnected and compassionate approach to care across the childbirth sphere are surmountable - and this begins with you and your mindful conscious intention.

References

Arendt, H. 1958. *The human condition*. Chicago: University of Chicago Press.

Bartlett, Whapio Diane. 2001. "Building sacred traditions in birth." *Midwifery Today with International Midwife* 58:24.

Buber, Martin. 2012. *I and thou*: eBookIt.com.

Crowther, S. 2020. "Ecology of birth." In *Joy at birth, an interpretive hermeneutic phenomenological inquiry*, edited by S. Crowther, 143–163. Abingdon, Oxon: Routledge.

Crowther, S., L. Smythe, and D. Spence. 2015. "Kairos time at the moment of birth." *Midwifery* 31:451–457. http://doi.org/10.1016/j.midw.2014.11.005.

Heidegger, M. 1927/1962. *Being and time*. Translated by J. Macquarrie and E Robinson. New York: Harper.

Hunter, B., Marie Berg, Ingela Lundgren, Ólöf Ásta Ólafsdóttir, and Mavis Kirkham. 2008. "Relationships: The hidden threads in the tapestry of maternity care." *Midwifery* 24 (2):132–137. http://doi.org/10.1016/j.midw.2008.02.003.

Kay, Lesley, Soo Downe, Gill Thomson, and Kenny Finlayson. 2017. ""Engaging with birth stories in pregnancy: A hermeneutic phenomenological study of women's experiences across two generations"." *BMC Pregnancy and Childbirth* 17 (1):283–283. https://doi.org/10.1186/s12884-017-1476-4.

Kazenshe, D. 2004. "Kairos time." FaithWriters, accessed October 2013. http://www.faithwriters.com/article-details.php?id=11461.

Liedloff, Jean. 1975. *The continuum concept*. London: Duckworth.

Merleau-Ponty, Maurice. 1962/2002. *Phenomenology of perception*. Atlantic Highlands, NJ: The Humanities Press.

van Manen, Max. 1990. *Researching lived experience: Human science for an action sensitive pedagogy*. Albany: State University of New York Press.

INDEX

Note: **Bold** page numbers refer to tables; *italic* page numbers refer to figures and page numbers followed by "n" denote endnotes.

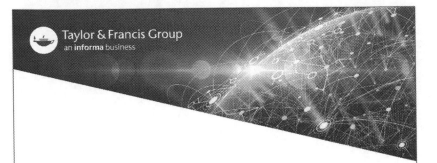

Printed in the United States
by Baker & Taylor Publisher Services